Handbook of Radiopharmaceuticals

Handbook of Radiopharmaceuticals

Editor: Aubree Hopkins

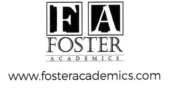

www.fosteracademics.com

www.fosteracademics.com

Cataloging-in-Publication Data

Handbook of radiopharmaceuticals / edited by Aubree Hopkins.
    p. cm.
Includes bibliographical references and index.
ISBN 978-1-64646-635-1
1. Radiopharmaceuticals. 2. Medical radiology. 3. Pharmacology. I. Hopkins, Aubree.
RM852 .H36 2023
616.075 75--dc23

Foster Academics,
118-35 Queens Blvd., Suite 400,
Forest Hills, NY 11375, USA

ISBN 978-1-64646-635-1 (Hardback)

Contents

Preface

This book aims to highlight the current researches and provides a platform to further the scope of innovations in this area. This book is a product of the combined efforts of many researchers and scientists, after going through thorough studies and analysis from different parts of the world. The objective of this book is to provide the readers with the latest information of the field.

Radiopharmaceuticals are a group of pharmaceutical drugs which contain radioactive isotopes. They are also referred to as medicinal radiocompounds. These agents are used to diagnose certain medical problems or treat certain diseases. Radiopharmaceuticals can be administered in patients through several different ways. They may be given by mouth, injection, or placed into the eye or into the bladder. The application of radiopharmaceuticals is classified into two principal areas, namely, diagnostic and therapeutic. There are several applications of diagnostic radiopharmaceuticals. They can be used to examine blood flow to the brain, functioning of the liver, lungs, heart or kidneys, to assess bone growth, and to confirm other diagnostic procedures. This book includes some of the vital pieces of work being conducted across the world, on various topics related to radiopharmaceuticals. Scientists and students engaged in radiopharmaceutical research will find it full of crucial and unexplored concepts.

I would like to express my sincere thanks to the authors for their dedicated efforts in the completion of this book. I acknowledge the efforts of the publisher for providing constant support. Lastly, I would like to thank my family for their support in all academic endeavors.

Editor

A Fast and Simple Method for the Determination of TBA in ^{18}F-Labeled Radiopharmaceuticals

Nils Erik Halvorsen and Ole Heine Kvernenes *⬤

Center for Nuclear medicine/PET, Department of Radiology, Haukeland University Hospital, Jonas Lies vei 65, N-5021 Bergen, Norway; nils.erik.halvorsen@helse-bergen.no
* Correspondence: ole.heine.kvernenes@helse-bergen.no

Abstract: A simple color spot test for determining the presence of residual tetrabutylammonium (TBA) in various ^{18}F-radiopharmaceuticals is described. The test can be performed in less than five minutes. Iodoplatinate-saturated TLC plates are initially spotted with the ^{18}F-radiopharmaceutical to be tested and TBA, then with deionized water or hydrogen peroxide (H_2O_2) solution, depending on if an antioxidant stabilizer is part of the pharmaceutical matrix. A distinct brown spot is visible at TBA concentrations of 50 µg/mL and up.

Keywords: tetrabutylammonium; TBA; PET; quality control; spot test; radiopharmaceuticals; PSMA; FDOPA; FDG; iodoplatinate

1. Introduction

Tetrabutylammonium (TBA) is a quaternary ammonium cation often used as a phase-transfer catalyst in the ^{18}F-labeling reactions of many common ^{18}F-radiopharmaceuticals. Due to TBA being labeled as a specified impurity in Pharm Eur. ^{18}F-radiopharmaceutical monographs, residual TBA in the finished pharmaceutical must be determined before release and use [1]. In Pharm Eur., the limit for TBA is ≤ 2.6 mg/V. V is defined as the maximum injected dose, in milliliters [1], and this volume defines the final quality control (QC) limits before release. Each producer is free to set V according to their own production and needs, and typically V is often set in the region between 10–20 mL, depending on the radiotracer and on the production site. This value should not be confused with the final production volume. For [^{18}F]FLT, [^{18}F]PSMA, and [^{18}F]FDOPA, we have chosen V = 10. The implications of this are that the maximum limit of TBA should be ≤ 0.26 mg/mL, in our QC of [^{18}F]FLT. If V was set to 20mL, the maximum limit of TBA would be ≤ 0.13 mg/mL.

The method for determining TBA content described in Pharm Eur. is based on ion-pairing HPLC [1]. Some shortcomings of this method and possible workarounds have been mentioned in the literature in recent times [2,3], and although modified methods work for determining TBA in [^{18}F]FLT, ion-pairing HPLC offers some significant drawbacks, like very long equilibration times for stable peak areas (12 h in our hands), which means it is almost a necessity to have two HPLC-systems for routine quality control when using this methodology. A further complication is that ion-pairing HPLC does not seem to work (no peak for TBA is observed) when analyzing TBA in more complex ^{18}F-radiopharmaceutical formulations, like [^{18}F]PSMA-1007 and [^{18}F]FDOPA, most likely due to matrix effects disturbing the ion-pairing relationship. Other described procedures for determining TBA are based on treating or eluting TLC-spots with MeOH/NH$_4$OH and staining with iodine vapors [4,5], but these procedures are, in our experience, time-consuming due to long TLC elution times (10–15 min) and hard to consistently reproduce because of the many variables (application of the spot, drying of the plate, amount of iodine vapor, time in the iodine chamber) that can affect the outcome of the test. We have been able to use the iodine staining methods to visualize TBA with no antioxidant present in the matrix. However, when an antioxidant is present, these tests have been unable to produce a spot for TBA in our hands. Lastly, some new, quantitative methods for determining TBA have been proposed [6]. Of these methods, the spectrophotometric method seems to be the most promising, and would allow for unbiased and accurate determination of TBA, whilst producing analytical data that could be easily incorporated in electronic batch reports. However, at present time, this equipment is not commercially available, and the cost is unknown.

Iodoplatinate is a well-known staining solution for visualizing tertiary amines, and is used as the standard Pharm Eur. method for determining the Kryptofix® 2.2.2 (Kryptofix) content in [¹⁸F]FDG [1,7]. In the literature, there are several descriptions of iodoplatinate being used to visualize quaternary ammonium compounds [8,9]. However, one of the problems with iodoplatinate-stained TLC plates is that they yield a false-negative result if the formulation to be tested contains an antioxidant stabilizer, such as sodium ascorbate, which is frequently used in ¹⁸F-radiopharmaceutical formulations [10]. As none of the methods described in the literature yield satisfactory results for determining the presence of TBA in all common ¹⁸F-radiopharmaceutical formulations, we decided to explore whether TBA content could be determined by the same general methodology as described in Pharm Eur. for Kryptofix, and to mend the antioxidant problem, thereby producing a standard methodology that would work for every ¹⁸F-radiopharmaceutical. We herein report a successful analysis of limit level TBA in ¹⁸F-radiopharmaceuticals, using easily available iodoplatinate-stained TLC plates, commonly in use in most PET-tracer quality control labs. The test is also found to work for antioxidant containing ¹⁸F-radiopharmaceuticals.

2. Results

Initial testing showed that a 2.5 µL application of TBA (0.26 mg/mL) produces a brown spot in the middle of a white circle in contact with iodoplatinate-stained TLC plates (Figure 1a, (1)). The addition of 2.5 µL of water on top of the same TBA spot made the spot appear brighter, thereby increasing the detection limit (Figure 1a, (2)). When an antioxidant was present in the ¹⁸F-radiopharmaceutical formulation, a bright white spot would occur on the iodoplatinate plate, without any coloration due to TBA (0.26 mg/mL), despite TBA being present (Figure 1b, (1)). By adding 2.5 µL of hydrogen peroxide (H₂O₂) on top of the false-negative TBA spot around 30 s after the initial application of the TBA spot, the brown spot from TBA complexing with iodoplatinate was revealed, with an orange and white-colored circle around it as a result of the oxidation (Figure 1b, (2)). Consequently, it was found that the time it took for the brown coloration in the middle of the spot to appear depended both on the amount of antioxidant present in the formulation and the concentration of H₂O₂ used. For the maximum amount of sodium ascorbate (20 mg/mL) in [¹⁸F]PSMA-1007 that was tested, it was found that a 1% (w/w) solution of H₂O₂ was sufficient to produce a distinct, brown and concentric spot in about one minute (Figure 2b). Some differences in the brown color of the spot depending on the matrix with antioxidant added were observed. TBA spots in the [¹⁸F]FDOPA matrix were a lighter shade of brown than spots from the [¹⁸F]PSMA matrix, this however, did not affect the visibility. To be certain that these effects are true and reliable it was decided to validate the method according to ICH Q2(R1) [11]. For a limit test, the specificity and limit of detection (LoD) must be proven. To determine that the method was specific, the following criteria needed to be fulfilled:

- Spots from the matrix and the ¹⁸F-radiopharmaceutical sample are identical.
- Spots from TBA can be clearly distinguished from spots from the matrix and the ¹⁸F-radiopharmaceutical sample.
- Spots from the matrix spiked with TBA and spots from the ¹⁸F-radiopharmaceutical sample spiked with TBA are identical.
- Spots from TBA in the allowable pH range for the ¹⁸F-radiopharmaceutical in question must be identical.

The LoD was determined by diluting the TBA solution until a concentration where the spots could no longer be identified as a distinct brown coloration. All validation experiments were run three times (n = 3). The experiments with hot ^{18}F-radiopharmaceuticals were run immediately after release of the quality control sample following production. The TBA dilution and pH experiments were prepared as "cold" solutions, i.e., without hot [^{18}F]PSMA, [^{18}F]FLT or [^{18}F]FDOPA. This was done to protect the operators from unnecessary radiation, according to the ALARA (as low as reasonably achievable) principle. Due to low concentrations of actual [^{18}F]fluorine compounds in the final solution, it is highly unlikely that these compounds will interfere with the spot test, and as a result, the main potential influencing factors are determined to be matrix excipients like buffers and stabilizers. In order to prove this to be true, hot [^{18}F]PSMA was spiked with TBA and a spot from the hot sample was compared visually with a spot from a cold [^{18}F]PSMA matrix (Figure 3a,b).

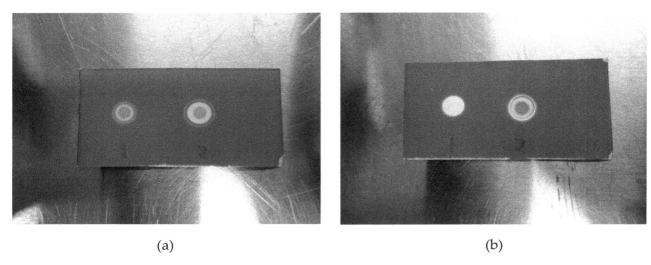

(a)   (b)

Figure 1. (a) Initial test without antioxidant: (1) Tetrabutylammonium (TBA) standard (0.26 mg/mL), (2) TBA standard (0.26 mg/mL) + water. **(b)** Initial test with antioxidant: (1) TBA standard (0.26 mg/mL), (2) TBA standard (0.26 mg/mL) + H_2O_2.

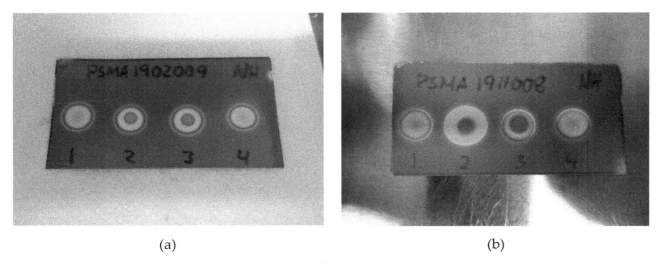

(a)   (b)

Figure 2. (a) Specificity without antioxidant: (1) [^{18}F]PSMA-1007 + water, (2) TBA standard (0.26 mg/mL) + [^{18}F]PSMA-1007, (3) TBA standard (0.26 mg/mL) + water, (4) matrix + water. **(b)** Specificity with antioxidant: (1) [^{18}F]PSMA-1007 + H_2O_2, (2) TBA standard (0.26 mg/mL) + [^{18}F]PSMA-1007 + H_2O_2, (3) TBA standard (0.26 mg/mL) + H_2O_2, (4) matrix + H_2O_2.

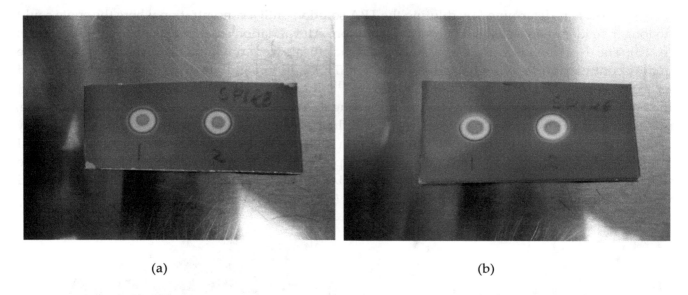

(a)   (b)

Figure 3. (**a**): Spike without antioxidant: (1) Matrix spiked with TBA, (2) [18F]PSMA-1007 spiked with TBA. (**b**): Spike with antioxidant: (1) Matrix spiked with TBA, (2) [18F]PSMA-1007 spiked with TBA.

3. Discussion

The purpose of the study was twofold. It had to show that the iodoplatinate plates were suitable for the analysis of TBA and to find a solution for the problem with ascorbate/antioxidant containing matrixes. The false-negative effect that the ascorbate induces is thought to be due to ascorbate reducing the platinum (IV) species to a platinum (II) species. By the addition of H_2O_2, the platinum (II) species is oxidized back to a platinum (IV) species, which can then form a colored complex with TBA. Findings to support this notion were observed when an ascorbate solution (5 mg/mL) was added dropwise to the standard iodoplatinate solution, until a color change from deep purple to golden yellow occurred. The consequent dropwise addition of a H_2O_2 solution (1% w/w) resulted in a rapid color change back to the deep purple color of the original iodoplatinate solution.

Figure 2a,b show a typical spot test for TBA, both with and without the ascorbate-containing matrix. The spot test is constructed in an identical manner to the spot test of Kryptofix in [18F]FDG, i.e., spot (1) is the radiotracer sample, spot (2) is the sample + reference standard, to show that there is no interference with the two, spot (3) is the reference standard in a concentration representing the acceptance limit. Spot (4) is water or matrix, representing a blank test. From the test it is evident that spot (2) and (3) containing a reference standard are clearly and distinctly different from spot (1) and (4), unequivocally showing the efficiency of the test. Figure 3a, b show that the spiked sample and spiked matrix yield identical spots, and therefore that [18F]PSMA-1007 has no interference on the test.

Due to the nature of the spot test and the dependence of TBA creating a colored complex with platinum, pH might be of relevance. To examine the effect of pH on the test, the matrices with pH varying from 4.5 to 8.5 were prepared and analyzed. As depicted in Figure 4a,b, no effect was found from changes in pH, neither with nor without ascorbate in the matrix, thus, TBA spots are unaffected by pH in the allowable range.

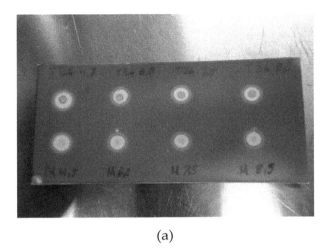
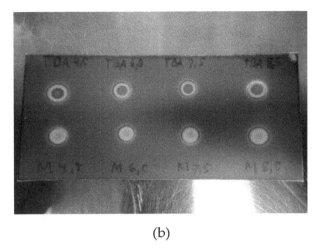

(a)

(b)

Figure 4. (**a**): TBA and matrix spots pH-range 4.5–8–5 for [^{18}F]PSMA-1007 without antioxidant and (**b**): TBA and matrix spots pH-range 4.5–8–5 for [^{18}F]PSMA-1007 with antioxidant.

In order to examine the range of the spot test, a linearity test was constructed. Five different concentrations of TBA in the matrix, ranging from 25 µg/mL to 260 µg/mL, were prepared, both with and without ascorbate. As expected, the difference between the TBA-containing matrix and the blank matrix became smaller with decreasing concentrations of TBA, and at 25 µg/mL, the trained eye might see the difference, but it is no longer striking. Three different QC operators, not familiar with the test, agreed that 50 µg/mL of TBA was visually distinct, thus, LoD was found to be around 50 µg/mL for all the tested matrix solutions (Figure 5a,b). There was a clear and distinct difference in the intensity of the spots depending on the concentration of TBA. No false-positive or false-negative results were observed during validation or later during routine usage of the method.

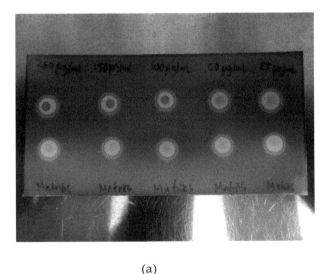
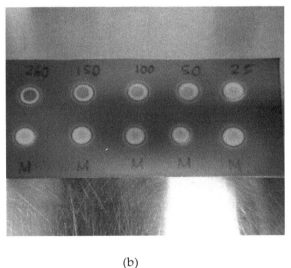

(a)

(b)

Figure 5. (**a**) LoD determination for TBA in the [^{18}F]PSMA-1007 matrix without antioxidant and. (**b**) LoD determination for TBA in the [^{18}F]PSMA-1007 matrix with antioxidant.

The concentration of antioxidant present in the matrix was found to only have one significant effect on the spot test, and this effect was that higher concentrations increased the time it took for the brown coloration to appear after the addition of H_2O_2 (1% w/w). As an example, when the concentration was 5 mg/mL, it took about 30 s for coloration, while at a concentration of 20 mg/mL, it took a little over a minute. Higher concentrations of H_2O_2 sped up the coloration process without affecting the test in any other way (Figure 6). Therefore, it is possible to increase H_2O_2 concentration if necessary.

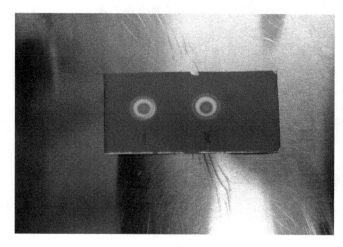

Figure 6. (1) TBA standard (0.26 mg/mL) + H_2O_2 (1% w/w), (2) TBA standard (0.26 mg/mL) + H_2O_2 (3% w/w).

Initial testing (Figure 7a,b) with Kryptofix (0.22 or 0.11 mg/mL) in a PBS matrix with either 20 mg/mL ascorbate or 5 mg/mL ascorbate indicates that the test also works for determining if Kryptofix is present in an antioxidant containing a ^{18}F-radiopharmaceutical formulation. It is evident from Figure 7a,b that ascorbate also affects the Kryptofix spot test, however, the addition of H_2O_2 (1% w/w) in a similar manner as for the TBA spot test, remedies the issue.

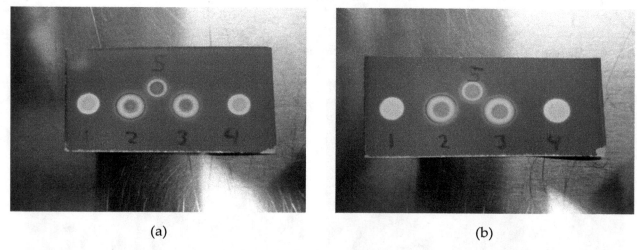

(a)   (b)

Figure 7. (**a**) Test with Kryptofix. (1) Kryptofix (0.22 mg/mL in 20 mg/mL ascorbate matrix), (2) Kryptofix (0.22 mg/mL in 20 mg/mL ascorbate matrix) + H_2O_2, (3) Kryptofix (0.22 mg/mL in 5 mg/mL ascorbate matrix) + H_2O_2, (4) Kryptofix (0.22 mg/mL in 5 mg/mL ascorbate matrix), (5) Kryptofix (0.22 mg/mL in matrix without ascorbate). (**b**) Test with Kryptofix at lower concentration. (1) Kryptofix (0.11 mg/mL in 20 mg/mL ascorbate matrix), (2) Kryptofix (0.11 mg/mL in 20 mg/mL ascorbate matrix) + H_2O_2, (3) Kryptofix (0.11 mg/mL in 5 mg/mL ascorbate matrix) + H_2O_2, (4) Kryptofix (0.11 mg/mL in 5 mg/mL ascorbate matrix), (5) Kryptofix (0.11 mg/mL in matrix without ascorbate).

A simple test for determining if TBA is present in ^{18}F-radiopharmaceuticals has been developed and validated. The test is fast (less than five minutes), consistent and robust. Matrix effects were only observed when the final formulation contained an antioxidant, and a solution to reverse the matrix effect was developed. The test is similar to the spot test for Kryptofix described in Pharm Eur. and it is therefore easy to implement in laboratories already running that test for routine [^{18}F]FDG productions. The test has successfully been implemented in our quality control facility.

4. Materials and Methods

4.1. General

Chemicals of the highest available grade were purchased from Sigma-Aldrich Norway AS (Oslo, Norway) or VWR International AS (Oslo, Norway).

Specified chemicals with article number and manufacturer in brackets:
Tetrabutylammonium hydroxide 30-hydrate ($\geq 99.0\%$) (Sigma-Aldrich, 86859)
Hexachloroplatinic (IV) acid hexahydrate (~40% Pt) (Merck, 8073400005)
Potassium iodide ($\geq 99.5\%$) (Sigma-Aldrich, 30315)
Silica gel 60 F_{254} TLC plates 50×100mm (Merck, 116834)

4.2. Production of [^{18}F]Fluoride

No-carrier-added [^{18}F]fluoride was produced on a PETtrace cyclotron 840 (GE Healthcare, Uppsala, Sweden) via $^{18}O(p,n)^{18}F$ nuclear reaction. 2.8 mL enriched [^{18}O]water (>97%, Rotem, Be'er Sheva, Israel) was irradiated with 16.5 MeV protons in a niobium target body with Havar® foils.

4.3. ^{18}F-Radiopharmaceuticals

[^{18}F]FLT was produced on a FASTlab 2 synthesizer (GE Healthcare, Oslo, Norway) with cassettes and reagent kits from GE Healthcare (Oslo, Norway), yielding 22 mL of product in water for injection and ethanol (~10%) with an average pH of 5.5–6.0. 0.8 mL of 0.14M tetrabutylammonium hydrogen carbonate was used as a source for TBA in the synthesis. The average activity of the product was 600 MBq/mL.

[^{18}F]FDOPA was produced on a FASTlab 2 synthesizer (GE Healthcare, Oslo, Norway) with cassettes and reagent kits from ABX (Radeberg, Germany), through nucleophilic pathway, yielding 28 mL of product in a phosphate buffer containing ascorbic acid, ethylenediaminetetraacetic acid disodium and ethanol (specification limit 10%, average content ~ 3%), with an average pH of 5.0–5.5. In this study, 0.75 mL of 0.075M tetrabutylammonium hydrogen carbonate was used as a source for TBA in the synthesis. The average activity of the product was 200 MBq/mL.

[^{18}F]PSMA-1007 was produced on a Mosaic-RS synthesizer (Neptis, Philippeville, Belgium) with cassettes and reagent kits from ABX (Radeberg, Germany), yielding 20 mL of product in phosphate-buffered saline (PBS) containing ethanol (~10%), with an average pH of 7.4. For testing antioxidant effects, 400 mg sodium ascorbate was added to the final product elution vial to yield a concentration of 20 mg/mL sodium ascorbate in the final product for select productions of [^{18}F]PSMA-1007. Then, 1.05 mL of 0.075M tetrabutylammonium hydrogen carbonate was used as a source for TBA in the synthesis. The average activity of the product was 1400 MBq/mL.

4.4. Preparation of Standard Solutions

TBA in [^{18}F]PSMA-1007 matrix without antioxidant stabilizer: TBA stock solution (10 mg/mL) was prepared by dissolving 330 mg tetrabutylammonium hydroxide 30-hydrate in 10 mL matrix solution (PBS (pH 7.4) and ethanol (10% V/V)). Standard solutions of 0.5, 0.26, 0.150, 0.100, 0.05 and 0.025 mg/mL TBA were prepared by diluting 500, 260, 150, 100, 50 and 25 µL of stock solution to 10 mL with matrix solution. [^{18}F]PSMA-1007 spike solution was prepared by adding 26 µL TBA stock solution (10 mg/mL) to 974 µL [^{18}F]PSMA-1007 solution, resulting in a concentration of 0.26 mg/mL TBA. The solutions for testing pH dependency were prepared by adjusting the pH of the matrix by adding 1M NaOH or 1M HCl to yield matrix solutions with pH 4.5, 6.0, 7.5 and 8.5.

TBA in [^{18}F]PSMA-1007 matrix with antioxidant stabilizer: TBA stock solution (10 mg/mL) was prepared by dissolving 330 mg tetrabutylammonium hydroxide 30-hydrate in 10 mL matrix solution (PBS (pH 7.4), ethanol (10% (V/V) and sodium ascorbate (20 mg/mL))). Standard solutions of 0.5, 0.26,

0.150, 0.100, 0.05 and 0.025 mg/mL TBA were prepared by diluting 500, 260, 150, 100, 50 and 25 µL of stock solution to 10 mL with matrix solution.

TBA in [^{18}F]FLT matrix: [^{18}F]FLT formulation does not contain any other excipients than ethanol diluted in water for injection. Therefore, it was unnecessary to test this solution for matrix effects. The method was validated by spiking cold [^{18}F]FLT batches with TBA and verifying the method with warm [^{18}F]FLT batches. Then, [^{18}F]FLT spike solution was prepared by adding 26 µL TBA stock solution (10 mg/mL) to 974 µL [^{18}F]FLT solution, resulting in a concentration of 0.26 mg/mL TBA.

TBA in [^{18}F]FDOPA matrix: TBA stock solution (10 mg/mL) was prepared by dissolving 330 mg tetrabutylammonium hydroxide 30-hydrate in matrix solution (Phosphate buffer (pH 6.1), ascorbic acid (1 mg/mL), ethylenediaminetetraacetic acid disodium salt dihydrate (1.5 mg/mL) and ethanol (10% V/V)). Standard solutions of 0.26, 0.150, 0.100, 0.05 and 0.025 mg/mL TBA were prepared by diluting 260, 150, 100, 50 and 25 µL of stock solution to 10 mL with matrix solution. [^{18}F]FDOPA spike solution was prepared by adding 26 µL TBA stock solution (10 mg/mL) to 974 µL [^{18}F]FDOPA solution, resulting in a concentration of 0.26 mg/mL TBA. The solutions for testing pH dependency were prepared by adjusting the pH of the matrix by adding 1M NaOH or 1M HCl to yield matrix solutions with pH 4.0, 4.5, 5.0 and 5.5.

H_2O_2 solution: (1% w/w) was prepared by weighing in 3.33 g H_2O_2 (3% w/w) and diluting to 10 g with deionized water.

Preparation of the iodoplatinate indicator strips: Iodoplatinate reagent was prepared by mixing 2.5 mL hexachloroplatinic (IV) acid hexahydrate in water (5% w/v) with 22.5 mL potassium iodide in water (10% w/v) and diluting with an additional 50 mL of water. The spot test plates were prepared by immersing TLC plates (50 × 100 mm) in the iodoplatinate reagent solution for 10 s, applying a gentle stream of air to dry off excess reagent and leaving to dry overnight in a vented container at room temperature, protected from light. For routine quality control spot test use, the plates are cut into four identical sized pieces (50 × 25 mm).

4.5. Test Protocol for Routine Quality Control

4.5.1. TBA without Antioxidant Stabilizer

An iodoplatinate-stained TLC plate is spotted with 2.5 µL [^{18}F]PSMA-1007 or [^{18}F]FLT (1), and 0.26 mg/mL TBA twice ((2) and (3)) and also on the matrix (4) to give four spots (Figure 2a). After 1 min of air drying, 2.5 µL of water was applied on top of previous spots (1, 3 and 4) while 2.5 µL [^{18}F]PSMA-1007 or [^{18}F]FLT was applied on top of the second TBA spot (2). After 1 min of air drying the plate was visually analyzed for TBA content.

4.5.2. Acceptance Criteria:

System suitability

- Spot (2) and (3) are similar in that they consist of a brown circle in the center with a white circle around. The intensity of the brown circle is proportional to the concentration of the impurity (TBA).
- Spot (4) consists of a pink area in the middle of a white circle.
- Spot (4) is clearly different from spot (2) and (3).

Limit
The central part of spot (1) is no more intense than the central part of spot (2) and (3).

4.5.3. TBA with Antioxidant Stabilizer

An iodoplatinate-stained TLC plate is spotted with 2.5 µL [^{18}F]PSMA-1007 or [^{18}F]FDOPA(1), 0.26 mg/mL TBA two times (2) and (3) and matrix (4) to give four spots (Figure 2b). After 1 min of air drying 2.5 µL of H_2O_2 solution was applied on top of previous spots (1, 3 and 4) while 2.5 µL

[^{18}F]PSMA-1007 or [^{18}F]FDOPA was applied on top of the second TBA spot (2), followed by 2.5 µL H$_2$O$_2$. After 1 min of air-drying, the plate was visually analyzed for TBA content.

Acceptance criteria:

System suitability

- Spots (2) and (3) are similar in that they consist of a brown circle in the center with an orange and white circle around it. The intensity of the brown circle is proportional to the concentration of the impurity (TBA).
- Spot (4) consists of a pink area in the middle of an orange and white circle.
- Spot (4) is clearly different from spot (2) and (3).

Limit

The central part of spot (1) is no more intense than the central parts of spots (2) and (3).

Author Contributions: Methodology, N.E.H. and O.H.K.; writing—review and editing, N.E.H. and O.H.K. All authors have read and agreed to the published version of the manuscript.

Acknowledgments: We would like to thank the Trond Mohn Foundation for their continuous contributions to Haukeland University Hospital and the Center of Nuclear medicine/PET-Center in Bergen.

References

1. *The European Pharmacopoeia, 8.0*; European Directorate for the Quality of Medicines (EDQM): Strasbourg, France, 2014.

2. Bogni, A.; Laera, L.; Cucchi, C.; Seregni, E.; Pascali, C. Tetrabutylammonium HPLC analysis: Shortcomings in the Ph. Eur. method. *J. Labelled Compd. Radiopharm.* **2020**, 1–6. [CrossRef] [PubMed]

3. Poon, J.; Katsifis, A.; Fulham, M. Alternate HPLC method for analysis of tetrabutylammonium hydroxide in [^{18}F]fluorodeoxythymidine (FLT). *J. Liq. Chromatogr. Related Technol.* **2017**, *40*, 667–670. [CrossRef]

4. Kuntzsch, M.; Lamparter, D.; Brüggener, N.; Müller, M.; Kienzle, G.J.; Reischl, G. Development and Successful Validation of Simple and Fast TLC Spot Tests for Determination of Kryptofix® 2.2.2 and Tetrabutylammonium in ^{18}F-Labeled Radiopharmaceuticals. *Pharmaceuticals* **2014**, *7*, 621–633. [CrossRef] [PubMed]

5. Cardinale, J.; Martin, R.; Remde, Y.; Schäfer, M.; Hienzsch, A.; Hübner, S.; Zerges, A.-M.; Marx, H.; Hesse, R.; Weber, K.; et al. Procedures for the GMP-Compliant Production and Quality Control of [^{18}F]PSMA-1007: A Next Generation Radiofluorinated Tracer for the Detection of Prostate Cancer. *Pharmaceuticals* **2017**, *10*, 77. [CrossRef] [PubMed]

6. Blevins, D.W.; Rigney, G.H.; Fang, M.Y.; Akula, M.R.; Osborne, D.R. Novel methods for quantification of toxic, residual phase transfer catalysts in fluorine-18 labeled radiotracers. *Nucl. Med. Biol.* **2019**, *74*, 41–48. [CrossRef] [PubMed]

7. Mock, B.H.; Winkle, W.; Vavrek, M.T. A color spot test for detection of Kryptofix 2.2.2 in [^{18}F]FDG preparation. *Nucl. Med. Biol.* **1997**, *24*, 193–195. [CrossRef]

8. Randerath, K. *Thin-Layer Chromatography*, 2nd ed.; Verlag Chemie, Academic Press: Weinheim, Germany, 1968; p. 89.

9. Spangenberg, B.; Poole, C.F.; Weins, C. *Quantitative Thin-Layer Chromatography: A Practical Survey*; Springer: Berlin/Heidelberg, Germany, 2011; pp. 189–190.

10. Scott, P.J.; Kilbourne, M.R. Determination of residual Kryptofix 2.2.2 levels in [^{18}F]-labeled radiopharmaceuticals for human use. *Appl. Radiat. Isot.* **2007**, *65*, 1359–1362. [CrossRef] [PubMed]

11. ICH Harmonized Tripartite Guideline: Validation of Analytical Procedures: Text and Methodology Q2(R1). In Proceedings of the International Conference of Harmonization of Technical Requirements for Registration of Pharmaceuticals for Human Use, Geneva, Switzerland, November 2005.

^{188}Re(V) Nitrido Radiopharmaceuticals for Radionuclide Therapy

Alessandra Boschi ^{1,*}, Petra Martini ^{1,2} and Licia Uccelli ^{1}

^{1} Department of Morphology, Surgery and Experimental Medicine, University of Ferrara, Ferrara 44121, Italy; petra.martini@unife.it (P.M.); licia.uccelli@unife.it (L.U.)
^{2} Italy and Legnaro National Laboratories, Italian National Institute for Nuclear Physics (LNL-INFN), Legnaro (PD) 35020, Italy
* Correspondence: alessandra.boschi@unife.it

Academic Editors: Klaus Kopka and Elisabeth Eppard

Abstract: The favorable nuclear properties of rhenium-188 for therapeutic application are described, together with new methods for the preparation of high yield and stable ^{188}Re radiopharmaceuticals characterized by the presence of the nitride rhenium core in their final chemical structure. ^{188}Re is readily available from an ^{188}W/^{188}Re generator system and a parallelism between the general synthetic procedures applied for the preparation of nitride technetium-99m and rhenium-188 theranostics radiopharmaceuticals is reported. Although some differences between the chemical characteristics of the two metallic nitrido fragments are highlighted, it is apparent that the same general procedures developed for the labelling of biologically active molecules with technetium-99m can be applied to rhenium-188 with minor modification. The availability of these chemical strategies, that allow the obtainment, in very high yield and in physiological condition, of ^{188}Re radiopharmaceuticals, gives a new attractive prospective to employ this radionuclide for therapeutic applications.

Keywords: rhenium-188; theranostics; radiopharmaceuticals; radionuclide therapy; peptides; bioconjugates

1. Introduction

The increase of malignant tumors has led to a dramatic surge in the development of new clinical procedures for cancer treatments, including the radionuclide based therapies employed in nuclear medicine. Ionizing radiation is commonly used by external radiotherapy of cancer patients. In this approach, only a limited area around the primary tumor is treated through irradiation with high energy X rays. Targeted radionuclide therapy, instead, is a systemic treatment that involves the injection of radioactive substances (radiopharmaceuticals) into the blood circulation [1]. The radiopharmaceuticals suited for this purpose are vehicle molecule radionuclide constructs with high tumor affinity, which can transport toxic doses of radiation to tumors and metastases. The tumor specificity of the vehicle molecule is determined by its affinity to target structures, whereas the ionizing radiation emitted by radionuclides is used to kill cancer cells. An ideal radiopharmaceutical for therapeutic purposes must have high specificity and act exclusively in the malignant tumors cells; must have accurate targeting capacity to reach all the tumor cells wherever they are localized; bring maximum doses of radiation to the tumor leaving healthy tissues and organs unscathed; eliminate malignant tumor cells with great effectiveness. This last point, essentially, depends on the radio physical properties and the ionizing radiation emitted by the radionuclide [2]. While imaging procedures in nuclear medicine require radionuclides that will emit γ radiation that can penetrate the body, a different class of radionuclides possessing optimal relative biological effectiveness (RBE) is needed for radionuclide therapy. The RBE depends on linear energy transfer (LET), which is defined as the amount of energy transferred to the material penetrated by an ionizing particle per unit distance (measured in keV·μm^{-1}). In principle, the most suitable radionuclides for tumor therapy are those emitting radiation with short penetration into the tissue, high LET and RBE, such as α emitters or nuclides producing the Auger effect. These will also cause more intense radiation induced side effects on accumulation outside the tumor. Moreover, β emitting radioisotopes with their directly ionizing electron radiation, still offer a higher LET and RBE than γ radiation and represent an acceptable compromise between therapeutic efficacy and levels of adverse side effects (Table 1).

Table 1. Selected β emitters for radionuclide therapy [1,3,4].

Radionuclides	Half-Life (T$_{1/2}$)	E$_{\beta max}$ (keV) *	R$_{\beta max}$ (mm) #
^{67}Cu	61.9 h	575	2.1
^{165}Dy	2.3 h	1285	5.9
^{166}Ho	28.8 h	1854	9.0
^{131}I	8.0 d	606	2.3
^{90}Y	64.1 h	2284	11.3
^{177}Lu	6.7 d	497	1.8
^{32}P	14.3 d	1710	8.2
^{186}Re	3.8 d	1077	4.8
^{188}Re	17.0 h	2120	10.4
^{89}Sr	50.5 d	1491	7.0

* Maximum energy of β particles emitted; # Maximum range of β particles emitted.

For several years, the development of therapeutic radiopharmaceuticals has been limited by the availability of suitable β emitter radionuclides, and even now, most therapeutic procedures are based on the use of radiopharmaceuticals containing iodine-131, yttrium-90. Samarium-153, a mixed emitter of β; γ radiation and strontium-89, a pure β emitter, are used for palliative treatment of bone metastases. Another highly promising radionuclide is lutetium-177, which is gradually replacing yttrium-90 for modern peptide based radio receptor therapy [5,6].

In the last years, the increased knowledge of radiochemical procedures has prompted the possibility to develop new radiopharmaceuticals preparation strategies for therapy using radio- metals with peculiar radionuclides properties [4]. The availability of therapeutic radionuclides with high specific activity and high radionuclidic and chemical purity is important for radionuclide therapy applications. In this context, ^{188}Re is a radionuclide with excellent properties that can be used to label many therapeutic molecules, including small molecules, peptides and despite its short half-life, monoclonal antibodies [7]. In particular, the short half-life of rhenium-188 would seem an unfavorable characteristic for therapeutic applications in view of the fact that a radionuclide with long physical half-life will deliver more decay energy than one with a short half-life having the same initial activity and biokinetics in the target tissue. Conversely, it was reported that higher dose rates delivered over shorter treatment times in biological tissues are more effective than lower dose rates delivered over longer periods [8]. Thus, a radionuclide with a shorter half-life will tend to be more biologically effective than one with similar emission energy but with a longer half-life; both have the same initial activity and biokinetics in the target tissue. In this context, rhenium-188 has the advantage over lutetium-177 and iodine-131 during the first day of a treatment, and it has been rated that 5 days after, the total dose delivered to the target by these radionuclides is quite similar [8]. Moreover, patients could be undergoing several treatment cycles until the absorbed dose is high enough for a therapeutic effect. Finally, in order to improve the pharmacokinetic and dosimetric properties of ^{188}Re, labeled big biological substrates such as antibodies, the use of locoregional applications and the pretargeting approaches can be used [8].

One potential advantage of rhenium-188 over other therapeutic radionuclides, such as yttrium-90, lutetium-177 and copper-67, is its routine availability because of the ^{188}W/^{188}Re generator.

Nevertheless, preclinical and clinical studies have demonstrated favorable pharmacokinetic and dosimetric properties for several [188]Re-based therapeutics; the simpler and most known chemistry of yttrium-90, lutetium-177 and copper-67 may be the principal reason for which [188]Re is less used in clinical practice [9].

Some perspectives and achievements on the radiochemical procedure proposed in the last years for the preparation of very stable high yield [188]Re radiopharmaceuticals are reported in this review. A special gaze is turned to the description of the synthetic procedures available for the preparation of [188]Re(V) nitrido radiopharmaceuticals, that for their high stability provide a very attractive outlook for clinical applications.

2. Rhenium-188

The β-emitting radionuclide, rhenium-188, is attracting interest as a suitable radionuclide for therapeutic applications due to its peculiar nuclear properties and chemical similarities with the most used diagnostic radionuclide technetium-99m. Rhenium-188 decays through the emission of a high-energy β particle ($E_{\beta max}$ = 2.1 MeV) with a half-life of 17.0 h. Associated at this decay mode, there is also a γ-emission of 155 keV that can be conveniently utilized to monitor the course of therapy using a conventional γ camera. Another important advantage comes from the easy availability of this radio-metal, which is available through a transportable [188]W/[188]Re generator system that offers the prospect of cost-effective radiopharmaceuticals preparation for cancer treatment.

The Parallelism between Technetium-99m and Rhenium-188 Radiopharmaceuticals Preparation

Technetium and Rhenium belong to the same group 7 of transition metals of the Periodic Table and possess a rich coordination chemistry. The organometallic chemistry of the two elements is well established [10]. In particular, due to the lanthanide contraction, the elements with the atomic numbers 43 (Tc) and 75 (Re), have comparable ionic radii. From the chemical point of view, this means that Tc and Re complexes, prepared by the reaction of the peculiarly coordinating ligands with the transition metal, give rise to analog complexes having exactly the same chemical structure and stability and differ only by the nature of the radio metal center. In these conditions, it is reasonable to expect that these analog complexes of technetium-99m and rhenium-188 have the same biological behavior; a fundamental aspect for theranostic applications in nuclear medicine. The first parallelism between the two radio metals is found in the method of production of the tetraoxo ions $[^{99m}Tc][TcO_4]^-$ and $[^{188}Re][ReO_4]^-$ based on the use of an alumina column onto which the corresponding parent nuclide, [99]Mo or [188]W, is adsorbed as tetraoxo molybdate $[^{99}Mo][MoO_4]^{2-}$ or wolframate anion $[^{188}W][WO_4]^{2-}$ respectively. The radioactive β decay of the [99]Mo nuclide yields the daughter nuclide ^{99m}Tc in the chemical form pertechnetate $[^{99m}Tc][TcO_4]^-$ which is successively eluted with a saline solution. This situation parallels completely that of [188]Re, which is obtained after the radioactive β decay of the [188]W nuclide and eluted through the alumina column, in the chemical form of perrhenate $[^{188}Re][ReO_4]^-$ with a physiological solution. However, due to the low specific activity of [188]W, the [188]Re obtained from [188]W/[188]Re generators is eluted with low radioactivity concentration. For this reason, it often needs an additional concentration step for therapeutic applications [11–16]. Alternative pathways such as [188]W/[188]Re gel generators based on zirconium or titanium wolframate, have also been exploited [17,18], however nowadays most of the commercial [188]W/[188]Re generators are based on alumina as sorbent on the column. Starting from the above considerations and taking into account the recent progress in the development of the coordination chemistry of technetium, that is directly related with the extended use of ^{99m}Tc compounds in diagnostic nuclear medicine [19], it can be expected that the same well established procedure developed for the preparation of ^{99m}Tc radiopharmaceuticals (^{99m}Tc-RPs) could be applied for the preparation of the corresponding [188]Re radiopharmaceuticals ([188]Re-RPs). The generator produced $[^{188}Re][ReO_4]^-$ represents the starting material for the preparation of rhenium-188 radiopharmaceuticals exactly likewise; $[^{99m}Tc][TcO_4]^-$ is the ubiquitous starting material for the preparation of ^{99m}Tc-RPs [20,21]. Unfortunately, it was found that the methods utilized for the preparation of high yield ^{188}Re-RPs cannot simply follow routes employed for ^{99m}Tc-RPs production, and more drastic conditions, such as very acidic pH, high amount of reduction agents and prolonged reaction time, are required [22]. This fact always constitutes a fundamental challenge for the efficient development of new ^{188}Re-RPs. The reason for this is the fundamental difference between the values of the standard reduction potentials of the redox reaction involving rhenium and technetium compounds. In particular, E° of a redox process that involves technetium is, on average, 200 mV higher than that of the corresponding rhenium process. This means that, in the same reaction conditions, the perrhenate reduction is more difficult than the pertechnetate one. Recently, a solution to this problem based on the use of an oxalate ion $(C_2O_4)^{2-}$ has been proposed [16]. The results demonstrated that the addition of $Na_2C_2O_4$ to radiopharmaceutical preparations starting from generator-eluted $[^{188}Re][ReO_4]^-$ dramatically improved the yield of the final ^{188}Re-compound. By the use of the above mentioned strategy, the high-yield production of $[^{188}Re][ReO(DMSA)_2]^-$ radiopharmaceutical in physiological conditions was performed [16]. This general procedure allows, theoretically, the application of the standard and well known procedure used for the preparation of ^{99m}Tc-RPs to the preparation of analog ^{188}Re-RPs with minor modification (Figure 1).

$$[^{99m}Tc][TcO_4]^- + Sn^{2+} + L \longrightarrow [^{99m}Tc][Tc(L)n]$$

$$[^{188}Re][ReO_4]^- + Sn^{2+} + L + oxalate \longrightarrow [^{188}Re][Re(L)n]$$

Figure 1. Scheme of the general procedure used for the preparation of high yield ^{99m}Tc and ^{188}Re radiopharmaceuticals. L represents a particular ligand able to coordinate the metal in a low oxidation state. The addition of oxalate in the ^{188}Re procedure allows the preparation of the analogs' compound in physiological solution.

3. Design of ^{188}Re Radiopharmaceuticals

A fundamental prerequisite for developing a therapeutic agent with some potential clinical utility is to produce a final metallic compound showing high chemical stability and inertness under physiological conditions. The design of a highly stable ^{188}Re conjugate can be achieved through a careful selection of the most stable rhenium cores. A rhenium atom tightly bound to some characteristic ligand gains functional groups that usually are strongly resistant to hydrolysis by water molecules. The rhenium(V) nitride, $[Re\equiv N]^{2+}$ and the rhenium(I) triscarbonyl, $[Re(CO)_3]^+$ cores are among the most stable chemical fragments [23–25]. In particular, the $[Re\equiv N]^{2+}$ constitutes a characteristic functional moiety in which the Re^{+5} ion is multiply bonded to a nitride nitrogen atom (N^{3-}). The resulting arrangement of atoms exhibits a very high chemical stability towards both oxidation-reduction reactions involving the rhenium ion and pH variations. This suggests that the synthesis of rhenium(V) nitride radiopharmaceuticals containing the Re≡N multiple bond would allow the facile variation of the other ancillary ligands coordinated to the metal center and hence make possible the fine tuning of the biological properties of the resulting compounds.

3.1. The Preparation of ^{188}Re(V) Nitrido Radiopharmaceuticals

Starting from the original method developed for the tracer-level preparation of the $[^{99m}Tc][Tc\equiv N]^{2+}$ radiopharmaceuticals [25], the oxalate-based method has been then utilized to develop the first efficient procedure for producing the $[^{188}Re][Re\equiv N]^{2+}$ core from $[^{188}Re][ReO_4]^-$, at tracer level and under physiological conditions [26]. The above mentioned approach involves the reaction of the generator eluted $[^{99m}Tc][TcO_4]^-$ with a reducing agent and a particular chemical species source of the nitride nitrogen atoms N^{3-}, able to produce in solution intermediate nitride ^{99m}Tc complexes. This intermediate mixture is converted in a single final product due to the addition of a strong bidentate coordinating ligand. Initially, the method was based on the reaction of $[^{99m}Tc][TcO_4]^-$ with $[H_2NN(CH_3)C(=S)SCH_3]$ (DTCZ), that behaves as an efficient donor of nitride nitrogen atoms N^{3-}

to yield the $[Tc\equiv N]^{2+}$ group, in acidic conditions and in the presence of triphenylphosphine. Then, it was observed that the formation of the $[Tc\equiv N]^{2+}$ group is independent of both the choice of the reducing agent and pH conditions, and that it also takes place at neutral pH using $SnCl_2$ as reductant. This method was utilized for the development of bis(dithiocarbamato) nitrido technetium-99m radiopharmaceuticals, a new class of neutral myocardial imaging agents [27,28]. A different donor of nitride nitrogen atoms N^{3-}, succinic dihydrazide (SDH), was also used in the lyophilized kit formulation for the preparation of the new cardiac tracer [99mTc]N-DBODC [29].

Starting from these procedures and adding sodium oxalate to the first step of the reaction, 188ReN-RPs have been prepared in high yields and in physiological solutions. Bis(dithiocarbamato) nitrido rhenium-188 complexes were carried out using a two-step procedure. In the first step, generator eluted [188Re][ReO_4]$^-$ was reacted in the presence of acetic acid with $SnCl_2$, oxalate and DTCZ to form nitride 188ReN-intermediate complexes with chemical nature not fully determined which, after the addition of carbonate buffer and the corresponding R_2NCS_2Na (R= alkyl group) ligand, completely converted in the final nitride complex [188Re][Re(N)(R_2NCS_2)_2] (Figure 2).

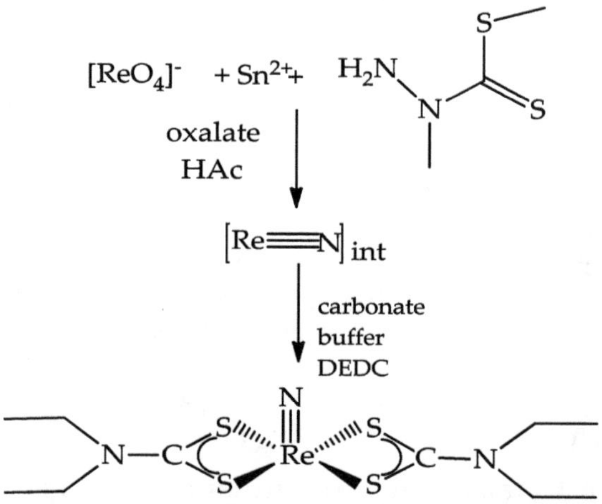

Figure 2. Two step procedure for the preparation of the nitride complex [188Re][Re(N)(R_2NCS_2)_2], R = –CH_2CH_3.

The highly lipophilic complex bis(diethyldithiocarbamato) nitride rhenium-188, 188ReN-DEDC, has been successively utilized for labelling lipiodol an iodinated ethyl ester of the poppy-seed fatty oil for the treatment of the Hepatocellular carcinoma (HCC). HCC is one of the most frequent cancerous diseases in Asiatic and South American areas; it often appears late and successful surgical resection in most cases is difficult or impossible. Carriers of therapeutic agents, such as lipiodol, treat hepatoma without damage to normal tissues. The strategy used for the lipiodol labelling is the dissolution of the strongly lipophilic 188ReN-DEDC compound into lipiodol, which constitutes a highly hydrophobic material [30]. Using this strategy, 188Re is tightly retained into the fatty oil as a consequence of its strong hydrophobic interaction with the lipophilic metal complex. Similar procedures have been attempted with lipophilic oxo complexes of 188Re, but the failure of these methods may be attributed to the difficulty in producing the required lipophilic 188Re complex in high yield [31–35]. This result reflects the difficulty in obtaining 188Re complexes in satisfactory yield and the intrinsic instability of oxo rhenium compounds in comparison with that of nitride rhenium complexes. Whole-body SPECT images of HCC patients after intrahepatic arterial administration of the nitride 188ReN-DEDC labeled lipiodol demonstrated excellent uptake in the lesion without significant activity in the gut and lungs and stable retention of activity in hepatoma was revealed at 20 h after administration with minimal increase in colonic activity and some uptake in the spleen [36].

An automated synthesis module for 188ReN-DEDC, labeled lipiodol preparation, has been also reported [37]. The system allows the easy preparation of sterile and pyrogen-free samples of 188Re lipiodol ready to be administered to the patient with a dramatic decrease of operator's radiation exposure. Application of the automated apparatus could be also extended to the preparation of other small therapeutic radiopharmaceuticals molecules labelled with different β-emitting radionuclides.

The strategy used for labelling lipiodol with the ^{188}ReN-DEDC compound could also be applied to the labelling of nanostructured lipid carriers (NLC). Recently, a new NLC production protocol has allowed one to firmly encapsulate a lipophilic nitride technetium-99m dithiocarbamate compound, ^{99m}TcN-DBODC$_2$, within nanoparticles (Figure 3) [38]. In vivo studies have evidenced that NLC remains stable in vivo, suggesting their suitability as a drugs-controlled release system for therapeutic and diagnostic purposes. It is reasonable to assume that similar procedures could be applied to the labelling of NLC with the analog ^{188}ReN compound and used in radionuclide-targeted cancer therapy.

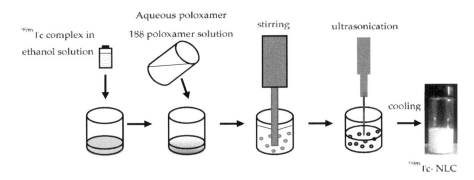

Figure 3. Production of ^{99m}Tc-NLC by the 3-step procedure schematized in the figure. The lipid mixture, constituted of the tristearin/miglyol plus ^{99m}TcN-DBODC$_2$ complex is melted at 80 °C; an aqueous poloxamer 188 solution is added. The two-phase system is high-speed stirred and subsequently ultrasonicated. After cooling at room temperature, the nanoparticle suspension has a homogeneous milky appearance [38].

3.2. The Labelling of Bioactive Molecules with the ^{188}ReN Core

In the last years, the labelling of biologically active molecules has become the most efficient tool to generate affinity of ^{99m}Tc and ^{188}Re complexes for a specific biological target. The most common design of this type of diagnostic and therapeutic agents is based on the so-called "bifunctional approach" [39]. This strategy consists firstly of the selection of an appropriate biologically active molecule having affinity for a specific biological substrate, and the choice of a convenient chelating system that allows one to stably bind the metal. The connection of these two different molecular blocks, which can be realized though a suitable chemical linker, results in a bifunctional ligand. The corresponding conjugate complex, which is formed by the coordination of the bifunctional ligand to the metal, will incorporate the biologically active molecule within its structure as an appended side chain. Various chelate systems of the type "N$_2$S$_2$" or "N$_3$S" have been investigated for the stable labelling of different biomolecules according to the bifunctional approach [40]. Unfortunately, these tetradentate chelating systems rapidly bind the [ReO]$^{3+}$ core to form stable five-coordinate complexes, however the resulting oxo ^{188}Re complexes frequently degrade much more rapidly than the technetium analogs, limiting further development of rhenium-based therapeutic agents.

In recent years, an alternative approach, called "metal fragment" strategy, to the biologically active labelling, has emerged. The new strategy is based on the preparation of a precursor metal complex, formed by the coordination of specific ligands that stably bind the metal, resulting in a striking inertness towards oxidation-reduction reactions. In addition, this "robust" metal fragment possesses a few substitution-labile coordination positions where transient ligands are easily replaced by a stronger coordination system without reacting with the more stable part of the molecular fragment. If in the chemical structure of the incoming chelating ligand, a bioactive molecule is present, its selective interaction with the metal fragment would result in the formation of a stable final compound incorporating the bioactive substrate. On the basis of this strategy, different technetium and rhenium mixed-ligand compounds have been proposed for the development of target specific radiopharmaceuticals, among which the most representative examples are the $[M(CO)_3]^+$ [41] system, the $[M(N)(PNP)]^{2+}$ (M = Tc, Re; PNP = phosphinoamine ligand) system [42], and the so-called "3+1" mixed-ligand system [43]. In particular, based on the "3+1" system, a new class of nitride ^{99m}Tc and [188]Re theranostic agents was recently described [43]. These nitrido rhenium radiopharmaceuticals can be prepared following a specific molecular design grounded on the chemical properties of the $[M\equiv N]^{2+}$ functional group (M = [188]Re, ^{99m}Tc). This group exhibits a predictable chemistry characterized by different structural arrangements whose formation is strongly controlled by the chemical nature of the coordinating ligands. In particular, the chemical characterization of technetium and rhenium nitrido complexes carried out at macroscopic level showed a highly stable arrangement provided by the combination of the π-donor ligand having the set of [X, Y, Z] as coordinating atoms and a monodentate π-acceptor monophosphine ligand (PR_3) coordinated around the $[M\equiv N]^{2+}$ (M = [188]Re, ^{99m}Tc) core [44]. This combination, commonly dubbed as "3+1 complexes" has also been observed in mono oxo complexes [45–47], however, with the metal nitrido core, the chemical requirements are structurally more restrictive because only a selected set of coordinating atoms can give rise to this molecular arrangement. The essential point here is that the tridentate XYZ ligand should be composed by a combination of three donor atoms that have to be selected from the restricted set of S and N donor atoms. On the contrary, the monodentate ligandhas to be selected from the category of the π -acceptor ligand, e.g., the monophosphines. A list of a monophosphines that are commercially available or can be easily prepared are reported in Figure 4.

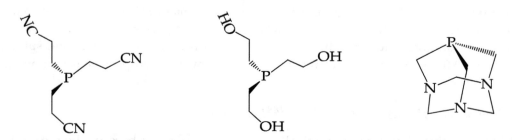

Figure 4. Examples of monophosphine ligands.

The highest structural stabilization was achieved when these two different types of ligands were simultaneously added to the intermediate $[^{99m}Tc][TcN]^{2+}$ fragment where the resulting "3+1" coordination environment was exclusively formed. On the other hand, marked differences were observed with [188]Re-nitrido complexes for which the same set of coordinating atoms was not as selective as that for analog nitrido ^{99m}Tc complexes. In particular, reactions performed with a monothiol ligand, such as 2-mercaptoethanol (HS = $HSCH_2CH_2OH$), revealed once again some differences between the chemical characteristics of the two metallic nitrido fragments, in contradiction to the conventional view that these two elements always exhibit superimposable properties. Indeed, when HS was used as coligand in place of a monophosphine ligand, monoanionic [188]Re complexes of the type $[^{188}Re][Re(N)(SNS)(S)]^-$ were isolated in satisfactory yields. On the contrary, no ^{99m}Tc complexes of the same type were obtained under similar experimental conditions. The proposed structure for $[^{188}Re][Re(N)(SNS)(S)]^-$ complexes comprises a SNS-type ligand in the usual tridentate coordination arrangement around the $[^{188}Re][ReN]^{2+}$ core, and a monodentate thiol ligand bound to the same group through the deprotonated thiol sulfur atom. Despite these differences, the so-called "3+1" strategy may provide a convenient route to the labelling of bioactive molecules with the $[^{188}Re][ReN]^{2+}$ core. In particular, the same SNS-type ligand can be easily prepared by the combinations of two basic amino acids or pseudoamino acids such as cysteine–cysteine, cysteine–isocysteine or cysteine–mercaptoacetic acid to yield potential tridentate chelating systems having [S, N, S] as a set of π-donor atoms [43]. This tridentate model peptide provides an almost 'natural' and straightforward method for labelling peptides with [188]Re since it only requires lengthening of the original peptidic sequence with a pair of these chelating amino acids and it also provides a convenient substrate for conjugation of biomolecules and pharmacophores to the metallic nitrido fragment (Figure 5).

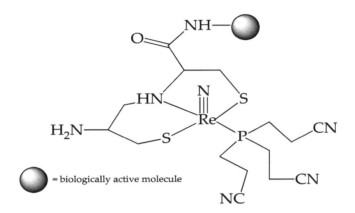

Figure 5. Schematic nitrido ^{188}Re "3+1" complex. The circle represents a general bioactive molecule that may be chemically conjugated to the π-donor SNS-type ligand.

Smilkov et al. [48] applied the nitride rhenium [^{188}Re][ReN]$^{2+}$ "3+1" strategy to label the undecapeptide substance-P (SP), an endogenous ligand for the NK1 receptor type, that plays an important role in modulating pain transmission and may be also involved in the pathogenesis of inflammatory diseases [49]. The presence of functional NK1 receptors has been documented in malignant brain tumors of glial origin, medullary thyroid cancer, non-small cell lung cancer and pancreatic carcinoma and targeting specific SP-NK1 receptors might provide a potential strategy for developing a new radionuclide-based anti-cancer therapy [50]. Based on this consideration, the complex [^{188}Re][Re(N)(Cys-Cys-SP)(PCN)], where PCN is (triscyanoethyl)phosphine, has been successfully prepared by applying the "3+1" strategy using the [^{188}Re][ReN]$^{2+}$ metal fragment. Incubation of ^{188}Re-SP radioconjugate with U-87 MG cells resulted in a pronounced cell surface binding, which reflects the expression level of NK1 receptors on these cells, thus suggesting the affinity of the ^{188}Re-compound for the surface membrane receptors.

The [^{188}Re][Re≡N]$^{2+}$ core has been also selected as a basic functional motif for the preparation of biotinylated ^{188}Re derivatives for the Intra Avidination for Radionuclide Therapy (IART) approach [51]. IART is a therapeutic approach recently proposed for the treatment of residual malignancies after surgical removal of a primary breast cancer lesion. This therapeutic strategy involves local deposition of avidin in the surgical bed followed by intravenous injection of labeled biotin that is, subsequently, captured by cancerous cells after selective uptake of avidin (Figure 6).

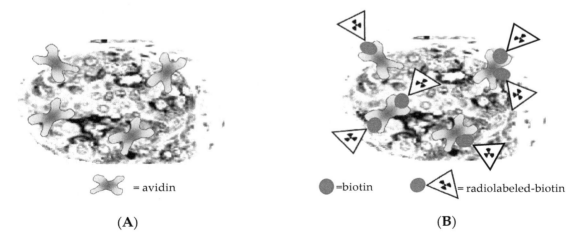

(**A**)   (**B**)

Figure 6. *Cont.*

(C)

PCN   PTA

(D)

Figure 6. (**A**) Uptake of avidin by tumor cells (schematic representation). Avidin is a charged protein and is avidly taken up by tumor cells because these latter have a strong electrical gradient across their membranes. Avidin is administered in situ by the surgeon after removal of the primary tumor [51]; (**B**) Interaction of radiolabeled biotin with avidin. The subsequent injection of radiolabeled biotin intravenously 16–48 h after surgery led this compound to reach tumor cells and to interact specifically with avidin deposited on the outer membrane; (**C**) [188]ReN-biotin "3+1" compounds; (**D**) (triscyanoethyl)phosphine (PCN) and 1,3,5-triaza-7 phosphaadamantane (PTA).

The IART procedure, that consists of a three steps protocol, can be summarized as follows: (1) In the operating theatre, after tumor resection, the surgeon injects directly into the tumor bed 100 mg of avidin diluted in saline; (2) from 16 to 48 h later, 20 mg of biotinylated human serum albumin (HAS) is intravenous (i.v.) injected to mop up any circulating avidin before administration of the radiolabelled biotin; (3) after 5–10 min, radiolabeled biotin is injected i.v. Several studies attempting to prepare [188]Re biotin derivatives, and various publications on this subject have previously appeared in the scientific literature [52–55]. However, none of these works reported convincing evidence that the chemical procedures employed were able to afford a stable [188]Re biotin conjugate in high radiochemical yield (>98%). This result is of extreme importance to avoid unnecessary and dangerous radiation burden to the patient caused by radioactivity not associated with the required chemical form. For this aim, a class of "3 + 1" complexes composed of an apical [188]Re≡N group surrounded by a tridentate dianionic ligand possessing the 2,2'-dimercapto diethylamine (SNS){[S(CH$_2$)$_3$NH(CH$_2$)$_3$S]$^{-2}$} set of coordinating atoms and a monodentate tertiary phosphine ligand (PR$_3$) spanning the four coordination positions on the basal plane of a distorted square pyramidal geometry, has been prepared [51,56]. The SNS-type tridentate chelating system utilized was obtained by tethering two cysteine residues (cys–cys), as shown in Figure 6C, whereas the monodentate phosphines were (triscyanoethyl)phosphine (PCN) and 1,3,5-triaza-7 phosphaadamantane (PTA) Figure 6D. The resulting compounds exhibited high in vitro stability and in vivo inertness towards biotin degradation enzymes. Binding affinity of these derivatives towards avidin was determined in vitro. Data indicated that affinity remained almost unchanged after labelling with respect to the free biotin. A model experiment aimed at elucidating the in vivo selective uptake by avidin was carried out in mice. This involved the preliminary intramuscular deposition of colloidal particles embedded with avidin, followed by intravenous injection of [188]Re labelled biotin. Biodistribution and imaging studies clearly showed that labelled biotin selectively concentrates in the area where avidin colloidal particles were previously distributed. A lyophilized ready-to-use kit formulation was successfully developed to allow easy on-site hospital preparation of this new therapeutic agent.

4. Conclusions

It is obvious from the previous sections that the development of new chemical strategies to obtain [188]ReN-RPs in very high yield and in physiological condition gives a new attractive prospective to the use of [188]Re for therapy. In particular, simple and efficient procedures are available and could be applied for the labelling of biologically active molecules such as peptides, steroids or other receptor-seeking molecules. Furthermore, the possibility of obtaining [188]Re in-house and on-demand in high specific activity make this radio metal ideal for nuclear medicine application. Finally, the simplicity of the reported chemical procedures suggests that lyophilized ready-to-use kit formulations could be conveniently developed to allow easy on-site hospital preparations of new therapeutic agents.

Acknowledgments: The authors would like to thank Elisabetta Esposito and Claudio Nastruzzi of the University of Ferrara for helpful suggestions for the paper.

References

1.   Dash, A.; Knapp, F.F.; Pillai, M.R. Targeted radionuclide therapy-an overview. *Curr. Radiopharm.* **2013**, *6*, 152–180. [CrossRef] [PubMed]
2.   Preston, R.J. Radiation biology: Concepts for radiation protection. *Health Phys.* **2005**, *88*, 545–556. [CrossRef] [PubMed]
3.   Sledge, C.B.; Zuckerman, J.D.; Zalutsky, M.R.; Atcher, R.W.; Shortkroff, S.; Lionberger, D.R.; Rose, H.A.; Hurson, B.J.; Lankenner, P.A.; Anderson, R.J., Jr.; et al. Treatment of rheumatoid synovitis of the knee with intraarticular injection of dysprosium 165-ferric hydroxide macroaggregates. *Arthrits Rheum.* **1986**, *29*, 153–159. [CrossRef]
4.   Brans, B.; Linden, O.; Giammarile, F.; Tenvall, J.; Punt, C. Clinical applications of newer radionuclide therapies. *Eur. J. Cancer* **2006**, *42*, 994–1003. [CrossRef] [PubMed]
5.   Cremonesi, M.; Ferrari, M.; Di Dia, A.; Botta, F.; De Cicco, C.; Bodei, L.; Paganelli, G. Recent issues on dosimetry and radiobiology for peptide receptor radionuclide therapy. *Q. J. Nucl. Med. Mol. Imaging* **2011**, *55*, 155–167. [PubMed]
6.   Zaknun, J.J.; Bodei, L.; Mueller-Bran, J.; Pavel, M.E.; Baum, R.P.; Hörsch, D.; O'Dorisio, M.S.; O'Dorisiol, T.M.; Howe, J.R.; Cremonesi, M.; et al. The joint IAEA, EANM, and SNMMI practical guidance on peptide receptor radionuclide therapy (PRRNT) in neuroendocrine tumours. *Eur. J. Nucl. Med. Mol. Imaging* **2013**, *40*, 800–816. [CrossRef] [PubMed]
7.   Ferro-Flores, G.; de Murphy, C.A. Pharmacokinetics and dosimetry of [188]Re-pharmaceuticals. *Adv. Drug Deliv. Rev.* **2008**, *60*, 1389–1401. [CrossRef] [PubMed]
8.   Kassis, A.I.; Adelstein, J. Considerations in the selection of radionuclides for cancer therapy. In *Handbook of Radiopharmaceuticals, Radiochemistry and Applications*; Welch, M.J., Redvanly, C.S., Kassis, A.I., Adelstein, S.J., Eds.; Wiley & Sons: London, UK, 2003; pp. 767–793.
9.   Frier, M. Rhenium-188 and Copper-67 Radiopharmaceuticals for the Treatment of Bladder Cancer. *Mini. Rev. Med. Chem.* **2004**, *4*, 61–68. [CrossRef] [PubMed]
10.   Sattelberger, A.P.; Bryan, J.C. *Comprehensive Organometallic Chemistry II*; Elsevier: Amsterdam, The Netherlands, 1994; Volume 4.
11.   Jackel, B.; Cripps, R.; Guntay, S.; Bruchertseifer, H. Development of semiautomated system for the preparation of [188]Re aqueous solutions of high and reproducible activity concentrations. *Appl. Radiat. Isot.* **2005**, *63*, 299–304. [CrossRef] [PubMed]
12.   Mansur, M.S.; Mushtaq, A.; Jehangir, M. Concentration of ^{99m}Tc-pertechnate and [188]Re-perrrhenate. *Radiochim. Acta* **2006**, *94*, 107–111. [CrossRef]

13. Mushtaq, A. Concentration of $^{99m}TcO_4^-/^{188}ReO_4^-$ by a single, compact, anion exchange cartridge. *Nucl. Med. Commun.* **2004**, *25*, 957–962. [CrossRef] [PubMed]

14. Sarkar, S.K.; Venkatesh, M.; Ramamoorthy, N. Evaluation of two methods of concentrating perrhanate (^{188}Re) eluates from ^{188}W-^{188}Re generator. *Appl. Radiat. Isot.* **2009**, *67*, 234–239. [CrossRef] [PubMed]

15. Tanase, M.; Tatenuma, K.; Ishikawa, K.; Kurosawa, K.; Nishino, M.; Hasegawa, Y. A ^{99m}Tc generator using a new inorganic polymer adsorbent for (n,γ)^{99}Mo. *Appl. Radiat. Isot.* **1997**, *48*, 607–611. [CrossRef]

16. Boschi, A.; Uccelli, L.; Pasquali, M.; Duatti, A.; Taibi, A.; Pupillo, G.; Esposito, J. ^{188}W/^{188}Re Generator System and Its Therapeutic Applications. *J. Chem.* **2014**, *2014*, 529406. [CrossRef]

17. Dadachov, M.; Lambrecht, R.M. ^{188}W-^{188}Re gel generators based on metal tungstates. *J. Radioanal. Nucl. Chem.* **1995**, *200*, 211–221. [CrossRef]

18. Dadachov, M.; Lambrecht, R.M.; Hetheringtion, E. An improved tungsten-188/rhenium-188 gel generator based on zirconium tungstate. *J. Radioanal. Nucl. Chem.* **1994**, *184*, 267–278. [CrossRef]

19. Arano, Y. Recent advances in ^{99m}Tc radiopharmaceuticals. *Ann. Nucl. Med.* **2002**, *16*, 79–93. [CrossRef] [PubMed]

20. Uccelli, L.; Boschi, A.; Pasquali, M.; Duatti, A.; Di Domenico, G.; Pupillo, G.; Esposito, J.; Giganti, M.; Taibi, A.; Gambaccini, M. Influence of the generator in-growth time on the final radiochemical purity and stability of Tc-99m radiopharmaceuticals. *Sci. Technol. Nucl. Ins.* **2013**, *2013*, 379283. [CrossRef]

21. Esposito, J.; Vecchi, G.; Pupillo, G.; Taibi, A.; Uccelli, L.; Boschi, A.; Gambaccini, M. Evaluation of ^{99}Mo and ^{99m}Tc productions based on a high-performance cyclotron. *Sci. Technol. Nucl. Ins.* **2013**. [CrossRef]

22. Deutsch, E.; Libson, K.; Vanderheyden, J.-L.; Ketring, A.R.; Maxon, H.R. The chemistry of rhenium and technetium as related to the use of isotopes of these elements in therapeutic and diagnostic nuclear medicine. *Nucl. Med. Biol.* **1986**, *13*, 465–477. [CrossRef]

23. Xia, J.; Wang, Y.; Yu, J.; Li, S.; Tang, L.; Zheng, M.; Liu, X.; Li, G.; Cheng, D.; Liang, S.; Yin, D. Synthesis, in vitro and in vivo behavior of $^{188}Re(I)$-tricarbonyl complexes for the future functionalization of biomolecules. *J. Radioanal. Nucl. Chem.* **2008**, *275*, 325–330. [CrossRef]

24. Fernandes, C.; Monteiro, S.; Belchior, A.; Marques, F.; Gano, L.; Correia, J.D.; Santos, I. Novel ^{188}Re multi-functional bone-seeking compounds: Synthesis, biological and radiotoxic effects in metastatic breast cancer cells. *Nucl. Med. Biol.* **2016**, *43*, 150–157. [CrossRef] [PubMed]

25. Pasqualini, R.; Comazzi, V.; Bellande, E.; Duatti, A.; Marchi, A. A new efficient method for the preparation of ^{99m}Tc radiopharmaceuticals containing the TcN multiple bond. *Appl. Radiat. Isot.* **1992**, *43*, 1329–1333. [CrossRef]

26. Boschi, A.; Bolzati, C.; Uccelli, L.; Duatti, A. High-yield synthesis of the terminal ^{188}ReN multiple bond from generator produced $[^{188}ReO_4]^-$. *Nucl. Med. Biol.* **2003**, *30*, 381–387. [CrossRef]

27. Pasqualini, R.; Bellande, E.; Comazzi, V.; Duatti, A. Improved synthesis of ^{99m}Tc nitrido dithiocarbamate myocardial imaging agents. *J. Nucl. Med.* **1992**, *33*, 989–990.

28. Pasqualini, R.; Duatti, A.; Bellande, E.; Comazzi, V.; Brucato, V.; Hoffschir, D.; Fagret, D.; Comet, M. A Class of Neutral Myocardial Imaging Agents. *J. Nucl. Med.* **1994**, *35*, 334–341. [PubMed]

29. Cittanti, C.; Uccelli, L.; Pasquali, M.; Boschi, A.; Flammia, C.; Bagatin, E.; Casali, M.; Stabin, M.G.; Feggi, L.; Giganti, M.; et al. Whole-Body Biodistribution and Radiation Dosimetry of the New Cardiac Tracer ^{99m}Tc-N-DBODC. *J. Nucl. Med.* **2008**, *49*, 1299–1304. [CrossRef] [PubMed]

30. Keng, G.H.; Sundram, F.X. Radionuclide therapy of hepatocellular carcinoma. *Ann. Acad. Med. Singap.* **2003**, *32*, 518–524. [PubMed]

31. Lee, Y.S.; Jeong, J.M.; Kim, Y.J.; Chung, J.W.; Park, J.H.; Suh, Y.G.; Lee, D.S.; Chung, J.K.; Lee, M.C. Synthesis of ^{188}Re-labelled long chain alkyl diaminedithiol for therapy of liver cancer. *Nucl. Med. Commun.* **2002**, *23*, 237–242. [CrossRef] [PubMed]

32. Jeong, J.M.; Kim, Y.J.; Lee, Y.S.; Ko, J.I.; Son, M.; Lee, D.S.; Chung, J.K.; Park, J.H.; Lee, M.C. Lipiodol solution of a lipophilic agent, ^{188}Re-TDD, for the treatment of liver cancer. *Nucl. Med. Biol.* **2001**, *28*, 197–204. [CrossRef]

33. Sundram, F.X.; Yu, S.W.; Jeong, J.M.; Somanesan, S.; Premaraj, J.; Saw, M.M.; Tan, B.S. $^{188}Rhenium$-TDD-lipiodol in treatment of inoperable primary hepatocellular carcinoma—A case report. *Ann. Acad. Med. Singap.* **2001**, *30*, 542–545. [PubMed]

34. Paeng, J.C.; Jeong, J.M.; Yoon, C.J.; Lee, Y.S.; Suh, Y.G.; Chung, J.W.; Park, J.H.; Chung, J.K.; Son, M.; Lee, M.C. Lipiodol solution of [188]Re-HDD as a new therapeutic agent for transhepatic arterial embolization in liver cancer: Preclinical study in a rabbit liver cancer model. *J. Nucl. Med.* **2003**, *44*, 2033–2038.

35. Keng, G.H.; Sundram, F.X.; Yu, S.W.; Somanesan, S.; Premaraj, J.; Oon, C.J.; Kwok, R.; Htoo, M.M. Preliminary experience in radionuclide therapy of hepatocellular carcinoma using hepatic intra-arterial radio-conjugates. *Ann. Acad. Med. Singap.* **2002**, *31*, 382–386. [PubMed]

36. Boschi, A.; Uccelli, L.; Duatti, A.; Colamussi, P.; Cittanti, C.; Filice, A.; Rose, A.H.; Martindale, A.A.; Claringbold, P.G.; Kearney, D.; et al. A kit formulation for the preparation of [188]Re-lipiodol: Preclinical studies and preliminary therapeutic evaluation in patients with unresectable hepatocellular carcinoma. *Nucl. Med. Commun.* **2004**, *25*, 691–699. [CrossRef] [PubMed]

37. Uccelli, L.; Pasquali, M.; Boschi, A.; Giganti, M.; Duatti, A. Automated preparation of Re-188 lipiodol for the treatment of hepatocellular carcinoma. *Nucl. Med. Biol.* **2011**, *38*, 207–213. [CrossRef] [PubMed]

38. Esposito, E.; Boschi, A.; Ravani, L.; Cortesi, R.; Drechsler, M.; Mariani, P.; Moscatelli, S.; Contado, C.; Di Domenico, G.; Nastruzzi, C.; et al. Biodistribution of nanostructured lipid carriers: A tomographic study. *Eur. J. Pharm. Biopharm.* **2015**, *89*, 145–156. [CrossRef] [PubMed]

39. Hom, R.K.; Katzenellenbogen, J.A. Technetium-99m-labeled receptor-specific small-molecule radiopharmaceuticals (Recent developments and encouraging results). *Nucl. Med. Biol.* **1997**, *24*, 485–498. [CrossRef]

40. Guozheng, L.; Hnatowich, D.J. Labeling biomolecules with radiorhenium—A review of the bifunctional chelators. *Anticancer Agents Med Chem.* **2007**, *7*, 367–377.

41. Alberto, R.; Schibli, R.; Angst, D.; Schubiger, P.A.; Abram, U.; Abram, S.; Kaden, T.A. Application of technetium and rhenium carbonyl chemistry to nuclear medicine. Preparation of $[NEt_4]_2[TcCl_3(CO)_3]$ from $[NBu_4][TcO_4]$ and structure of $[NEt_4][Tc-2(mu-Cl)_3(CO)_6]$; structures of the model complexes $[NEt_4][Re-2(mu-OEt)_2(mu-OAc)(CO)_6]$ and $[ReBr(\{-CH_2S(CH_2)_2Cl\}_2)(CO)_3]$. *Transit. Metal Chem.* **1997**, *2*, 97–601.

42. Thieme, S.; Agostini, S.; Bergmann, R.; Pietzsch, J.; Pietzsch, H.-J.; Carta, D.; Salvarese, N.; Refosco, F.; Bolzati, C. Synthesis, characterization and biological evaluation of $[^{188}Re(N)(cys\sim)(PNP)]^{+/0}$ mixed-ligand complexes as prototypes for the development of [188]Re(N)-based target-specific radiopharmaceuticals. *Nucl. Med. Biol.* **2011**, *38*, 399–415. [CrossRef] [PubMed]

43. Boschi, A.; Uccelli, L.; Pasquali, M.; Pasqualini, R.; Guerrini, R.; Duatti, A. Mixed tridentate π-donor and monodentate π-acceptor ligands as chelating systems for rhenium-188 and technetium-99m nitride radiopharmaceuticals. *Curr. Radiopharm.* **2013**, *6*, 137–145. [CrossRef] [PubMed]

44. Boschi, A.; Cazzola, E.; Uccelli, L.; Pasquali, M.; Ferretti, V.; Bertolasi, V.; Duatti, A. Rhenium(V) and technetium(V) nitride complexes with mixed tridentate π-donor and monodentate π-acceptor ligands. *Inorg. Chem.* **2012**, *51*, 3130–3137. [CrossRef] [PubMed]

45. Giglio, J.; Rey, A.; Cerecetto, H.; Pirmettis, I.; Papadopoulos, M.; León, E.; Monge, A.; López de Ceráin, A.; Azqueta, A.; González, M.; et al. Design and evaluation of "3 + 1" mixed ligand oxorhenium and oxotechnetium complexes bearing a nitroaromatic group with potential application in nuclear medicine oncology. *Eur. J. Med. Chem.* **2006**, *41*, 1144–1152. [CrossRef] [PubMed]

46. Pirmettis, I.C.; Papadopoulos, M.S.; Chiotellis, E. Novel ^{99m}Tc aminobisthiolato/monothiolato "3 + 1" mixed ligand complexes: structure-activity relationships and preliminary in vivo validation as brain blood flow imaging agents. *J. Med. Chem.* **1997**, *40*, 2539–2546. [CrossRef] [PubMed]

47. Pirmettis, I.C.; Papadopoulos, M.S.; Mastrostamatis, S.G.; Raptopoulou, C.P.; Terzis, A.; Chiotellis, E. Synthesis and characterization of oxotechnetium(V) mixed-ligand complexes containing a tridentate N-substituted bis(2-mercaptoethyl)amine and a monodentate thiol. *Inorg. Chem.* **1996**, *35*, 1685–1691. [CrossRef] [PubMed]

48. Smilkov, K.; Janevik, E.; Guerrini, R.; Pasquali, M.; Boschi, A.; Uccelli, L.; Di Domenico, G.; Duatti, A. Preparation and first biological evaluation of novel Re-188/Tc-99m peptide conjugates with substance-P. *Appl. Radiat. Isot.* **2014**, *92*, 25–31. [CrossRef] [PubMed]

49. Van Hagen, P.M.; Breeman, W.A.P.; Reubi, J.C.; Postema, P.T.E.; Van den AnkerLugtenburg, P.J.; Kwekkeboom, D.J.; Laissue, J.; Waser, B.; Lamberts, S.W.J.; Visser, T.J.; et al. Visualization of the thymus by substance P receptor scintigraphy in man. *Eur. J. Nucl. Med.* **2005**, *23*, 1508–1513. [CrossRef]

50. Ansquer, C.; Kraeber-Bodéré, F.; Chatal, J. Current status and perspectives in peptide receptor radiation therapy. *Curr. Pharm. Des.* **2009**, *15*, 2453–2462. [CrossRef] [PubMed]

51. Pasquali, M.; Janevik, E.; Uccelli, L.; Boschi, A.; Duatti, A. Labelling of biotin with ^{188}Re. In *IAEA Radioisotopes and Radiopharmaceuticals Series, Yttrium-90 and Rhenium-188 Radiopharmaceuticals for Radionuclide Therapy*; IAEA: Vienna, Austria, 2015; pp. 120–133.

52. James, S.; Maresca, K.P.; Allis, D.G.; Valliant, J.F.; Eckelman, W.; Babich, J.W.; Zubieta, J. Extension of the single amino acid chelate concept (SAAC) to bifunctional biotin analogues for complexation of the M(CO)3+1 core (M = Tc and Re): Syntheses, characterization, biotinidase stability, and avidin binding. *Bioconjugate Chem.* **2006**, *17*, 579–589. [CrossRef] [PubMed]

53. Rudolf, B.; Makowska, M.; Domagala, A.; Rybarczyk-Pirek, A.; Zakrzewski, J. Metallo-carbonyl conjugates of biotin and biocytin. *J. Organomet. Chem.* **2003**, *668*, 95–100. [CrossRef]

54. Kam-Winglo, K.; Hui, W.K.; Chun-Ming, N.G.D. Novel rhenium(I) polypyridine biotin complexes that show luminescence enhancement and lifetime elongation upon binding to avidin. *J. Am. Chem. Soc.* **2002**, *124*, 9344–9345.

55. Kam-Winglo, K.; Hui, W.K. Design of rhenium(I) polypyridine biotin complexes as a new class of luminescent probes for avidin. *Inorg. Chem.* **2005**, *44*, 1992–2002.

56. Duatti, A.; Boschi, A.; Pasquali, M.; Janevik, E.; Guerrini, R.; Trapella, C.; Uccelli, L. Might Re-188 be more effective for boosting therapy of breast cancer using the IART approach? *Eur. J. Nucl. Med. Mol. Imaging* **2010**, *37*, S363.

3

Novel Radiolabeled Bisphosphonates for PET Diagnosis and Endoradiotherapy of Bone Metastases

Nina Pfannkuchen [1], Marian Meckel [1], Ralf Bergmann [2], Michael Bachmann [2,3], Chandrasekhar Bal [4], Mike Sathekge [5], Wolfgang Mohnike [6], Richard P. Baum [7] and Frank Rösch [1,*]

[1] Institute of Nuclear Chemistry, Johannes Gutenberg University Mainz, Fritz-Strassmann-Weg 2, 55128 Mainz, Germany; pfannkuchen@uni-mainz.de (N.P.); marian.meckel@itg-garching.de (M.M.)

[2] Helmholtz-Zentrum Dresden-Rossendorf, Institute of Radiopharmaceutical Cancer Research, Bautzner Landstrasse 400, 01328 Dresden, Germany; r.bergmann@hzdr.de (R.B.); m.bachmann@hzdr.de (M.B.)

[3] University Cancer Center (UCC) Carl Gustav Carus, Tumorimmunology, Technical University Dresden, Fetscherstr. 74, 01307 Dresden, Germany

[4] Department of Nuclear Medicine & PET, All India Institute of Medical Sciences, Ansari Nagar, New Delhi 110029, India; csbal@hotmail.com

[5] Department of Nuclear Medicine, University of Pretoria & Steve Biko Academic Hospital, Private Bag X169, Pretoria 0001, South Africa; mike.sathekge@up.ac.za

[6] Diagnostisch Therapeutisches Zentrum, DTZ am Frankfurter Tor, Kadiner Straße 23, 10243 Berlin, Germany; info@berlin-dtz.de

[7] Department of Nuclear Medicine, Center for PET/CT, Zentralklinik Bad Berka, Robert-Koch-Allee 9, 99438 Bad Berka, Germany; richard.baum@zentralklinik.de

* Correspondence: frank.roesch@uni-mainz.de

Academic Editors: Klaus Kopka and Elisabeth Eppard

Abstract: Bone metastases, often a consequence of breast, prostate, and lung carcinomas, are characterized by an increased bone turnover, which can be visualized by positron emission tomography (PET), as well as single-photon emission computed tomography (SPECT). Bisphosphonate complexes of ^{99m}Tc are predominantly used as SPECT tracers. In contrast to SPECT, PET offers a higher spatial resolution and, owing to the ^{68}Ge/^{68}Ga generator, an analog to the established ^{99m}Tc generator exists. Complexation of Ga(III) requires the use of chelators. Therefore, DOTA (1,4,7,10-tetraazacyclododecane-1,4,7,10-tetraacetic acid), NOTA (1,4,7-triazacyclododecane-1,4,7-triacetic acid), and their derivatives, are often used. The combination of these macrocyclic chelators and bisphosphonates is currently studied worldwide. The use of DOTA offers the possibility of a therapeutic application by complexing the β-emitter ^{177}Lu. This overview describes the possibility of diagnosing bone metastases using [^{68}Ga]Ga-BPAMD (^{68}Ga-labeled (4-{[bis-(phosphonomethyl))carbamoyl]methyl}-7,10-bis(carboxymethyl)-1,4,7,10-tetraazacyclododec-1-yl)acetic acid) as well as the successful application of [^{177}Lu]Lu-BPAMD for therapy and the development of new diagnostic and therapeutic tools based on this structure. Improvements concerning both the chelator and the bisphosphonate structure are illustrated providing new ^{68}Ga- and ^{177}Lu-labeled bisphosphonates offering improved pharmacological properties.

Keywords: bisphosphonates; bone metastases; diagnosis; therapy; ^{68}Ga; ^{177}Lu

1. Introduction

Malignant tumors, especially carcinomas of the breast, prostate, and lung, often lead to painful bone metastases. Since complications, like severe bone pain, pathological fractures, spinal cord compression, or hypercalcaemia, distinctly influence the quality of life and, therefore, result in a shorter survival, diagnosis of bone metastases at an early stage, as well as subsequent therapy is of great importance for patients [1,2]. Bone-seeking radiopharmaceuticals are currently used for diagnostic and therapeutic purposes [3].

Bone lesions are characterized by an increase in bone turnover. This increased metabolism of the bone material can be visualized via both single-photon emission computed tomography (SPECT) and positron emission tomography (PET). In contrast to SPECT, PET offers a higher spatial, as well as temporal, resolution [4]. As a SPECT nuclide, ^{99m}Tc is predominantly used in the form of ^{99m}Tc-labeled bisphosphonate complexes. For PET [^{18}F]NaF is used as bone-seeking compound [5,6].

The ^{68}Ge/^{68}Ga generator system provides a distinguished PET analog of the established ^{99m}Tc generator. The daughter nuclide ^{68}Ga offers appropriate decay properties ($t_{1/2}$ = 67.7 min, β^+ = 89%, $E_{\beta max}$ = 1.9 MeV) and the generator ensures a long shelf-life with a continuous supply of ^{68}Ga [7]. In addition to [^{18}F]NaF, ^{68}Ga-labeled PSMA radioligands have emerged recently and are currently used for diagnosis of bone metastases as a consequence of prostatic cancer [8]. However, further ^{68}Ga-based bone-seeking PET-radiopharmaceuticals have not been established clinically.

The development of radiometal-labeled bisphosphonate-based tracers requires the use of chelators for complexation of trivalent metals. Many research groups across the world are currently undertaking research into complexing bisphosphonate compounds to radionuclides using macrocyclic chelators and aim at identifying a labeled product that has high affinity for bone and offers a high thermodynamic and kinetic stability. For the complexation of Ga(III), DOTA (1,4,7,10-tetraazacyclododecane-1,4,7,10-tetraacetic acid), NOTA (1,4,7-triazacyclododecane-1,4,7-triacetic acid), as well as their derivatives, are commonly used.

For the treatment of disseminated bone metastases, there are two classes of therapeutic bone-seeking radiopharmaceuticals: calcimimetic- and phosphonate-based radiopharmaceuticals. The simplest bone binding radiopharmaceuticals for palliative endoradiotherapy, belonging to the class of calcium mimetics, for example, ^{89}Sr, ^{32}P, and ^{223}Ra. Their localization underlies the same mechanisms as calcium and, therefore, may be unpredictable [9].

Due to the short range of the α-rays emitted by ^{223}Ra, an impairment of the red bone marrow can be avoided, while allowing deposition of high-energy doses into the target tissue. The first successful clinical phase III studies showed a low haemotoxicity and prolonged survival in metastatic prostate cancer [10]. However, the consequences of the ^{223}Ra decay chain for the body, as well as the influence of the α-rays on the sensitive gastrointestinal tract, remain uncertain [9]. The longer half-lives of nuclides such as ^{89}Sr and ^{32}P have discouraged their use and have favored nuclides such as ^{153}Sm and ^{177}Lu with shorter half-lives and lower bone marrow toxicity. The use of ^{177}Lu is particularly promising due to its suitable decay properties ($t_{1/2}$ = 6.71 d, β^- = 89%, $E_{\beta max}$ = 0.5 MeV) and its carrier-free production route [11]. These trivalent nuclides reach regions of increased bone turnover in the form of complexes with phosphonate-containing chelators, like EDTMP (ethylenediamine tetra(methylene phosphonic acid)) (Figure 1). These phosphonate-containing chelators exhibit high thermodynamic stabilities with trivalent nuclides, the acyclic ligands, however, possess lower kinetic stabilities [12]. Nevertheless, radiopharmaceuticals based on phosphonates like EDTMP and HEDP (1,1-hydroxyethylidene diphosphonate) (Figure) show good results in palliative therapy of painful bone metastases in combination with ^{153}Sm, ^{177}Lu, ^{186}Re, and ^{188}Re [13]. ^{188}Re has also been shown to have good properties as a therapeutic nuclide due to its appropriate decay characteristics ($t_{1/2}$ = 0.7 d, $E_{\beta max}$ = 2.12 MeV) and its generator-based production [14].

However, EDTMP complexes have shown low in vivo stability and an excess of the ligand is routinely applied in order to avoid decomplexation in vivo (>1.5 mg/kg body weight of EDTMP vs. approximately 0.05–0.250 mg BPAMD (4-{[bis-(phosphonomethyl))carbamoyl]methyl}-7,10-bis(car-boxymethyl)-1,4,7,10-tetraazacyclododec-1-yl)acetic acid)) [12,15]. This excess may lead to a blocking of the biological target which could reduce the radiotracer uptake. Furthermore, high amounts of ^{152}Sm due to the production route of ^{153}Sm can cause a reduction of the dose rate deposited on osseous metastases and, therefore, a lower therapeutic efficiency [16,17]. Using ^{177}Lu instead of ^{153}Sm increases the specific activity due to the carrier-free production [17], but the low kinetic stability of EDTMP complexes remains problematic.

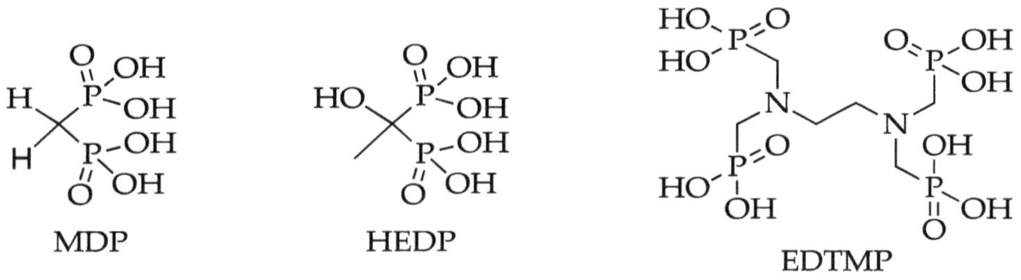

Figure 1. Structures of MDP (methylene diphosphonate), HEDP (1,1-hydroxyethylidene diphosphonate), and EDTMP (ethylenediamine tetra(methylene phosphonic acid)).

This review describes the concept of macrocyclic chelate-conjugated bisphosphonates, which are able to circumvent the disadvantages of open-chain chelators, and possible improvements concerning the chosen chelator, as well as the bisphosphonate structure, based on the DOTA bisphosphonate BPAMD.

2. Design and Development of Radiolabeled Bisphosphonates

2.1. Status Quo

During the last 10 years, the clinical application of bisphosphonates, especially for the treatment of patients with osseous metastases, distinctly increased. Bisphosphonates are analogs of naturally-occurring pyrophosphate. In contrast to pyrophosphate, they are resistant to chemical, as well as enzymatic, hydrolysis due to the substitution of the central oxygen atom by a carbon atom. Their effect is based on two characteristics: they show high affinity for bone material and inhibitory effects on osteoclasts [18]. Binding of bisphosphonates to bone material probably relies on bidentate or tridentate complexation of calcium atoms in the hydroxyapatite depending on the bisphosphonate structure [19].

The two side chains on the carbon atom are replaceable and responsible for the activity of the particular bisphosphonate (Figure 2). Substitution of R1 by a hydroxyl or amino group enhances the affinity to hydroxyapatite. Varying the R2 side chain influences the antiresorptive potency [18]. Nitrogen atoms, especially aromatic nitrogen atoms, considerably raise the antiresorptive potency. This is linked to another hydrogen bond between the amine and the hydroxyapatite and the ability to act on biochemical activities, for example, the inhibition of farnesyl pyrophosphate synthase (FPPS) [18].

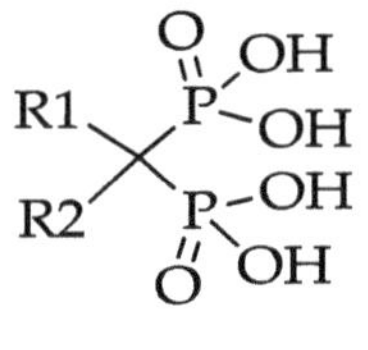

Figure 2. Bisphosphonate structure with variable side chains R1 and R2.

In SPECT tracers like [^{99m}Tc]Tc-MDP (^{99m}Tc-labeled methylene diphosphonate) the phosphonates are responsible for complexation of the radionuclide, as well as binding to the target tissue, which may lead to a decreased uptake in bone metastases [20]. This drawback can be circumvented by complete separation of the chelating unit and the targeting vector, using a macrocyclic chelator for complexation of the radiometal and a coupled bisphosphonate as targeting vector. Figure 3 shows the concept of the combination of a macrocyclic chelator with a bisphosphonate. Depending on the chelator various radionuclides can be complexed, also allowing the combination of diagnosis and therapy in one and the same compound. This theranostic concept already showed excellent results concerning diagnosis and treatment of neuroendocrine tumors using DOTA-TOC (1,4,7,10-tetraazacyclododecan-4,7,10-tricarboxy-methyl-1-yl-acetyl-D-Phe[1]-Tyr[3]-octreotide) radiolabeled with ^{68}Ga and [177]Lu [21].

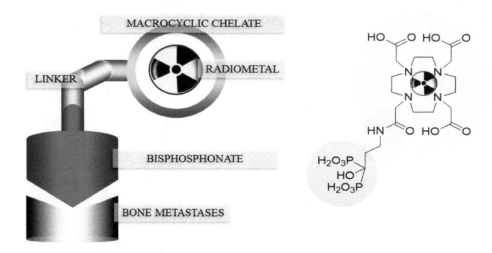

Figure 3. Concept of the combination of a macrocyclic chelator with a bisphosphonate illustrated with DOTA[ZOL].

One of these so-called macrocyclic bisphosphonates is BPAMD (Figure 4), which was initially able to show its high potential in terms of high bone accumulation in ^{68}Ga small animal PET experiments [22].

BPAMD

NO2AP[BP]

DOTA[ZOL]

Figure 4.   Structures of macrocyclic bisphosphonates BPAMD, NO2AP[BP] (2,2'-(7-(((2,2-diphosphonoethyl)(hydroxy)phosphoryl)methyl)-1,4,7-triazonane-1,4-diyl)diacetic   acid)   and DOTA[ZOL] (2,2',2''-(10-(2-(2-(1-(2-hydroxy-2,2-diphosphonoethyl)-1H-imidazol-4-yl)ethylamino)-2-oxoethyl)-1,4,7,10-tetraazacyclododecane-1,4,7-triyl)triacetic acid).

Later, it also showed good results in the first human applications [23] (Figure 5). The bisphosphonate revealed very high target-to-soft tissue ratios combined with a fast renal clearance. SUVs (standardized uptake values) were comparable with those of the [^{18}F]NaF scan, and some metastases even showed higher accumulation of the bisphosphonate. These promising diagnostic examinations finally led to the first therapeutic applications using the β-emitter ^{177}Lu instead of [68]Ga.

[^{177}Lu]Lu-BPAMD was successfully applied in several patients (Figure 6). It showed a comparable biodistribution as [^{68}Ga]Ga-BPAMD, including a good target-to-background ratio and a fast renal clearance. The radiopharmaceutical's long half-life in the metastases provided high tumor doses which led to a significant reduction in osteoblastic activity of the bone metastases. Furthermore, the therapy did not cause any significant adverse effects [21,24].

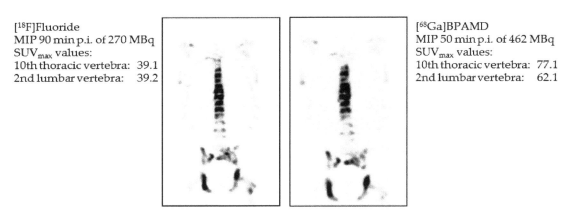

[^{18}F]Fluoride
MIP 90 min p.i. of 270 MBq
SUV$_{max}$ values:
10th thoracic vertebra: 39.1
2nd lumbar vertebra: 39.2

[^{68}Ga]BPAMD
MIP 50 min p.i. of 462 MBq
SUV$_{max}$ values:
10th thoracic vertebra: 77.1
2nd lumbar vertebra: 62.1

Figure 5. Maximum intensity projection (MIP) 90 min post injection (p.i.) of 270 MBq [^{18}F]NaF (**left**) and maximum intensity projection 50 min p.i. of 462 MBq [^{68}Ga]Ga-BPAMD (**right**). Comparison of standardized uptake values (SUV) of Th10 and L2 [23].

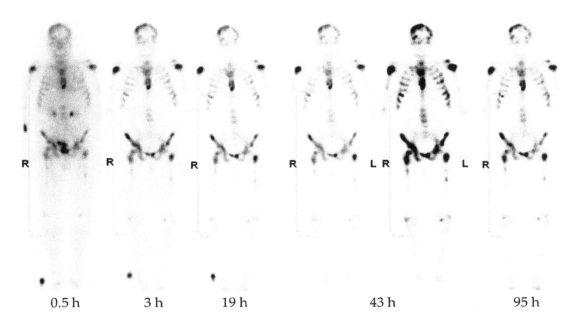

0.5 h   3 h   19 h   43 h   95 h

Figure 6. Anterior whole-body scintigraphs of a prostate cancer patient 30 min, 3 h, 19 h, 43 h, and 95 h after application of 3.5 GBq [^{177}Lu]Lu-BPAMD, demonstrating abnormal accumulation in the skull, both humeri, ribs, sternum, vertebrae, pelvis, and both femora. The best target-to-background ratio is demonstrated at 43 h p.i.

A comparative biodistribution study between [^{177}Lu]Lu-BPAMD and [^{177}Lu]Lu-EDTMP indicated higher bone uptake for [^{177}Lu]Lu-BPAMD, as well as a higher target-to-background ratio [25]. This may be attributed to the already-mentioned much higher amount of ligand used for the preparation of [^{177}Lu]Lu-EDTMP and the conceivable target blocking.

Despite those promising clinical results, there is still much potential for improvements with regard to radiosynthesis, raising the accumulation in bone metastases and reducing the uptake in healthy tissue. According to Figure 3, both the bisphosphonate and the chelator should be optimized.

2.2. Chelator

Chelators based on a polyamino polycarboxylic structure belong to the most efficient ligands and are widely used for the complexation of metal ions. They can be divided into two categories, open chain ligands, such as EDTA (ethylenediaminetetraacetic acid), and DTPA (diethylenetriaminepentaacetic acid) and macrocyclic chelates, such as DOTA or NOTA [26].

DOTA is the most commonly used macrocyclic chelator for PET applications. It is able to complex a variety of isotopes, e.g., [44/47]Sc, ^{111}In, ^{177}Lu, [86/90]Y, and [225]Ac. It is also used broadly with [67/68]Ga, which offers the possibility of a theranostic application, as already mentioned using the example of [68]Ga- and ^{177}Lu-labeled DOTA-TOC [27,28]. Nevertheless, DOTA has a comparatively low stability constant for gallium (log K = 21.3) resulting in temperatures of about 95 °C needed for radiolabeling. NOTA, by contrast, exhibits a smaller ring structure and a higher stability constant (log K = 31.0) due to the smaller gallium fitting cavity [28].

Figure 7 shows the fast and quantitative ^{68}Ga-labeling of the NOTA bisphosphonate NO2AP[BP] (Figure 4). Comparison with the DOTA-based BPAMD shows the expected faster labeling of NOTA derivatives.

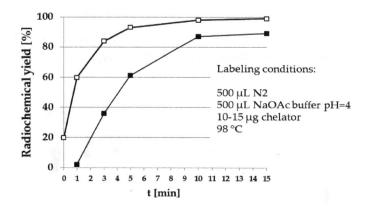

Figure 7. Radiosynthesis of [^{68}Ga]Ga-NO2AP[BP] (□) in comparison to [^{68}Ga]Ga-BPAMD (■). The NOTA-based derivative clearly shows higher radiochemical yields within a shorter reaction time.

Interestingly, using this NOTA derivative not only provides an improved radiosynthesis, it also exhibits a significantly higher femur accumulation in rats compared with the DOTA derivative BPAMD (Figure 8). This may be explained by differences in charge and physical properties of both complexes. It is a recurrent phenomenon that different chelators provide different in vivo properties with the same target vector [27].

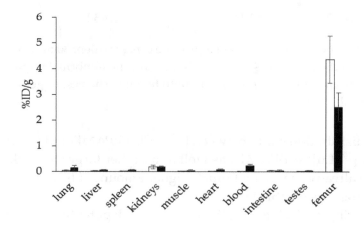

Figure 8. Ex vivo biodistribution of [^{68}Ga]Ga-NO2AP[BP] (□) (3.0 ± 0.1 MBq, n = 4) and [^{68}Ga]Ga-BPAMD (■) (9.7 ± 1.3 MBq, n = 8) in healthy Wistar rats 60 min p.i.

These positive results were also confirmed in a prospective patient study by Passah et al. comparing [68Ga]Ga-NO2AP^{BP}, [18F]NaF, and [99mTc]Tc-MDP in female breast cancer patients with osseous metastases [29]. Within this study, the NOTA-based bisphosphonate was able to underline its high diagnostic efficiency. Figure 9 shows the PET and SPECT scans of a breast cancer patient. Generally, the PET tracers are able to detect more, as well as smaller, metastases. [68Ga]Ga-NO2AP^{BP} revealed a similar detection capability as the gold standard [18F]NaF. In selected metastases bisphosphonate uptake was even higher.

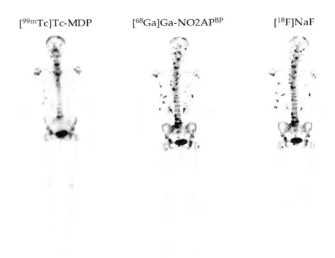

Figure 9. Comparison of [99mTc]Tc-MDP, [68Ga]Ga-NO2AP^{BP}, and [18F]NaF in a breast cancer patient with bone metastases [29]. [99mTc]Tc-MDP demonstrates abnormal uptake only in the skull, cervical vertebra, sternum, two ribs on the right side, and pelvis, while both [68Ga]Ga-NO2AP^{BP} and [18F]NaF distinctly show more lesions in the skull, cervical, thoracic, lumbar and sacral vertebrae, pelvis, and both femorae. [68Ga]Ga-NO2AP^{BP} and [18F]NaF are equivalent regarding the number of detected lesions and far superior than [99mTc]Tc-MDP [29].

In addition to the well-established NOTA derivatives, there is another class of bifunctional chelators appropriate for labeling with ^{68}Ga. These so-called DATA chelators are based on 6-amino-1,4-diazepine-triacetic acid and enable more rapid quantitative radiolabeling under milder conditions [30]. The combination of this chelator with next-generation bisphosphonates is also conceivable and might provide a compound of high diagnostic efficiency, as well [31].

2.3. Pharmacophoric Group

As mentioned above, the side chains on the central carbon atom are responsible for the bisphosphonate's activity, i.e., in terms of affinity to hydroxyapatite. Using a hydroxybisphosphonate, bearing a hydroxyl group as R1, could lead to higher bone accumulation due to increased affinity for bone material. Furthermore, an aromatic nitrogen atom in the R2 side chain could cause building of another hydrogen bond and thereby also raise bone accumulation (Figure 10) [18].

Such a bisphosphonate, like risedronate or zoledronate, would also influence biochemical processes. They possess an inhibiting effect on the FPPS and inhibition of this enzyme causes an increased apoptosis rate [18]. A DOTA-conjugated zoledronate (DOTA^{ZOL}, Figure 4) was already labeled with ^{68}Ga and ^{177}Lu and examined in in vitro and ex vivo biodistribution studies, as well as small animal PET and SPECT studies. [68Ga]Ga-DOTA^{ZOL} was compared to [18F]NaF and a known DOTA-α-H-bisphosphonate ([68Ga]Ga-BPAPD (68Ga-labeled (4-{[(bis-phosphonopropyl)carba-moyl]methyl}-7,10-bis-(carboxy-methyl)-1,4,7,10-tetraazacyclododec-1-yl)-acetic acid) (Figures 11 and 12) [32]. [68Ga]Ga-DOTA^{ZOL} showed the highest bone accumulation and very low uptake in soft tissue. [177Lu]Lu-DOTA^{ZOL} revealed a comparable femur accumulation in ex vivo biodistribution studies in healthy Wistar rats (Figure 13) [32]. Figure 14 shows its high bone accumulation, especially in the high metabolic epiphyseal plates and other joint regions.

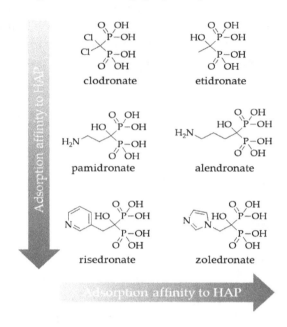

Figure 10. Classification of bisphosphonates according to their adsorption affinity to hydroxyapatite (HAP).

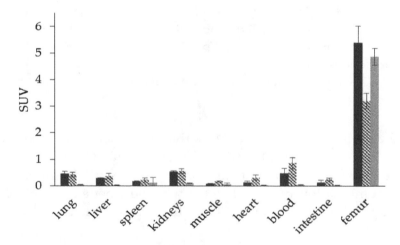

Figure 11. Ex vivo biodistribution of [^{68}Ga]Ga-DOTA^{ZOL} (■) (6.9 ± 0.1 MBq, $n = 4$), [^{68}Ga]Ga-BPAPD (▨) (9.8 ± 0.2 MBq, $n = 8$), and [^{18}F]NaF (■) (10.9 ± 0.4, $n = 4$) in healthy Wistar rats 60 min p.i.

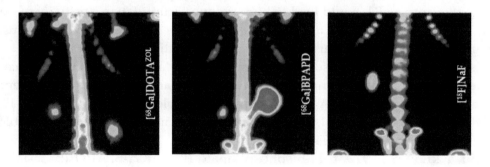

Figure 12. Maximum intensity projection of the thorax region of Wistar rats 60 min p.i. [32].

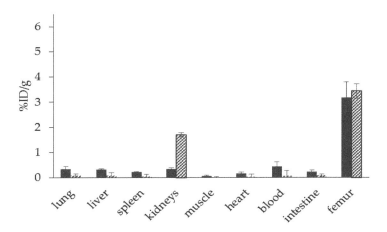

Figure 13. Ex vivo biodistribution of [^{68}Ga]Ga-DOTA^{ZOL} (■) (6.9 ± 0.1 MBq, n = 4) and [^{177}Lu]Lu-DOTA^{ZOL} (▨) (3.7 ± 0.1 MBq, n = 4) in healthy Wistar rats 60 min p.i.

Figure 14. Whole body scintigraphy 60 min p.i. of [^{177}Lu]Lu-DOTA^{ZOL} in a healthy Wistar rat [32].

Considering the good results of both the ^{68}Ga- and the ^{177}Lu-labeled derivatives in small animal studies, ^{68}Ga- and ^{177}Lu-labeled DOTA^{ZOL} seem to offer high potential for theranostic applications. This potential now needs to be proven in clinical studies.

Figure 15 shows a comparison of [^{68}Ga]Ga-PSMA-11 and [^{68}Ga]Ga-DOTA^{ZOL} in one and the same prostate cancer patient. Both tracers detected multiple skeletal lesions in thoracic and lumbar vertebrae, as well as in the pelvis. Comparison of SUVs revealed an approximately three-fold higher uptake of the bisphosphonate in bone metastases and an approximately three-fold lower uptake in normal tissue organs, exemplifying the bisphosphonate's better target-to-background ratio.

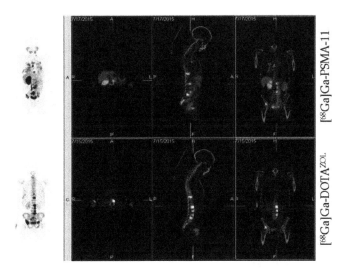

Figure 15. Whole-body PET/CT 60 min p.i. 170 MBq [^{68}Ga]Ga- PSMA-11 and 155 MBq [^{68}Ga]Ga-DOTA^{ZOL}, respectively, in a prostate cancer patient (71 years old, Gleason 4 + 4).

[^{177}Lu]Lu-DOTA^{ZOL} has been used in ten patients with bone metastases for dosimetry studies (data to be published). Whole body scintigraphic images were acquired at different time points after injection. Within this study it showed a fast renal clearance and a high target-to-background ratio, and was able to confirm the results of the ex vivo biodistribution studies (Figure 16).

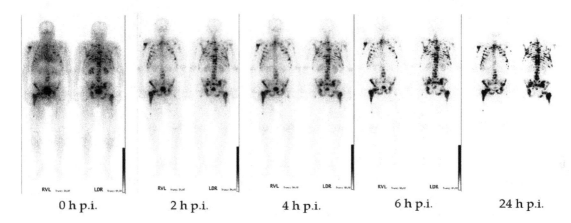

0 h p.i.   2 h p.i.   4 h p.i.   6 h p.i.   24 h p.i.

Figure 16. Anterior and posterior whole-body scintigraphs of [^{177}Lu]Lu-DOTA^{ZOL} in a prostate cancer patient. 0 min, 2 h, 4 h, 6 h, and 24 h after application of 1 GBq [^{177}Lu]Lu-DOTA^{ZOL} demonstrating multiple intense accumulation in the axial skeleton and both humerae and femorae. The target-to-background ratio is progressively better in later images and best at 24 h p.i.

3. Conclusions

The combination of novel bisphosphonates with macrocyclic chelators provides promising tracers for diagnosis, therapy, and also theranostics of bone metastases.

Currently, the most potent ^{68}Ga-bisphosphonate is [^{68}Ga]Ga-NO2AP^{BP}, which enables quantitative radiolabeling and exhibits very high accumulation in bone metastases 30–60 min after injection, as well as a fast blood clearance and very low uptake in soft tissue. It is superior to [^{99m}Tc]Tc-MDP and comparable to [^{18}F]NaF.

DOTA bisphosphonates are eminently suitable for labeling with ^{177}Lu. [^{177}Lu]Lu-BPAMD has proved valuable in clinical application. The low-energy β^- emission hardly reaches the bone marrow and only a low or no haematotoxicity was observed. The good target-to-background ratio, that all examined bisphosphonates have in common, is also advantageous for therapeutic applications due to reduced radiation dose for non-target tissue.

Due to further developments regarding the chemical structure of these macrocyclic bisphosphonates, new ^{68}Ga- and ^{177}Lu-labeled bisphosphonates possessing improved pharmacological properties are expected. Zoledronate based bisphosphonates appear to be the most potent radiotracers with regard to bone lesions. Thus, DOTA^{ZOL} for example may be a potent conjugate for theranostics of bone metastases.

Acknowledgments: The authors thank Matthias Miederer, Nicole Bausbacher, and Barbara Biesalski (University Hospital Mainz) for processing of the biodistribution studies. Thanks are given to ITG Munich for supplying ^{177}Lu. This work was partially supported by the Deutsche Forschungsgemeinschaft (grant BE-2607/1-1/1-2 (Ralf Bergmann).

References

1. Rubens, R. Bone metastases—The clinical problem. *Eur. J. Cancer* **1998**, *34*, 210–213. [CrossRef]
2. Nørgaard, M.; Jensen, A.Ø.; Jacobsen, J.B.; Cetin, K.; Fryzek, J.P.; Sørensen, H.T. Skeletal Related Events, Bone Metastasis and Survival of Prostate Cancer: A Population Based Cohort Study in Denmark (1999 to 2007). *J. Urol.* **2010**, *184*, 162–167. [CrossRef] [PubMed]

3. Sartor, O.; Hoskin, P.; Bruland, Ø.S. Targeted radio-nuclide therapy of skeletal metastases. *Cancer Treat. Rev.* **2013**, *39*, 18–26. [CrossRef] [PubMed]

4. Rahmim, A.; Zaidi, H. PET versus SPECT: Strengths, limitations and challenges. *Nucl. Med. Commun.* **2008**, *29*, 193–207. [CrossRef] [PubMed]

5. Love, C.; Din, A.S.; Tomas, M.B.; Kalapparambath, T.P.; Palestro, C.J. Radionuclide Bone Imaging: An Illustrative Review. *RadioGraphics* **2003**, *23*, 341–358. [CrossRef] [PubMed]

6. Harmer, C.L.; Burns, J.E.; Sams, A.; Spittle, M. The value of fluorine-18 for scanning bone tumours. *Clin. Radiol.* **1969**, *20*, 204–212. [CrossRef]

7. Rösch, F. Past, present and future of 68Ge/68Ga generators. *Appl. Radiat. Isot.* **2013**, *76*, 24–30. [CrossRef] [PubMed]

8. Benesova, M.; Schafer, M.; Bauder-Wust, U.; Afshar-Oromieh, A.; Kratochwil, C.; Mier, W.; Haberkorn, U.; Kopka, K.; Eder, M. Preclinical Evaluation of a Tailor-Made DOTA-Conjugated PSMA Inhibitor with Optimized Linker Moiety for Imaging and Endoradiotherapy of Prostate Cancer. *J. Nucl. Med.* **2015**, *56*, 914–920. [CrossRef] [PubMed]

9. Lange, R.; Ter Heine, R.; Knapp, R.F.; de Klerk, J.M.; Bloemendal, H.J.; Hendrikse, N.H. Pharmaceutical and clinical development of phosphonate-based radiopharmaceuticals for the targeted treatment of bone metastases. *Bone* **2016**, *91*, 159–179. [CrossRef] [PubMed]

10. Hoskin, P.; Sartor, O.; O'Sullivan, J.M.; Johannessen, D.C.; Helle, S.I.; Logue, J.; Bottomley, D.; Nilsson, S.; Vogelzang, N.J.; Fang, F.; et al. Efficacy and safety of radium-223 dichloride in patients with castration-resistant prostate cancer and symptomatic bone metastases, with or without previous docetaxel use: A prespecified subgroup analysis from the randomised, double-blind, phase 3 5ALSYMPCA6 trial. *Lancet Oncol.* **2014**, *15*, 1397–1406. [PubMed]

11. Lebedev, N.A.; Novgorodov, A.F.; Misiak, R.; Brockmann, J.; Rösch, F. Radiochemical separation of no-carrier-added 177Lu as produced via the 176Yb(n,γ)177Yb→177Lu process. *Appl. Radiat. Isot.* **2000**, *53*, 421–425. [CrossRef]

12. Kálmán, F.K.; Király, R.; Brücher, E. Stability Constants and Dissociation Rates of the EDTMP Complexes of Samarium(III) and Yttrium(III). *Eur. J. Inorg. Chem.* **2008**, *2008*, 4719–4727. [CrossRef]

13. Pandit-Taskar, N.; Batraki, M.; Divgi, C.R. Radiopharmaceutical Therapy for Palliation of Bone Pain from Osseous Metastases. *J. Nucl. Med.* **2004**, *45*, 1358–1365. [PubMed]

14. Pillai, M.R.A.; Dash, A.; Knapp, F.F. Rhenium-188: Availability from the 188W/188Re generator and status of current applications. *Curr. Radiopharm.* **2012**, *5*, 228–243. [CrossRef] [PubMed]

15. Fellner, M.; Riss, P.; Loktionova, N.S.; Zhernosekov, K.P.; Thews, O.; Geraldes, C.F.G.C.; Kovacs, Z.; Lukes, I.; Rösch, F. Comparison of different phosphorus-containing ligands complexing 68Ga for PET-imaging of bone metabolism. *Radiochim. Acta* **2011**, *99*, 43–51. [CrossRef]

16. Awang, M.B.; Hardy, J.G.; Davis, S.S.; Wilding, I.R.; Parry, S.J. Radiolabelling of pharmaceutical dosage forms by neutron activation of samarium-152. *J. Label. Compd. Radiopharm.* **1993**, *33*, 941–948. [CrossRef]

17. Yousefnia, H.; Zolghadri, S.; Shanehsazzadeh, S. Estimated human absorbed dose of 177Lu-BPAMD based on mice data: Comparison with 177Lu-EDTMP. *Appl. Radiat. Isot.* **2015**, *104*, 128–135. [CrossRef] [PubMed]

18. Russell, R.G.G.; Watts, N.B.; Ebetino, F.H.; Rogers, M.J. Mechanisms of action of bisphosphonates: Similarities and differences and their potential influence on clinical efficacy. *Osteoporos. Int.* **2008**, *19*, 733–759. [CrossRef] [PubMed]

19. Papapoulos, S.E. Bisphosphonates: How do they work? *Best Pract. Res. Clin. Endocrinol. Metab.* **2008**, *22*, 831–847. [CrossRef] [PubMed]

20. Ogawa, K.; Mukai, T.; Inoue, Y.; Ono, M.; Saji, H. Development of a Novel 99mTc-Chelate–Conjugated Bisphosphonate with High Affinity for Bone as a Bone Scintigraphic Agent. *J. Nucl. Med.* **2006**, *47*, 2042–2047. [PubMed]

21. Baum, R.P.; Kulkarni, H.R. THERANOSTICS: From Molecular Imaging Using Ga-68 Labeled Tracers and PET/CT to Personalized Radionuclide Therapy—The Bad Berka Experience. *Theranostics* **2012**, *2*, 437–447. [CrossRef] [PubMed]

22. Fellner, M.; Biesalski, B.; Bausbacher, N.; Kubícek, V.; Hermann, P.; Rösch, F.; Thews, O. 68Ga-BPAMD: PET-imaging of bone metastases with a generator based positron emitter. *Nucl. Med. Biol.* **2012**, *39*, 993–999. [CrossRef]

23. Fellner, M.; Baum, R.P.; Kubíček, V.; Hermann, P.; Lukeš, I.; Prasad, V.; Rösch, F. PET/CT imaging of osteoblastic bone metastases with 68Ga-bisphosphonates: First human study. *Eur. J. Nucl. Med. Mol. Imaging* **2010**, *37*, 834. [CrossRef]

24. Rösch, F.; Baum, R.P. Generator-based PET radiopharmaceuticals for molecular imaging of tumours: On the way to Theranostics. *Dalton Trans.* **2011**, *40*, 6104–6111. [CrossRef] [PubMed]

25. Yousefnia, H.; Zolghadri, S.; Sadeghi, H.R.; Naderi, M.; Jalilian, A.R.; Shanehsazzadeh, S. Preparation and biological assessment of 177Lu-BPAMD as a high potential agent for bone pain palliation therapy: Comparison with 177Lu-EDTMP. *J. Radioanal. Nucl. Chem.* **2016**, *307*, 1243–1251. [CrossRef]

26. Lattuada, L.; Barge, A.; Cravotto, G.; Giovenzana, G.B.; Tei, L. The synthesis and application of polyamino polycarboxylic bifunctional chelating agents. *Chem. Soc. Rev.* **2011**, *40*, 3019–3049. [CrossRef] [PubMed]

27. Price, E.W.; Orvig, C. Matching chelators to radiometals for radiopharmaceuticals. *Chem. Soc. Rev.* **2014**, *43*, 260–290. [CrossRef]

28. Spang, P.; Herrmann, C.; Roesch, F. Bifunctional Gallium-68 Chelators: Past, Present, and Future. *Semin. Nucl. Med.* **2016**, *46*, 373–394. [CrossRef] [PubMed]

29. Passah, A.; Tripathi, M.; Ballal, S.; Yadav, M.P.; Kumar, R.; Roesch, F.; Meckel, M.; Sarathi Chakraborty, P.; Bal, C. Evaluation of bone-seeking novel radiotracer 68Ga-NO2AP-Bisphosphonate for the detection of skeletal metastases in carcinoma breast. *Eur. J. Nucl. Med. Mol. Imaging* **2017**, *44*, 41–49. [CrossRef]

30. Seemann, J.; Waldron, B.P.; Roesch, F.; Parker, D. Approaching 'Kit-Type' Labelling with 68Ga: The DATA Chelators. *ChemMedChem* **2015**, *10*, 1019–1026. [CrossRef] [PubMed]

31. Wu, Z.; Zha, Z.; Choi, S.R.; Plössl, K.; Zhu, L.; Kung, H.F. New 68Ga-PhenA bisphosphonates as potential bone imaging agents. *Nucl. Med. Biol.* **2016**, *43*, 360–371. [CrossRef] [PubMed]

32. Meckel, M.; Bergmann, R.; Miederer, M.; Roesch, F. Bone targeting compounds for radiotherapy and imaging: *Me(III)-DOTA conjugates of bisphosphonic acid, pamidronic acid and zoledronic acid. *EJNMMI Radiopharm. Chem.* **2016**, *1*, 14. [CrossRef]

4

Ketamine and Ceftriaxone-Induced Alterations in Glutamate Levels Do Not Impact the Specific Binding of Metabotropic Glutamate Receptor Subtype 5 Radioligand [18F]PSS232 in the Rat Brain

Adrienne Müller Herde [1] 🆔, Silvan D. Boss [1], Yingfang He [1], Roger Schibli [1,2] 🆔, Linjing Mu [1,2] and Simon M. Ametamey [1,*]

[1] Center for Radiopharmaceutical Sciences of ETH, PSI, and USZ, Department of Chemistry and Applied Biosciences of ETH, 8093 Zurich, Switzerland; adrienne.herde@pharma.ethz.ch (A.M.H.); silvanboss@hotmail.com (S.D.B.); yingfang.he@pharma.ethz.ch (Y.H.); roger.schibli@pharma.ethz.ch (R.S.); linjing.mu@pharma.ethz.ch (L.M.)

[2] Department of Nuclear Medicine, University Hospital Zurich, 8091 Zurich, Switzerland

* Correspondence: simon.ametamey@pharma.ethz.ch

Abstract: Several studies showed that [11C]ABP688 binding is altered following drug-induced perturbation of glutamate levels in brains of humans, non-human primates and rats. We evaluated whether the fluorinated derivative [18F]PSS232 can be used to assess metabotropic glutamate receptor 5 (mGluR5) availability in rats after pharmacological challenge with ketamine, known to increase glutamate, or ceftriaxone, known to decrease glutamate. In vitro autoradiography was performed on rat brain slices with [18F]PSS232 to prove direct competition of the drugs for mGluR5. One group of rats were challenged with a bolus injection of either vehicle, racemic ketamine, S-ketamine or ceftriaxone followed by positron emission tomography PET imaging with [18F]PSS232. The other group received an infusion of the drugs during the PET scan. Distribution volume ratios (DVRs) were calculated using a reference tissue model. In vitro autoradiography showed no direct competition of the drugs with [18F]PSS232 for the allosteric binding site of mGluR5. DVRs of [18F]PSS232 binding in vivo did not change in any brain region neither after bolus injection nor after infusion. We conclude that [18F]PSS232 has utility for measuring mGluR5 density or occupancy of the allosteric site in vivo, but it cannot be used to measure in vivo fluctuations of glutamate levels in the rat brain.

Keywords: glutamate; metabotropic glutamate receptor subtype 5; [18F]PSS232; ketamine; ceftriaxone; positron emission tomography; allosteric modulator; MMPEP; ABP688

1. Introduction

Glutamate is the principle excitatory neurotransmitter in the nervous system, which elicits its action on ionotropic (N-methyl-D-aspartate receptor (NMDA), Kainate, α-amino-3-hydroxy-5-methyl-4-isoxazolepropionic acid receptor (AMPA)) and metabotropic (mGluR) receptors, especially in the mammalian brain [1]. Ionotropic receptors form ion channels and exhibit a fast relay. Metabotropic receptors are G protein-coupled, acting through a second messenger and produce stimuli that are more prolonged. Since glutamate is not degraded in the synaptic cleft, two major astrocytic transporters, the glutamate transporter-1 (GLT-1, EAAT2) and the glutamate aspartate transporter (GLAST, EAAT1), remove glutamate and provide the regulation to orchestrate receptor excitability [2]. Glutamate works not only as a point-to-point transmitter, but also through spill-over synaptic crosstalk between synapses in which summation of glutamate released from a neighboring synapse creates extrasynaptic signaling [3]. A disruption of these fine-tuning mechanisms can cause excitotoxicity, which is a driving force in the pathophysiology of various neuropsychological disorders. An important role of the glutamatergic system has been established in depression [4], schizophrenia [5], Parkinson's disease [6], Alzheimer's disease [7] and drug addiction [8]. Due to the involvement of the glutamatergic system in a large array of diseases, intense efforts have been made in recent years to visualize acute fluctuations in endogenous glutamate levels. Positron emission tomography (PET) using the highly selective allosteric antagonist of mGluR5, 3-(6-methyl-pyridin-2-ylethynyl)-cyclohex-2-enone-O-(11)C-methyl-oxime ([11C]ABP688) [9], has been used to measure in vivo receptor availability and fluctuations of endogenous glutamate. Several studies have shown that [11C]ABP688 binding is altered following drug-induced perturbation of glutamate levels in humans [10–12], baboons [13], rhesus monkeys [14] and rats [15]. In a pharmacological challenge study by Wyckhuys et al. [16], N-acetylcysteine (NAc), a compound which facilitates the activity of the cysteine–glutamate antiporter and indirectly increases extrasynaptic glutamate levels [17] did not affect the in vivo binding of [11C]ABP688 in the rat brain. In another pharmacological challenge study, Zimmer et al. [15] used the drug ceftriaxone, a potent GLT-1 activator [18], which induces a decrease in extracellular glutamate levels. Ceftriaxone selectively increases the expression of glial GLT-1 and protects neurons against ischemia via upregulation of GLT-1 following increased uptake of glutamate. This leads to diminished excitotoxicity of glutamate and protection of neurons against ischemia [19]. In their publication, Zimmer et al. reported an increase in [11C]ABP688 binding potential in the thalamic ventral anterior nucleus of the rat brain, however, the global binding potential (whole brain) was not changed under baseline and ceftriaxone challenge. No information was provided on any other rat brain compartment besides the thalamic ventral anterior nucleus.

We here present our study assessing the feasibility of using the novel ^{18}F-labelled mGluR5 antagonist [18F]PSS232 [20] to measure in vivo fluctuation of endogenous glutamate levels in the rat brain by PET imaging. The results of this study should potentially shed more light on the utility of [18F]PSS232 for measuring mGluR5 availability after drug-induced perturbation of glutamate levels in the rat brain. We already reported on the kinetics of [18F]PSS232 in the rat brain and established the model-independent area-under-the-curve ratio method for robust quantification of PET results [21].

Given the contradictory results obtained in rats using [11C]ABP688, we applied two different pharmacological challenges of altering glutamate levels. We used (i) subanesthetic doses of ketamine, an NMDA receptor antagonist known to increase glutamate release [22,23] and (ii) the GLT-1 activator ceftriaxone, known to reduce glutamate levels. Furthermore, we compared the effects of racemic and S-ketamine on mGluR5 availability since a number of studies have suggested a two-fold higher potency for S-ketamine compared to racemic or R-ketamine [24–26]. Finally, in contrast to previous studies that used bolus injections to modulate glutamate release, we compared the effect of bolus injection and infusion of the three drugs.

2. Results

2.1. In Vitro Effects of Racemic Ketamine, S-Ketamine or Ceftriaxone on [18F]PSS232 Binding

To exclude direct binding of either racemic ketamine, S-ketamine or ceftriaxone to mGluR5, we performed in vitro autoradiography using rat brain slices. Figure 1 shows [18F]PSS232 binding to mGluR5-rich regions such as the striatum, hippocampus, cortex, cortex cingulate and bulbus olfactorius. The cerebellum with low mGluR5 density showed less [18F]PSS232 binding. This binding pattern was not altered when the brain slices were co-incubated with either racemic ketamine, S-ketamine or ceftriaxone compared to the vehicle. This result indicates that there is no direct interference of these pharmaceuticals with the binding site of [18F]PSS232 to mGluR5. In addition, after co-incubation of rat brain slices with L-glutamate, we found no competition between L-glutamate and [18F]PSS232 binding to mGluR5. As expected, the binding of [18F]PSS232 was abolished upon co-incubation with the two mGluR5 antagonists, MMPEP and ABP688.

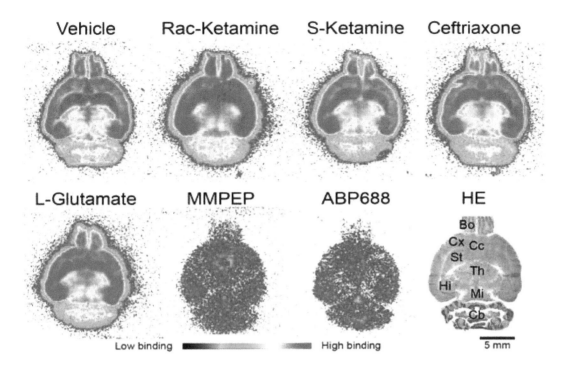

Figure 1. Representative in vitro autoradiograms of a rat brain incubated with 1 nM [^{18}F]PSS232 solution supplemented with vehicle (0.9% NaCl), racemic ketamine, S-ketamine, ceftriaxone, L-glutamate, MMPEP ((2-[2-(3-methoxyphenyl)ethynyl]-6-methylpyridine hydrochloride) or ABP688 ((Z)-N-methoxy-3-[2-(6-methylpyridin-2-yl)ethynyl]-cyclohex-2-en-1-imine) (each 1 μM). [^{18}F]PSS232 binding was strong to bulbus olfactorius (Bo), cortex (Cx), cortex cingulate (Cc), striatum (St) and hippocampus (Hi). Moderate binding was observed to thalamus (Th) and midbrain (Mi) and low binding to cerebellum (Cb). Color bar indicates low and high binding. Hematoxylin/eosin (HE) staining shows rat brain morphology. Scale bar: 5 mm.

2.2. In Vivo Effects of Racemic Ketamine, S-Ketamine or Ceftriaxone on [^{18}F]PSS232 Binding

To measure ketamine- or ceftriaxone-induced changes in mGluR5 availability as an index of glutamate release, we used [^{18}F]PSS232 PET imaging applying a bolus injection protocol. In Figure 2a, the mGluR5 distribution volume ratios (DVRs) for selected brain regions are depicted. For all three drugs, the highest mGluR5 DRVs were found in the striatum (2.6 ± 0.03) followed by the hippocampus (2.2 ± 0.04), cortex cingulate (2.2 ± 0.04) and cortex (2.1 ± 0.06). Global mGluR5 DVR for the three drugs, racemic ketamine, S-ketamine and ceftriaxone, did not change and was similar for the whole brain (1.7 ± 0.03). We found no significant between-group differences after bolus injections. Based on human studies with [^{11}C]ABP688 that reported reduced mGluR5 availability after infusion of ketamine [10,12], we adjusted our study protocol and infused ketamine or ceftriaxone after an initial bolus injection. Figure 2b shows the DVRs for different brain regions and the whole brain after the different challenges, which, however, did not significantly differ from each other. Similar to the bolus protocol, mGluR5 DVRs were highest in the striatum (2.6 ± 0.02) followed by the hippocampus (2.1 ± 0.08), cortex cingulate (2.2 ± 0.05) and cortex (2.0 ± 0.05). Global mGluR5 DVR (1.7 ± 0.01) was not affected by the different challenges and intergroup differences were also not significant. Figure 3a shows parametric DVR images of the rat brain using bolus and infusion protocols. There were no differences in [^{18}F]PSS232 binding in either ketamine- or ceftriaxone-induced glutamate fluctuations or injection protocols. Figure 3b shows the brain regions-of-interest defined to calculate the DVRs.

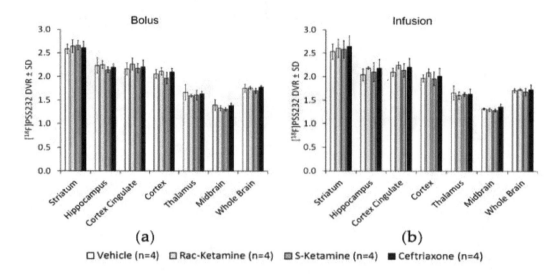

Figure 2. Influence of (**a**) bolus injection or (**b**) infusion of vehicle (0.9% NaCl), racemic ketamine, S-ketamine and ceftriaxone on [^{18}F]PSS232 distribution volume ratios (DVRs) in different rat brain regions. Number of animals as depicted. SD, standard deviations.

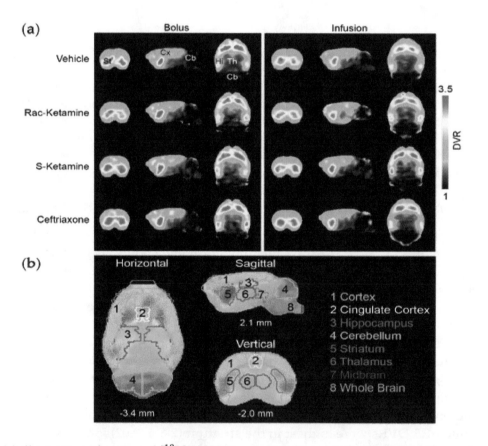

Figure 3. (**a**) illustration of averaged [^{18}F]PSS232 brain uptake as mGluR5 distribution volume ratios (DVRs) after vehicle (0.9% NaCl; $n = 4$), racemic ketamine ($n = 4$), S-ketamine ($n = 4$) and ceftriaxone ($n = 4$) challenge. PET images were derived after bolus injection (**left**) or infusion (**right**) and presented in axial, sagittal and coronal planes. St, striatum; Cx, cortex; Cb, cerebellum; Hi, hippocampus; Th, thalamus; (**b**) definition of brain regions-of-interest on PET images in horizontal (coronal), sagittal and vertical (axial) sections. Locations in mm are distance to the Bregma. The quantitative regions-of-interest analysis is shown in Figure 2.

In order to demonstrate reversibility of binding of [^{18}F]PSS232 in vivo, displacement studies, using MMPEP and ABP688, which were applied 40 min after [^{18}F]PSS232 injection, were performed. The results showed a rapid wash-out of radioactivity from mGluR5-rich brain regions (Figure 4a). Striatal radioactivity values decreased shortly after MMPEP or ABP688 administration to the cerebellar level and remained low (Figure 4b).

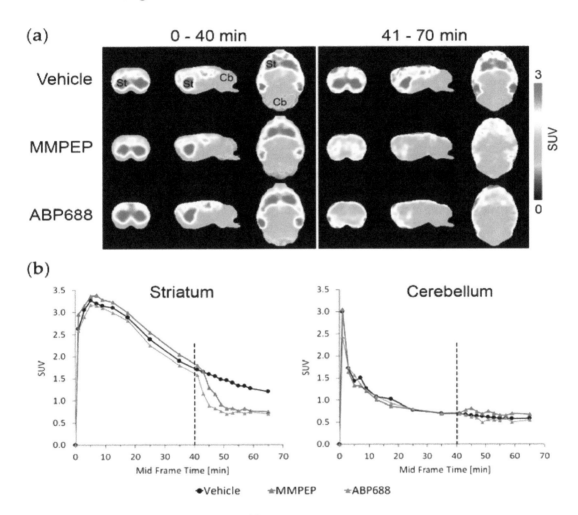

Figure 4. In vivo displacement study of [^{18}F]PSS232 with either vehicle ($n = 1$; 1:1 PEG200/aqua ad inject), 1 mg/kg MMPEP ($n = 1$) or 1 mg/kg ABP688 ($n = 1$) at 40 min post radiotracer injection. (**a**) [^{18}F]PSS232 PET images of rat brains averaged from 0–40 and 41–70 min after radiotracer injection. PET images are presented in axial, sagittal and coronal planes. St, striatum; Cb, cerebellum; (**b**) time–activity curves for [^{18}F]PSS232 in the mGluR5-rich striatum and mGluR5-low cerebellum. Dashed line at 40 min represents the time point of injection of the vehicle, MMPEP ((2-[2-(3-methoxyphenyl)ethynyl]-6-methylpyridine hydrochloride) or ABP688 ((Z)-N-methoxy-3 -[2-(6-methylpyridin-2-yl)ethynyl]-cyclohex-2-en-1-imine). SUV, standardized uptake values.

3. Discussion

The goal of this study was to investigate whether [^{18}F]PSS232 can be used to image glutamate fluctuations as was, to some extent, reported for [^{11}C]ABP688. [^{18}F]PSS232 is a fluorinated derivative of [^{11}C]ABP688, which binds to the same site in the transmembrane domain of mGluR5 as [^{11}C]ABP688. In our experimental setup, we induced glutamate increase by injection of ketamine and glutamate decrease by activating GLT-1 with ceftriaxone. Several publications report significant changes in endogenous extraneuronal glutamate levels by ketamine and ceftriaxone [12,15,22]. In our study, we used ketamine dosages (25 mg/kg bolus, 0.6 mg/kg/h infusion) known to be high enough to increase extraneuronal glutamate levels, as measured in vivo with microdialysis [12,22]. Ketamine increases glutamate directly by influencing mGluR5 functional status and through the antagonism of NMDA receptors. Furthermore, mGluR5 and NMDA receptors functionally interact and mutually potentiate their responses [27,28]. The dosage of the bolus-injected ceftriaxone (200 mg/kg) used in this study was also reported to be high enough to decrease glutamate levels, at least in the thalamic ventral anterior nucleus of the rat brain by micro-PET and microdialysis [15]. Changes in glutamate levels after infusion of ceftriaxone have not been reported yet. Although GLT-1 and mGluR5 are expressed in almost all brain regions, splice variants or differential expression of GLT-1 may explain the distinct activation by ceftriaxone. Our experiments demonstrated that the mGluR5-specific radiotracer, [18F]PSS232, was not able to detect changes in endogenous glutamate levels induced by ketamine or ceftriaxone in the rat brain in vivo. Our in vitro autoradiography results showed that neither ketamine nor ceftriaxone or glutamate itself competed with [18F]PSS232 for binding to mGluR5. However, the allosteric antagonists MMPEP and unlabeled ABP688 reduced [18F]PSS232 binding in vitro and in vivo. The in vivo displacement studies confirmed that [18F]PSS232 binds to the allosteric site of mGluR5. Our in vivo findings indicate that the altered levels of endogenous glutamate did not alter the capacity of [18F]PSS232 to bind to mGluR5 in the rat brain. We hypothesized that changes in endogenous glutamate would lead to conformational changes of mGluR5 resulting in an increased or decreased affinity of [18F]PSS232. However, our results indicated no affinity shift of [18F]PSS232 to mGluR5 in vivo. The binding of [18F]PSS232 to the allosteric site instead of the orthosteric binding site of mGluR5 might be dependent on the tertiary and quaternary receptor conformations [29]. Oligomeric and heteromeric forms of mGluR5 might influence the availability of the allosteric site [30,31]. Furthermore, changes of in vivo glutamate levels might alter mGluR5 conformational states, which were, however, not supported by our findings. On the other hand, affinity shift in receptor–radioligand interactions was described for dopamine D2 receptors, where amphetamine challenge altered the binding of a D2 PET radioligand [32,33].

To the best of our knowledge, this is the first study reporting on the potential of [18F]PSS232 to image glutamate fluctuations. In contrast to our results, a recent study in rats indicated that [11C]ABP688 was able to visualize acute fluctuation in endogenous glutamate levels after challenge with ceftriaxone [15]. Ceftriaxone administration increased [11C]ABP688 binding potential in the thalamic ventral anterior nucleus bilaterally, but not in the frontal cortex. The authors have, so far, no explanation why this thalamic region was the first to be affected by ceftriaxone and suggested further investigations. We investigated the thalamic area but found no changes in mGluR5 DVRs after vehicle, ceftriaxone or ketamine administration. To date, no publication is available that has reported on ketamine-induced glutamate fluctuations and consequent alterations in mGluR5 availability using PET imaging in the rat brain. Most of the ketamine challenges were performed in humans demonstrating a rapid and large (20%) reduction in [11C]ABP688 binding after ketamine infusion in healthy humans [10]. The ketamine-induced decrease in [11C]ABP688 binding was explained by a reduction in mGluR5 availability due to internalization. This internalization might be in response to glutamate release or a glutamate-induced conformational change in the receptor that reduces the likelihood of radioligand binding at the allosteric site. Other approaches to increase endogenous glutamate have been made with NAc in rats, rhesus monkeys and baboons. In baboons, NAc decreased [11C]ABP688 binding potential, which may be the result of an affinity shift in the binding to the allosteric site [13]. In rats [16] and rhesus monkeys [14], the binding of [11C]ABP688 was not affected after NAc challenge. In the rat study, the authors applied the NMDA receptor antagonist MK-801, which has a similar action as ketamine, and found no changes in [11C]ABP688 binding [16]. Although the authors used a different pharmacological approach, their results are in line with our findings. Discrepancies among the different studies could be species differences and variations in the methodology.

4. Materials and Methods

4.1. Animals

All procedures were performed according the Guide to the Care and Use of Experimental Animals of the Swiss legislation on animal welfare. All procedures fulfilled the ARRIVE guidelines on reporting animal experiments and complied with the commonly-accepted '3Rs'. The protocols for pharmacological administration and PET imaging were approved by the Veterinary Office of the Canton Zurich, Switzerland (permit number: ZH017/2015). Male Wistar (Crl:WI) rats were purchased from Charles River (Sulzfeld, Germany) and their body weights were between 350 g and 420 g at the time of the experiments. Rats were kept in a room with controlled temperature (21 °C) under a 12-h light/12-h dark cycle, with ad libitum access to food and water.

4.2. Radiosynthesis and Pharmaceuticals

The radiosynthesis of [18F]PSS232 was conducted as described previously [20]. The mean molar radioactivity at end of synthesis was 95.3 ± 6.2 GBq/μmol. Racemic ketamine hydrochloride was obtained from LGC (MM0144.00) (Teddington, UK), S-ketamine hydrochloride from Cayman Chemical (CAY-9001961) (Ann Arbor, MI, USA), ceftriaxone from Sigma Aldrich (C5793) (St. Louis, MO, USA), L-glutamate from Sigma Aldrich (128430), and 0.9% NaCl from B.Braun (Melsungen, Germany). MMPEP (2-[2-(3-methoxyphenyl)ethynyl]-6-methylpyridine hydrochloride) and ABP688 ((Z)-N-methoxy-3-[2-(6-methylpyridin-2-yl)ethynyl]-cyclohex-2-en-1-imine) were produced in-house. For in vivo administration, both forms of ketamine were dissolved in aqua ad inject and ceftriaxone in 0.9% NaCl. MMPEP and ABP688 were dissolved in 1:1 PEG200/aqua ad inject. Isoflurane (Isocare, Animalcare, York, UK) was used as an anesthetic agent. Scheme 1 shows the chemical structures of [18F]PSS232, ABP688 and MMPEP.

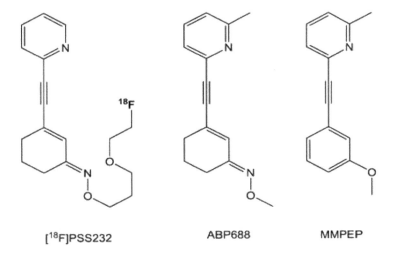

| [18F]PSS232 | ABP688 | MMPEP |

Scheme 1. Chemical structures of the mGluR5 radiotracer [18F]PSS232 and mGluR5 antagonists ABP688 ((Z)-N-methoxy-3-[2-(6-methylpyridin-2-yl)ethynyl]-cyclohex-2-en-1-imine) and MMPEP ((2-[2-(3-methoxyphenyl)ethynyl]-6-methylpyridine hydrochloride).

4.3. In Vitro Autoradiography

Coronal Wistar rat brain sections (10 μm) were cut on a cryostat (CryoStar NX50, Thermo Scientific, Waltham, MA, USA) and mounted on glass slides (Superfrost Plus, Thermo Scientific). Consecutive sections were thawed on ice for 10 min before pre-incubation in HEPES/BSA-buffer (4-(2-hydroxyethyl)-1-piperazineethanesulfonic acid/bovine serum albumin) (30 mM HEPES, 1.2 mM MgCl$_2$, 110 mM NaCl, 2.5 mM CaCl$_2$, 5 mM KCl, pH 7.4, 0.1% BSA) at 4 °C for another 10 min. Excess solution was carefully removed and tissue slices were incubated with 1 nM [18F]PSS232 supplemented with either vehicle (0.9% NaCl), 1 μM racemic ketamine, 1 μM S-ketamine, 1 μM ceftriaxone, 1 μM L-glutamate, 1 μM mGluR5 antagonist MMPEP or 1 μM mGluR5 antagonist ABP688. After incubation for 40 min at room temperature in a wet chamber, the slices were washed in ice cold HEPES/BSA-buffer for 5 min, twice in HEPES-buffer for 2 min each and finally dipped twice in distilled water. Dried slices were exposed to a phosphor imager plate (BAS-MS 2025, Fuji, Dielsdorf, Switzerland) for 15 min and the plate was scanned in a BAS-5000 reader (Fuji). A consecutive section was stained with hematoxylin (Gill No. 1, Sigma) and eosin (Eosin Y, Sigma) (HE) and digitalized by a slide scanner (Pannoramic 250, Sysmex, Horgen, Switzerland) to obtain brain morphology.

4.4. In Vivo PET Imaging

In vivo positron emission tomography/computed tomography (PET/CT) scans were performed with a calibrated Super Argus scanner (Sedecal, Madrid, Spain). Rats were anesthetized with isoflurane (2% isoflurane at 0.4 L/min oxygen:air (1:1) flow). Respiratory rate and temperature were controlled during the whole scan period (SA Instruments, Inc., Stony Brook, NY, USA). Rats were placed in a prone position and the brain was positioned in the center of the field of view. All intravenous (i.v.) injections were conducted via tail vein.

4.5. Bolus and Infusion Protocol

For the bolus injection protocol (Figure 5a), rats were injected with either 0.5 mL/kg vehicle i.v. (0.9% NaCl; n = 4), 25 mg/kg racemic ketamine (n = 4) intraperitoneal (i.p.), 25 mg/kg S-ketamine (n = 4) i.p. or 200 mg/kg ceftriaxone (n = 4) i.v. at 30 min before i.v. injection of [^{18}F]PSS232 (28.0 ± 2.1 MBq, 3.3 ± 2.0 nmol/kg, 87.8 ± 9.8 GBq/μmol). A short CT scout preceded the PET acquisition that lasted for 60 min and was followed by a CT scan to obtain anatomical orientation.

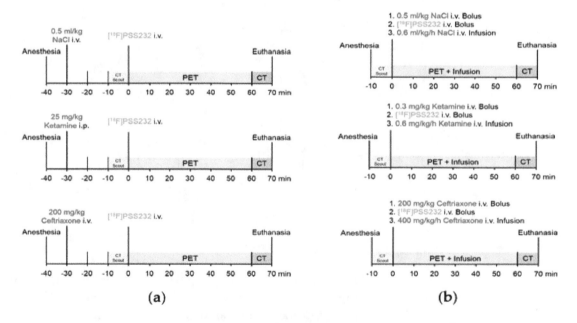

Figure 5. Glutamate challenge study design. (a) bolus protocol: anesthetized rats were injected either with 0.5 mL/kg vehicle intravenously (0.9% NaCl i.v.), 25 mg/kg racemic or S-ketamine intraperitoneally (i.p.) or 200 mg/kg ceftriaxone i.v. at 20 min before a short computed tomography (CT scout) or 30 min before injection of [^{18}F]PSS232 i.v., respectively. Positron emission tomography (PET) scans lasted for 60 min followed by CT scan; (b) infusion protocol: anesthetized rats received a short CT scout and were injected i.v. with either 0.5 mL/kg vehicle (0.9% NaCl), 0.3 mg/kg racemic or S-ketamine or 200 mg/kg ceftriaxone. Administration of [^{18}F]PSS232 i.v. preceded the infusion of either 0.6 mL/kg/h vehicle (0.9% NaCl), 0.6 mg/kg/h racemic or S-ketamine or 400 mg/kg/h ceftriaxone. PET acquisition and infusion lasted for 60 min followed by a CT scan.

For the infusion protocol (Figure 5b), rats received a short CT scout and were injected i.v. with either 0.5 mL/kg vehicle (0.9% NaCl; $n = 4$), 0.3 mg/kg racemic ketamine ($n = 4$), 0.3 mg/kg S-ketamine ($n = 4$) or 200 mg/kg ceftriaxone ($n = 4$). Administration of [^{18}F]PSS232 i.v. (28.5 $\pm$ 3.2 MBq, 3.6 $\pm$ 2.4 nmol/kg, 95.2 $\pm$ 7.8 GBq/μmol) preceded the infusion of either 0.6 mL/kg/h vehicle (0.9% NaCl), 0.6 mg/kg/h racemic ketamine, 0.6 mg/kg/h S-ketamine or 400 mg/kg/h ceftriaxone. PET acquisition lasted for 60 min followed by a CT scan. At the end of the scans, rats were euthanized.

4.6. In Vivo Displacement Study

For displacement studies of [^{18}F]PSS232 from mGluR5 binding sites either 1 mL/kg vehicle (1:1 PEG200/aqua ad inject), 1 mg/kg MMPEP or 1 mg/kg ABP688 was i.v. injected at 40 min after [^{18}F]PSS232 i.v. injection (30.1 $\pm$ 3.2 MBq, 3.0 $\pm$ 1.9 nmol/kg, 103.6 $\pm$ 4.8 GBq/μmol). We chose this relatively late time point to guarantee radiotracer equilibration in the brain. The total duration of the PET scan was 70 min followed by a CT scan.

4.7. Image Data Reconstruction, Analysis and Calculation of Distribution Volume Ratios (DVRs) as Well as Standardized Uptake Values (SUVs)

PET data were reconstructed in user-defined time frames with a voxel size of 0.3875 $\times$ 0.3875 $\times$ 0.775 mm^3 by two-dimensional-ordered subsets expectation maximization (2D-OSEM). Random and single but no attenuation correction was applied. Image files were analyzed with PMOD 3.8 software (PMOD Technologies Ltd., Zurich, Switzerland). For calculation of DVRs in regions-of-interest, specific brain regions were defined on the bases of the rat MRI T2 template (provided with PMOD software) (Figure 3b). Given that hardly any specific binding was found in rat cerebellum, this brain region was used as a reference region. DVRs were calculated from areas-under-the-curve as described recently [21]. Individual DVR images were calculated voxel-wise with the PXMod module of PMOD by means of the implemented reference Logan model and the cerebellum as reference region. Individual DVR images of the 4 animals per group were combined and averaged with the View module of PMOD.

For calculation of the time–activity curves for striatum and cerebellum, both regions were defined on the rat MRI T2 template. The tissue radioactivity values of both brain regions were decay-corrected and normalized to the injected radioactivity and body weight resulting in SUVs.

4.8. Statistical Analysis

Differences in mean values were evaluated by one-way analysis of variance (ANOVA) tests, followed by corrections for multiple testing (Bonferroni) using GraphPad Prism 6.0 software (GraphPad, La Jolla, CA, USA). A p-value < 0.05 was considered significant.

5. Conclusions

The present study verified that [^{18}F]PSS232 binds to delineated structures in the rat brain; however, [^{18}F]PSS232 does not seem to be a valuable tool for the in vivo assessment of acute endogenous glutamate fluctuations. Neither increased glutamate levels after ketamine challenge with changes in the functional status of mGluR5 through inhibition of the NMDA receptor nor decreased glutamate levels after challenge with GLT-1 activator ceftriaxone had any effect on the binding of [^{18}F]PSS232 to mGluR5. Whether [^{18}F]PSS232 will show similar effects in humans as demonstrated for [^{11}C]ABP688 remains to be validated in future clinical studies.

Author Contributions: A.M.H. designed the experiments, performed the in vitro experiments, analyzed the data and wrote the manuscript. S.D.B. and Y.H. performed [^{18}F]PSS232 productions and quality control. L.M. supervised [^{18}F]PSS232 productions and quality control, and contributed to the design of the in vivo displacement study and the syntheses of MMPEP and ABP688. S.D.B., Y.H., R.S. and L.M. reviewed the manuscript. S.M.A. conceived, designed and supervised the study and revised the manuscript.

Acknowledgments: We thank Claudia Keller for technical support with the infusion protocol and performing PET/CT scans. Selena Milicevic Sephton (Wolfson Brain Imaging Centre, University of Cambridge, UK) and Bruno Mancosu are acknowledged for their support during radiolabeling. We appreciate the fruitful discussions with Stefanie D. Krämer. The authors are grateful for the support of the Scientific Center for Optical and Electron Microscopy (ScopeM) of the ETH Zurich (Switzerland).

References

1. Pin, J.P.; Duvoisin, R. The metabotropic glutamate receptors: Structure and functions. *Neuropharmacology* **1995**, *34*, 1–26. [CrossRef]
2. Danbolt, N.C. Glutamate uptake. *Prog. Neurobiol.* **2001**, *65*, 1–105. [CrossRef]
3. Okubo, Y.; Sekiya, H.; Namiki, S.; Sakamoto, H.; Iinuma, S.; Yamasaki, M.; Watanabe, M.; Hirose, K.; Iino, M. Imaging extrasynaptic glutamate dynamics in the brain. *Proc. Natl. Acad. Sci. USA* **2010**, *107*, 6526–6531. [CrossRef] [PubMed]
4. Sanacora, G.; Zarate, C.A.; Krystal, J.H.; Manji, H.K. Targeting the glutamatergic system to develop novel, improved therapeutics for mood disorders. *Nat. Rev. Drug Discov.* **2008**, *7*, 426–437. [CrossRef] [PubMed]
5. Olney, J.W.; Farber, N.B. Glutamate receptor dysfunction and schizophrenia. *Arch. Gen. Psychiatry* **1995**, *52*, 998–1007. [CrossRef] [PubMed]
6. Chase, T.N.; Oh, J.D. Striatal dopamine- and glutamate-mediated dysregulation in experimental parkinsonism. *Trends Neurosci.* **2000**, *23*, S86–S91. [CrossRef]
7. Bruno, V.; Ksiazek, I.; Battaglia, G.; Lukic, S.; Leonhardt, T.; Sauer, D.; Gasparini, F.; Kuhn, R.; Nicoletti, F.; Flor, P.J. Selective blockade of metabotropic glutamate receptor subtype 5 is neuroprotective. *Neuropharmacology* **2000**, *39*, 2223–2230. [CrossRef]
8. Chiamulera, C.; Epping-Jordan, M.P.; Zocchi, A.; Marcon, C.; Cottiny, C.; Tacconi, S.; Corsi, M.; Orzi, F.; Conquet, F. Reinforcing and locomotor stimulant effects of cocaine are absent in mGluR5 null mutant mice. *Nat. Neurosci.* **2001**, *4*, 873–874. [CrossRef] [PubMed]
9. Ametamey, S.M.; Kessler, L.J.; Honer, M.; Wyss, M.T.; Buck, A.; Hintermann, S.; Auberson, Y.P.; Gasparini, F.; Schubiger, P.A. Radiosynthesis and preclinical evaluation of 11C-ABP688 as a probe for imaging the metabotropic glutamate receptor subtype 5. *J. Nucl. Med.* **2006**, *47*, 698–705. [PubMed]
10. DeLorenzo, C.; DellaGioia, N.; Bloch, M.; Sanacora, G.; Nabulsi, N.; Abdallah, C.; Yang, J.; Wen, R.; Mann, J.J.; Krystal, J.H.; et al. In vivo ketamine-induced changes in [^{11}c]ABP688 binding to metabotropic glutamate receptor subtype 5. *Biol. Psychiatry* **2015**, *77*, 266–275. [CrossRef] [PubMed]
11. DeLorenzo, C.; Sovago, J.; Gardus, J.; Xu, J.; Yang, J.; Behrje, R.; Kumar, J.S.; Devanand, D.P.; Pelton, G.H.; Mathis, C.A.; et al. Characterization of brain mGluR5 binding in a pilot study of late-life major depressive disorder using positron emission tomography and [^{11}c]ABP688. *Transl. Psychiatry* **2015**, *5*, e693. [CrossRef] [PubMed]
12. Esterlis, I.; DellaGioia, N.; Pietrzak, R.H.; Matuskey, D.; Nabulsi, N.; Abdallah, C.G.; Yang, J.; Pittenger, C.; Sanacora, G.; Krystal, J.H.; et al. Ketamine-induced reduction in mGluR5 availability is associated with an antidepressant response: An [^{11}c]ABP688 and pet imaging study in depression. *Mol. Psychiatry* **2018**, *23*, 824–832. [CrossRef] [PubMed]
13. Miyake, N.; Skinbjerg, M.; Easwaramoorthy, B.; Kumar, D.; Girgis, R.R.; Xu, X.; Slifstein, M.; Abi-Dargham, A. Imaging changes in glutamate transmission in vivo with the metabotropic glutamate receptor 5 tracer [^{11}c]ABP688 and n-acetylcysteine challenge. *Biol. Psychiatry* **2011**, *69*, 822–824. [CrossRef] [PubMed]
14. Sandiego, C.M.; Nabulsi, N.; Lin, S.F.; Labaree, D.; Najafzadeh, S.; Huang, Y.; Cosgrove, K.; Carson, R.E. Studies of the metabotropic glutamate receptor 5 radioligand [^{11}c]ABP688 with n-acetylcysteine challenge in rhesus monkeys. *Synapse* **2013**, *67*, 489–501. [CrossRef] [PubMed]
15. Zimmer, E.R.; Parent, M.J.; Leuzy, A.; Aliaga, A.; Aliaga, A.; Moquin, L.; Schirrmacher, E.S.; Soucy, J.P.; Skelin, I.; Gratton, A.; et al. Imaging in vivo glutamate fluctuations with [^{11}c]ABP688: a GLT-1 challenge with ceftriaxone. *J. Cereb. Blood Flow Metab.* **2015**, *35*, 1169–1174. [CrossRef] [PubMed]
16. Wyckhuys, T.; Verhaeghe, J.; Wyffels, L.; Langlois, X.; Schmidt, M.; Stroobants, S.; Staelens, S. N-acetylcysteine- and mk-801-induced changes in glutamate levels do not affect in vivo binding of metabotropic glutamate 5 receptor radioligand [^{11}c]ABP688 in rat brain. *J. Nucl. Med.* **2013**, *54*, 1954–1961. [CrossRef] [PubMed]

17. Rathinam, M.L.; Watts, L.T.; Stark, A.A.; Mahimainathan, L.; Stewart, J.; Schenker, S.; Henderson, G.I. Astrocyte control of fetal cortical neuron glutathione homeostasis: Up-regulation by ethanol. *J. Neurochem.* **2006**, *96*, 1289–1300. [CrossRef] [PubMed]

18. Rothstein, J.D.; Patel, S.; Regan, M.R.; Haenggeli, C.; Huang, Y.H.; Bergles, D.E.; Jin, L.; Dykes Hoberg, M.; Vidensky, S.; Chung, D.S.; et al. Beta-lactam antibiotics offer neuroprotection by increasing glutamate transporter expression. *Nature* **2005**, *433*, 73–77. [CrossRef] [PubMed]

19. Hu, Y.Y.; Xu, J.; Zhang, M.; Wang, D.; Li, L.; Li, W.B. Ceftriaxone modulates uptake activity of glial glutamate transporter-1 against global brain ischemia in rats. *J. Neurochem.* **2015**, *132*, 194–205. [CrossRef] [PubMed]

20. Milicevic Sephton, S.; Müller Herde, A.; Mu, L.; Keller, C.; Rudisuhli, S.; Auberson, Y.; Schibli, R.; Krämer, S.D.; Ametamey, S.M. Preclinical evaluation and test-retest studies of [^{18}F]PSS232, a novel radioligand for targeting metabotropic glutamate receptor 5 (mGlu5). *Eur. J. Nucl. Med. Mol. Imaging* **2015**, *42*, 128–137. [CrossRef] [PubMed]

21. Müller Herde, A.; Keller, C.; Milicevic Sephton, S.; Mu, L.; Schibli, R.; Ametamey, S.M.; Krämer, S.D. Quantitative positron emission tomography of mGluR5 in rat brain with [^{18}F]PSS232 at minimal invasiveness and reduced model complexity. *J. Neurochem.* **2015**, *133*, 330–342. [CrossRef] [PubMed]

22. Lorrain, D.S.; Baccei, C.S.; Bristow, L.J.; Anderson, J.J.; Varney, M.A. Effects of ketamine and N-methyl-D-aspartate on glutamate and dopamine release in the rat prefrontal cortex: Modulation by a group II selective metabotropic glutamate receptor agonist LY379268. *Neuroscience* **2003**, *117*, 697–706. [CrossRef]

23. Moghaddam, B.; Adams, B.; Verma, A.; Daly, D. Activation of glutamatergic neurotransmission by ketamine: A novel step in the pathway from NMDA receptor blockade to dopaminergic and cognitive disruptions associated with the prefrontal cortex. *J. Neurosci.* **1997**, *17*, 2921–2927. [CrossRef] [PubMed]

24. Doenicke, A.; Kugler, J.; Mayer, M.; Angster, R.; Hoffmann, P. Ketamine racemate or S-(+)-ketamine and midazolam. The effect on vigilance, efficacy and subjective findings. *Anaesthesist* **1992**, *41*, 610–618. [PubMed]

25. Domino, E.F. Taming the ketamine tiger. *Anesthesiology* **2010**, *113*, 678–684. [CrossRef] [PubMed]

26. Himmelseher, S.; Pfenninger, E. The clinical use of S-(+)-ketamine—A determination of its place. *Anasthesiol. Intensivmed. Notfallmed. Schmerzther.* **1998**, *33*, 764–770. [CrossRef] [PubMed]

27. Alagarsamy, S.; Marino, M.J.; Rouse, S.T.; Gereau, R.W.t.; Heinemann, S.F.; Conn, P.J. Activation of NMDA receptors reverses desensitization of mGluR5 in native and recombinant systems. *Nat. Neurosci.* **1999**, *2*, 234–240. [CrossRef] [PubMed]

28. Homayoun, H.; Moghaddam, B. Bursting of prefrontal cortex neurons in awake rats is regulated by metabotropic glutamate 5 (mGlu5) receptors: Rate-dependent influence and interaction with NMDA receptors. *Cereb. Cortex* **2006**, *16*, 93–105. [CrossRef] [PubMed]

29. Changeux, J.P.; Edelstein, S.J. Allosteric mechanisms of signal transduction. *Science* **2005**, *308*, 1424–1428. [CrossRef] [PubMed]

30. Cabello, N.; Gandia, J.; Bertarelli, D.C.; Watanabe, M.; Lluis, C.; Franco, R.; Ferre, S.; Lujan, R.; Ciruela, F. Metabotropic glutamate type 5, dopamine D2 and adenosine A2a receptors form higher-order oligomers in living cells. *J. Neurochem.* **2009**, *109*, 1497–1507. [CrossRef] [PubMed]

31. Canela, L.; Fernandez-Duenas, V.; Albergaria, C.; Watanabe, M.; Lluis, C.; Mallol, J.; Canela, E.I.; Franco, R.; Lujan, R.; Ciruela, F. The association of metabotropic glutamate receptor type 5 with the neuronal Ca^{2+}-binding protein 2 modulates receptor function. *J. Neurochem.* **2009**, *111*, 555–567. [CrossRef] [PubMed]

32. Seneca, N.; Finnema, S.J.; Farde, L.; Gulyas, B.; Wikstrom, H.V.; Halldin, C.; Innis, R.B. Effect of amphetamine on dopamine D2 receptor binding in nonhuman primate brain: A comparison of the agonist radioligand [^{11}c]MNPA and antagonist [^{11}c]raclopride. *Synapse* **2006**, *59*, 260–269. [CrossRef] [PubMed]

33. Wilson, A.A.; McCormick, P.; Kapur, S.; Willeit, M.; Garcia, A.; Hussey, D.; Houle, S.; Seeman, P.; Ginovart, N. Radiosynthesis and evaluation of [^{11}c]-(+)-4-propyl-3,4,4a,5,6,10b-hexahydro-2H-naphtho[1,2-b][1,4]oxazin-9-ol as a potential radiotracer for in vivo imaging of the dopamine D2 high-affinity state with positron emission tomography. *J. Med. Chem.* **2005**, *48*, 4153–4160. [CrossRef] [PubMed]

5

Comparative Study of Two Oxidizing Agents, Chloramine T and Iodo-Gen®, for the Radiolabeling of β-CIT with Iodine-131: Relevance for Parkinson's Disease

Ana Claudia R. Durante [1,2], Danielle V. Sobral [1], Ana Claudia C. Miranda [2], Érika V. de Almeida [2], Leonardo L. Fuscaldi [2], Marycel R. F. F. de Barboza [2,*] and Luciana Malavolta [1]

[1] Department of Physiological Sciences, School of Medical Sciences, Santa Casa de Sao Paulo, Rua Cesario Mota Junior 61, Sao Paulo 01221-020, Brazil; aninhapharma30@gmail.com (A.C.R.D.); danielle_sobral@hotmail.com (D.V.S.); luciana.malavolta@gmail.com (L.M.)

[2] Hospital Israelita Albert Einstein, Avenida Albert Einstein 627/701, Sao Paulo 05652-900, Brazil; ana.miranda@einstein.br (A.C.C.M.); eriquimika@yahoo.com.br (E.V.d.A.), leonardo.fuscaldi@hotmail.com (L.L.F.)

* Correspondence: marycelfigols@gmail.com

Abstract: Parkinson's disease (PD) is a neurodegenerative disease characterized by the loss of dopaminergic neurons in the *substantia nigra pars compacta*, leading to alteration of the integrity of dopaminergic transporters (DATs). In recent years, some radiopharmaceuticals have been used in the clinic to evaluate the integrity of DATs. These include tropane derivatives such as radiolabeled β-CIT and FP-CIT with iodine-123 (^{123}I), and TRODAT-1 with metastable technetium-99 (^{99m}Tc). Radiolabeling of β-CIT with radioactive iodine is based on electrophilic radioiodination using oxidizing agents, such as Chloramine T or Iodo-Gen®. For the first time, the present work performed a comparative study of the radiolabeling of β-CIT with iodine-131 (^{131}I), using either Chloramine T or Iodo-Gen® as oxidizing agents, in order to improve the radiolabeling process of β-CIT and to choose the most advantageous oxidizing agent to be used in nuclear medicine. Both radiolabeling methods were similar and resulted in high radiochemical yield (> 95%), with suitable ^{131}I-β-CIT stability up to 72 h. Although Chloramine T is a strong oxidizing agent, it was as effective as Iodo-Gen® for β-CIT radiolabeling with ^{131}I, with the advantage of briefer reaction time and solubility in aqueous medium.

Keywords: Chloramine T; electrophilic radioiodination; iodine-131; Iodo-Gen®; oxidizing agent; β-CIT.

1. Introduction

Dopamine transporters (DATs) are transmembrane proteins present on the presynaptic membrane of dopaminergic neurons, playing an important role in the regulation of intensity and duration of dopaminergic transmission [1,2].

The pathophysiology of Parkinson's disease (PD) is characterized by progressive loss of dopaminergic neurons in the *substantia nigra pars compacta* (SNpc), leading to a denervation of the nigrostriatal tract that emits its terminal projections to the putamen and caudate nucleus with significant reduction of dopamine and, consequently, loss of DAT integrity [3–5].

Since it is a chronic and progressive disease, it is very important to perform an early diagnosis based on clinical evaluation then confirmed by imaging techniques. The clinical relevance of DAT integrity evaluation by diagnostic imaging techniques, such as single photon emission computed tomography (SPECT) and positron emission tomography (PET), are based on the differentiation between degenerative parkinsonism and other conditions not associated with dopamine loss, such as essential tremor, drug-induced parkinsonism, vascular parkinsonism, and psychogenic parkinsonism [6,7].

DAT-SPECT radiopharmaceuticals available for clinical use are all tropane derivatives: (i) β-CIT (2β-carbomethoxy-3β-(4-iodophenyl)tropane) and FP-CIT (N-3-fluoropropyl-2β-carbomethoxy-3β-(4-iodophenyl)nortropane) radiolabeled with iodine-123 (^{123}I).; (ii) TRODAT-1 ([2-[[2-[[[3-(4-chlorophenyl)-8-methyl-8-azabicyclo[3.2 0.1]oct-2-yl]methyl](2-mercaptoethyl)amino]ethyl]amino]ethanethiolato(3-)-N2,N2′,S2,S2′]oxo-[1R-(exo-exo)]) radiolabeled with metastable technetium-99 (^{99m}Tc) [6,8,9].

β-CIT is a molecule that has been studied since the 90s [10]. Due to its binding affinity to presynaptic DATs, radioisotope-labeled β-CIT can differentiate PD from essential tremor with a sensibility of 95% and a specificity of 93% [8]. The proposed mechanism of β-CIT interaction with presynaptic DATs involves electrostatic interactions or hydrogen bonds [11]. In nuclear medicine, ^{123}I-β-CIT is a diagnostic agent for SPECT imaging used both in the initial phase (in individuals with uncertain diagnosis) and in the follow-up of PD [12].

The radiolabeling of molecules, including β-CIT, with radioactive iodine (^{123}I, ^{124}I, ^{125}I or ^{131}I) is frequently based on electrophilic aromatic substitution using several oxidizing agents such as Chloramine T (N-chloro-p-toluenesulfonamide sodium salt), Iodo-Gen® (1,3,4,6-tetrachloro-3α,6β-diphenylglycouril), lactoperoxidase, and the solid-state variants as pre-coated Iodo-Gen® tubes, Iodo-Beads®, or Enzymobeads®. The most commonly used are Chloramine T and Iodo-Gen®, at room temperature [13–16].

Chloramine T has been used since 1962 [17]. It is a strong oxidizing agent, demanding shorter reaction periods, and is soluble in aqueous solutions [15,18]. On the other hand, Iodo-Gen® is a moderate oxidizing agent, requiring longer reaction times, and is insoluble under aqueous conditions [19,20].

To the best of our knowledge, until now there have been no comparative studies between these two oxidizing agents in β-CIT radiolabeling with radioactive iodine. Therefore, the present study aims to evaluate the electrophilic radioiodination of β-CIT with iodine-131 (^{131}I), due to its 8.04 d half-life, using either Chloramine T trihydrate or Iodo-Gen®, in order to compare the radiolabeling efficiency and compound stability.

The importance of this work is based on the improvement of the radiolabeling process of β-CIT with radioactive iodine through the choice of the most advantageous oxidizing agent. This study may result in high quality radiopharmaceuticals labeled with ^{123}I for use in nuclear medicine and, consequently, higher quality SPECT images of the DATs.

2. Results and Discussion

The electrophilic radioiodination of β-CIT, using the precursor trimethylstannyl-β-CIT (TMS-β-CIT), was performed using either Chloramine T or Iodo-Gen® as an oxidizing agent (Figure 1). The final product, ^{131}I-β-CIT, was purified by solid-phase extraction (SPE) using Sep-Pak® C$_{18}$. Radiochemical purity was evaluated by both ascendant chromatography and reversed phase-high performance liquid chromatography (RP-HPLC).

Ascendant chromatography was performed on thin-layer chromatography on silica gel (TLC-SG; Al) strips using 95% acetonitrile (ACN) as an eluent (Figure 2). Results are summarized in Table 1. In this chromatographic system, Na^{131}I migrates with the solvent front (R_f = 0.9−1.0) and ^{131}I-β-CIT remains in the origin (R_f = 0.1−0.3). Radiochemical yield was over 95% for both radiolabeling methods. SPE purification did not significantly improve the radiochemical purity; however, this procedure is recommended in order to remove iodate ions (IO$_3$$^-$), which are not detected by this chromatographic system. In general, radiopharmaceuticals must present high radiochemical purity level (>90%). Therefore, this comparative study showed that both radiolabeling procedures, using either Chloramine

T or Iodo-Gen® as an oxidizing agent, yielded ^{131}I-β-CIT with suitable radiochemical features, and that no significant differences were observed between radiolabeling methods (Table 1).

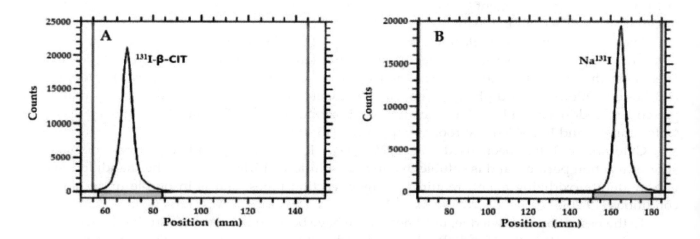

Figure 1. Simplified scheme of the electrophilic radioiodination of β-CIT.

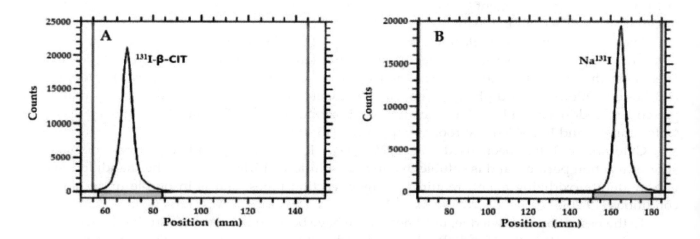

Figure 2. TLC-chromatograms: (**A**) ^{131}I-β-CIT (R$_f$ = 0.1—0.3) and (**B**) Na^{131}I (R$_f$ = 0.9—1.0).

Table 1. Radiolabeling yield and radiochemical purity of ^{131}I-β-CIT.

Oxidizing Agents	Radiolabeling Yield	Radiochemical Purity
Chloramine T	97.40 ± 1.17	98.48 ± 0.63
Iodo-Gen®	97.81 ± 0.99	98.24 ± 0.76

Values are expressed as mean ± SD (n = 9). No significant differences were observed for ^{131}I-β-CIT obtained by both radiolabeling methods (p > 0.05).

The radiochemical purity of ^{131}I-β-CIT was also evaluated by RP-HPLC analysis (Figure 3) in order to confirm ascendant chromatographic data. The unlabeled precursor TMS-β-CIT was analyzed and presented a retention time (RT) of 6.68 min (Figure 3A). Free Na^{131}I was also evaluated, showing a different chromatographic profile (RT = 1.16 min) when compared to unlabeled precursor TMS-β-CIT (Figure 3B). The final product, ^{131}I-β-CIT, obtained by both radiolabeling methods, using either Chloramine T or Iodo-Gen® as an oxidizing agent, showed high radiochemical purity (Figure 3C,D). Therefore, RP-HPLC analyses were in accordance with TLC-SG data, confirming that both radiolabeling methods yield ^{131}I-β-CIT with high radiochemical purity and similar chromatographic profiles.

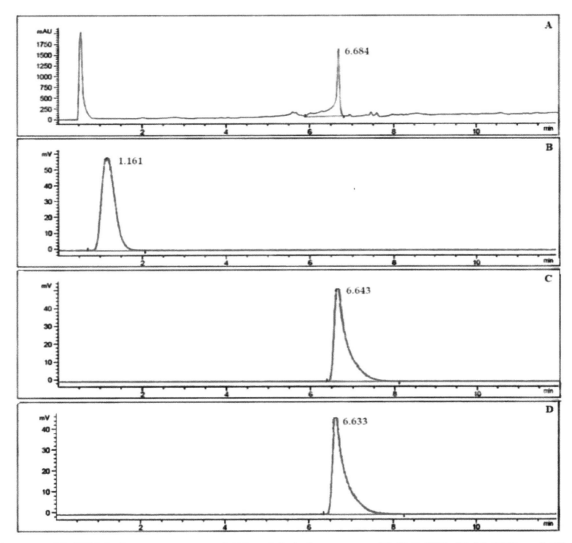

Figure 3. RP-HPLC chromatograms of (A) unlabeled precursor TMS-β-CIT, (B) Na131I, and (C, D) 131I-β-CIT obtained by both radiolabeling methods.

The stability of ^{131}I-β-CIT was analyzed by ascendant chromatography (Figure 4). The final product was stable up to 72 h. Although slight statistical differences in the stability were observed between both radiolabeling methods, radiochemical purity maintained over 94%, regardless of the storage way, at room temperature or at $2-8\,^{\circ}$C (Figure 4A, B). It is important to consider that these small variations in stability in reaction medium should not affect the application of ^{131}I-β-CIT. Moreover, ^{131}I-β-CIT serum stability was also evaluated, and data showed high stability (>94%) up to 24 h, with no significant statistical differences between the radiolabeling methods (Figure 4C).

The partition coefficient (P) of ^{131}I-β-CIT was determined at room temperature by the ratio between n-octanol and 0.9% NaCl. For both radioiodination processes, data showed P tending to the hydrophobic range (Table 2). The hydrophobicity of ^{131}I-β-CIT was also evaluated by the determination of the percentage of serum protein binding (SPB), incubating ^{131}I-β-CIT with serum at 37 °C for 30 min. The results showed approximately 45% of SPB in both cases (Table 2).

The physicochemical features of the final product are in agreement, once P tending to the hydrophobic range relates to high SPB [21]. Furthermore, these data are consistent with the intended ^{131}I-β-CIT clinical application, as a radiotracer for measuring presynaptic DAT density in order to provide information on the integrity of these terminals [12]. Therefore, ^{131}I-β-CIT must cross the blood—brain barrier, which is easier for lipophilic molecules. In addition, it has been reported that 45—85% of SPB is related to higher uptake by the brain [22].

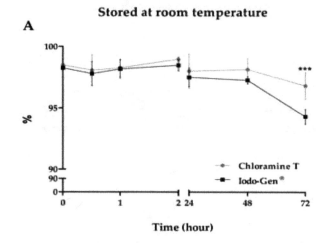

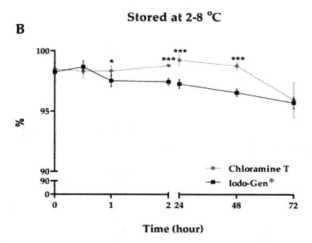

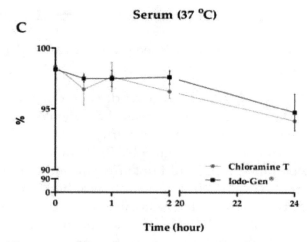

Figure 4. Evaluation of ^{131}I-β-CIT stability. Values are expressed as mean ± SD [(**A**) and (**B**): $n = 9$; (**C**): $n = 3$]. Asterisks indicate significant differences (*$p < 0.05$; ***$p < 0.001$).

Table 2. Partition coefficient and serum protein binding of ^{131}I-β-CIT.

Partition coefficient(P)	Chloramine T	0.12 ± 0.02
	Iodo-Gen®	0.13 ± 0.02
Serum protein binding (SPB)	Chloramine T	47.44 ± 1.31%
	Iodo-Gen®	44.99 ± 3.06%

Values are expressed as mean ± SD ($n = 5$). No significant differences were observed for ^{131}I-β-CIT obtained by both radiolabeling methods ($p > 0.05$).

3. Materials and Methods

3.1. Electrophilic Radioiodination of β-CIT and SPE Purification

The electrophilic radioiodination of β-CIT was performed using either Chloramine T or Iodo-Gen® as an oxidizing agent followed by SPE purification according to previous methods [14,15,23–25], with some modifications. The precursor TMS-β-CIT was purchased from ABX Advanced Biochemical Compounds GmbH (Radeberg, Germany).

For the Chloramine T method, an aliquot of Na^{131}I solution (7.4–14.8 MBq) was added to a vial containing the precursor TMS-β-CIT (0.12 µmol/50 µL EtOH). Next, 10 µL of Chloramine T trihydrate solution (1.5 mg·mL^{-1}) and 4 µL of HCl solution (0.1 mol·L^{-1}) were added. The mixture (pH = 3.0–3.5) was kept at room temperature for 3 min and the reaction was quenched with 40 µL of NaOH solution (0.01 mol·L^{-1}). The final pH was 6.0–6.5.

For the Iodo-Gen® method, an aliquot of Na^{131}I solution (37.0–44.4 MBq) was added to a vial containing the precursor TMS-β-CIT (0.12 µmol/50 µL EtOH). Next, 37.5 µL of Iodo-Gen® solution (6.2 mg·mL^{-1}) and 75 µL of H$_3$PO$_4$ solution (0.1 mol·L$^-$) were added. The mixture (pH = 3.0–3.5) was kept at room temperature for 15 min and the reaction was quenched with 20 µL of NaOH solution (0.1 mol·L^{-1}). The final pH was 6.0–6.5.

After each radiolabeling method, the final product (^{131}I-β-CIT) was purified by SPE using Sep-Pak® C$_{18}$, preconditioned with EtOH (5 mL) and 0.9% NaCl (5 mL). Free ^{131}I was removed in 0.9% NaCl (5 mL) and ^{131}I-β-CIT was eluted by EtOH (2 mL).

3.2. Radiochemical Purity Analysis

Radiochemical purity was evaluated by ascendant chromatography ($n = 9$) and RP-HPLC.

Ascendant chromatography was performed by TLC-SG (Al) strips (Merck) using 95% ACN as an eluent. The radioactivity was determined with an AR-2000 radio-TLC Imaging Scanner (Eckert & Ziegler, Germany).

RP-HPLC analyses were performed on a 1290 Infinity II UHPLC system (Agilent Technologies, Santa Clara, CA, USA) equipped with a radioactivity detector (Eckert & Ziegler, Germany) and Open Lab ECM data system (Agilent Technologies, Santa Clara, CA, USA). The analytical column was a Phenomenex Kinetex® Reversed Phase C$_{18}$ (100 mm × 3 mm; 2.6 µm) maintained at 30 °C. Mobile phase A was 0.1% (v:v) TFA in water. Mobile phase B was 0.1% (v:v) TFA in MeOH. The gradient of mobile phase B was: 10% (0.0–1.0 min); 10–90% (1.0–8.0 min); 90% (8.0–10.5 min); and 90–10% (10.5–12.0 min). The flow rate was 0.8 mL·min^{-1} and the UV detector was set at 284 nm.

3.3. Stability Studies

The stability of ^{131}I-β-CIT, stored at room temperature and at 2–8 °C, was evaluated at 0.5, 1, 2, 24, 48, and 72 h ($n = 9$). Beyond that, the serum stability of ^{131}I-β-CIT, incubated at 37 °C under slight agitation (500 rpm), was evaluated at 1, 2, and 24 h ($n = 3$). In both cases, the stability of ^{131}I-β-CIT was analyzed by ascendant chromatography, as described in the previous section.

3.4. Partition Coefficient

An aliquot of purified ^{131}I-β-CIT (50 µL) was added in a mixture of n-octanol and 0.9% NaCl (1:1) and submitted to agitation ($n = 5$). The mixture was centrifuged (825 g; 3 min). Aliquots of 100 µL of both aqueous and organic phases were collected, and their radioactivities were measured with a 2480 automatic gamma counter Wizard^{2}™ 3″ (PerkinElmer, Waltham, MA, USA).

3.5. Serum Protein Binding

An aliquot of ^{131}I-β-CIT (25 µL) was added to 475 µL of serum and incubated at 37 °C for 30 min ($n = 5$). Post-incubation, serum proteins were precipitated with 500 µL of 10% trichloroacetic acid and the content was centrifuged (825 g; 10 min; 3x). Pellets' and supernatants' radioactivities were measured with a 2480 automatic gamma counter Wizard^2™ 3″ (PerkinElmer, Waltham, MA, USA).

4. Conclusions

In summary, the data demonstrated that both radiolabeling methods, using either Chloramine T or Iodo-Gen® as an oxidizing agent, yield ^{131}I-β-CIT with similar radiochemical parameters. Although Chloramine T induces harder reaction conditions when compared to Iodo-Gen®, the results showed that it is possible to use Chloramine T instead of Iodo-Gen® without compromising the radiolabeling result and the final product stability, provided that the physicochemical parameters of each radiolabeling process are respected (pH, reaction time, temperature). Furthermore, it is important to highlight that Chloramine T is a water-soluble reagent with strong oxidizing properties requiring a briefer reaction time, simplifying the process in nuclear medicine. Therefore, this comparative study presents the possibility of alternating between Iodo-Gen® and Chloramine T in the radiolabeling process of β-CIT with $^{123/131}$I, depending on the availability and costs of the oxidizing agents, without changing the integrity of the final product, used for SPECT imaging diagnosis of PD in nuclear medicine.

Author Contributions: Conceptualization, M.R.F.F.d.B.; methodology, A.C.R.D., D.V.S., A.C.C.M. and E.V.d.A.; data analysis and statistics, A.C.R.D. and L.L.F.; writing—original draft preparation, A.C.R.D. and L.L.F.; writing—review and editing, all authors; supervision, L.M.; project administration, M.R.F.F.d.B.

Acknowledgments: The authors would like to thank Hospital Israelita Albert Einstein (HIAE), Coordenação de Aperfeiçoamento de Pessoal de Nível Superior (CAPES) and Fundação de Amparo à Pesquisa do Estado de São Paulo (FAPESP) for their grants and fellowships. Thanks are also due to Centro de Radiofarmácia (CR) of Instituto de Pesquisas Energéticas e Nucleares of Comissão Nacional de Energia Nuclear (IPEN-CNEN/SP) for the supply of Na^{131}I, Centro de Experimentação e Treinamento em Cirurgia (CETEC) for the infrastructure, and Associação Beneficente Alzira Denise Hertzog da Silva (ABADHS) for the donation.

References

1. Park, E. A new era of clinical dopamine transporter imaging using ^{123}I-FP-CIT. *J. Nucl. Med. Technol.* **2012**, *40*, 222–228. Available online: https://www.ncbi.nlm.nih.gov/pubmed/23160562 (accessed on 28 March 2017). [CrossRef] [PubMed]
2. Ba, F.; Martin, W.R.W. Dopamine transporter imaging as a diagnostic tool for parkinsonism and related disorders in clinical practice. *Parkinsonism Relat. Disord.* **2015**, *21*, 87–94. Available online: https://www.ncbi.nlm.nih.gov/pubmed/25487733 (accessed on 14 April 2017). [CrossRef] [PubMed]
3. Kalia, L.V.; Lang, A.E. Parkinson's disease. *Lancet* **2015**, *386*, 896–912. Available online: https://www.ncbi.nlm.nih.gov/pubmed/25904081 (accessed on 22 February 2018). [CrossRef]
4. Williams-Gray, C.H.; Worth, P.F. Parkinson's disease. *Medicine* **2016**, *44*, 542–546. [CrossRef]
5. Wei, Z.; Li, X.; Li, X.; Liu, Q.; Cheng, Y. Oxidative stress in Parkinson's disease: A systematic review and meta-analysis. *Front. Mol. Neurosci.* **2018**, *11*, 1–7. Available online: https://www.ncbi.nlm.nih.gov/pubmed/30026688 (accessed on 10 December 2018). [CrossRef] [PubMed]
6. Varrone, A.; Halldin, C. Molecular imaging of the dopamine transporter. *J. Nucl. Med.* **2010**, *51*, 1331–1334. Available online: https://www.ncbi.nlm.nih.gov/pubmed/20720060 (accessed on 5 March 2017). [CrossRef] [PubMed]
7. Cummings, J.L.; Henchcliffe, C.; Schaier, S.; Simuni, T.; Waxman, A.; Kemp, P. The role of dopaminergic imaging in patients with symptoms of dopaminergic system neurodegeneration. *Brain* **2011**, *134*, 3146–3166. [CrossRef]
8. Shen, L.; Liao, M.; Tseng, Y. Recent advances in imaging of dopaminergic neurons for evaluation of neuropsychiatric disorders. *J. Biomed. Biotechnol.* **2012**, *2012*, 1–14. [CrossRef]
9. Wang, L.; Zhang, Q.; Li, H.; Zhang, H. SPECT molecular imaging in Parkinson's disease. *J. Biomed. Biotechnol.* **2012**, *2012*, 1–11. [CrossRef]

10. Kägi, G.; Bhatia, K.P.; Tolosa, E. The role of DAT-SPECT in movement disorders. *J. Neurol. Neurosurg. Psychiatry* **2010**, *81*, 5–12. Available online: https://www.ncbi.nlm.nih.gov/pubmed/20019219 (accessed on 9 March 2017). [CrossRef]

11. Bois, F.; Baldwin, R.M.; Kula, N.S.; Baldessarini, R.J.; Innis, R.B.; Tamagnan, G. Synthesis and monoamine transporter affinity of 3′-analogs of 2β-carbomethoxy-3-β-(4′-iodophenyl)tropane (β-CIT). *Bioorg. Med. Chem. Lett.* **2004**, *14*, 2117–2120. [CrossRef] [PubMed]

12. Eerola, J.; Tienari, P.J.; Kaakkola, S.; Nikkinen, P.; Launes, J. How useful is [^{123}I]β-CIT SPECT in clinical practice? *J. Neurol. Neurosurg. Psychiatry* **2005**, *76*, 1211–1216. Available online: https://www.ncbi.nlm.nih.gov/pmc/articles/PMC1739796/ (accessed on 13 December 2016). [CrossRef]

13. Markwell, M.A.K. A new solid-state reagent to iodinate proteins: I. Conditions for the efficient labeling of antiserum. *Anal. Biochem.* **1982**, *125*, 427–432. [CrossRef]

14. Carpinelli, A.; Matarrese, M.; Moresco, R.M.; Simonelli, P.; Todde, S.; Magni, F.; Galli Kienle, M.; Fazio, F. Radiosynthesis of [^{123}I]βCIT, a selective ligand for the study of the dopaminergic and serotoninergic systems in human brain. *Appl. Radiat. Isotopes* **2001**, *54*, 93–95. [CrossRef]

15. Sihver, W.; Drewes, B.; Schulze, A.; Olsson, R.A.; Coenen, H.H. Evaluation of novel tropane analogues in comparison with the binding characteristics of [^{18}F]FP-CIT and [^{131}I]β-CIT. *Nucl. Med. Biol.* **2007**, *34*, 211–219. [CrossRef]

16. Blois, E.; Chan, H.S.; Breeman, W.A.P. Iodination and stability of somatostatin analogues: Comparison of iodination techniques. A practical overview. *Curr. Top. Med. Chem.* **2012**, *12*, 2668–2676. [CrossRef] [PubMed]

17. Hunter, W.M.; Greenwood, F.C. Preparation of iodine-131 labelled human growth hormone of high specific activity. *Nature* **1962**, *194*, 495–496. [CrossRef] [PubMed]

18. Tashtoush, B.M.; Traboulsi, A.A.; Dittert, L.; Hussain, A.A. Chloramine-T in radiolabeling techniques. IV. Penta-O-acetyl-N-chloro-N-methylglucamine as an oxidizing agent in radiolabeling techniques. *Anal. Biochem.* **2001**, *288*, 16–21. [CrossRef] [PubMed]

19. Fraker, P.J.; Speck, J.C., Jr. Protein and cell membrane iodinations with a sparingly soluble chloroamide, 1,3,4,6-tetrachloro-3a,6a-diphrenylglycoluril. *Biochem. Biophys. Res. Commun.* **1978**, *80*, 849–857. [CrossRef]

20. Amin, A.M.; Gouda, A.A.; El-Sheikh, R.; Seddik, U.; Hussien, H. Radioiodination, purification and bioevaluation of Piroxicam in comparison with Meloxicam for imaging of inflammation. *J. Radioanal. Nucl. Chem.* **2009**, *280*, 589–598. [CrossRef]

21. Lexa, K.W.; Dolghih, E.; Jacobson, M.P. A structure-based model for predicting serum albumin binding. *PLoS ONE* **2014**, *9*, 1–12. Available online: https://www.ncbi.nlm.nih.gov/pubmed/24691448 (accessed on 20 June 2018). [CrossRef]

22. Tavares, A.A.; Lewsey, J.; Dewar, D.; Pimlott, S.L. Radiotracer properties determined by high performance liquid chromatography: A potential tool for brain radiotracer discovery. *Nucl. Med. Biol.* **2012**, *39*, 127–135. Available online: https://www.ncbi.nlm.nih.gov/pubmed/21958855 (accessed on 29 July 2018). [CrossRef]

23. Katsifis, A.; Papazian, V.; Jackson, T.; Loc'h, C. A rapid and efficient preparation of [^{123}I]radiopharmaceuticals using a small HPLC (Rocket) column. *Appl. Radiat. Isotopes* **2006**, *64*, 27–31. [CrossRef]

24. Saji, H.; Iida, Y.; Kawashima, H.; Ogawa, M.; Kitamura, Y.; Mukai, T.; Shimazu, S.; Yoneda, F. In vivo imaging of brain dopaminergic neurotransmission system in small animals with high-resolution single photon emission computed tomography. *Anal. Sci.* **2003**, *19*, 67–71. [CrossRef]

25. Fuchigami, T.; Mizoguchi, T.; Ishikawa, N.; Haratake, M.; Yoshida, S.; Magata, Y.; Nakayama, M. Synthesis and evaluation of a radioiodinated 4,6-diaryl-3-cyano-2-pyridinone derivative as a survivin targeting SPECT probe for tumor imaging. *Bioorg. Med. Chem. Lett.* **2016**, *26*, 999–1004. Available online: https://www.ncbi.nlm.nih.gov/pubmed/26733475 (accessed on 21 January 2018). [CrossRef]

6

Design and Synthesis of ^{99m}TcN-Labeled Dextran-Mannose Derivatives for Sentinel Lymph Node Detection

Alessandra Boschi [1,*] ⓘ, **Micòl Pasquali** [2], **Claudio Trapella** [3] ⓘ, **Alessandro Massi** [3], **Petra Martini** [1], **Adriano Duatti** [3], **Remo Guerrini** [3], **Vinicio Zanirato** [3], **Anna Fantinati** [3] ⓘ, **Erika Marzola** [3], **Melchiore Giganti** [1] and **Licia Uccelli** [1]

[1]   Department of Morphology, Surgery and Experimental Medicine, University of Ferrara, Ferrara 44121, Italy; petra.martini@unife.it (P.M.); melchiore.giganti@unife.it (M.G.); licia.uccelli@unife.it (L.U.)

[2]   Department of Physic and Earth Science, University of Ferrara, Ferrara 44122, Italy; micol.pasquali@unife.it

[3]   Department of Chemical and Pharmaceutical Sciences, University of Ferrara, Ferrara 44121, Italy; claudio.trapella@unife.it (C.T.); alessandro.massi@unife.it (A.M.); adriano.duatti@unife.it (A.D.); remo.guerrini@unife.it (R.G.); vinicio.zanirato@unife.it (V.Z.); anna.fantinati@unife.it (A.F.); erika.marzola@unife.it (E.M.)

*   Correspondence: alessandra.boschi@unife.it

Abstract: Background: New approaches based on the receptor-targeted molecular interaction have been recently developed with the aim to investigate specific probes for sentinel lymph nodes. In particular, the mannose receptors expressed by lymph node macrophages became an attractive target and different multifunctional mannose derivate ligands for the labeling with ^{99m}Tc have been developed. In this study, we report the synthesis of a specific class of dextran-based, macromolecular, multifunctional ligands specially designed for labeling with the highly stable $[^{99m}Tc{\equiv}N]^{2+}$ core. Methods: The ligands have been obtained by appending to a macromolecular dextran scaffold pendant arms bearing a chelating moiety for the metallic group and a mannosyl residue for allowing the interaction of the resulting macromolecular ^{99m}Tc conjugate with specific receptors on the external membrane of macrophages. Two different chelating systems have been selected, S-methyl dithiocarbazate $[H_2N\text{-}NH\text{-}C(=S)SCH_3 = HDTCZ]$ and a sequence of two cysteine residues, that in combination with a monophosphine coligand, are able to bind the $[^{99m}Tc{\equiv}N]^{2+}$ core. Conclusions: High-specific-activity labeling has been obtained by simple mixing and heating of the $[^{99m}Tc{\equiv}N]^{2+}$ group with the new mannose-dextran derivatives.

Keywords: sentinel lymph node; dextran; mannose; ^{99m}Tc-radiopharmaceuticals

1. Introduction

The sentinel lymph node (SLN) is defined as the first lymph node that receives lymphatic drainage as well as metastatic cells from the primary tumor sites. An accurate identification and characterization of SLNs is very important as it helps the physician to decide the extension of surgery, the tumor staging, and the development of an appropriate treatment plan.

Sentinel lymph node detection (SLND) is a radionuclide-based technique for imaging regional lymph node drainage systems, performed by injecting small radiolabeled particles (20 to 500 nm). This technique has become the standard of care in breast cancer [1,2] and melanoma [3,4], and is increasingly being applied to other solid cancers with high metastatic potential in lymph nodes, such as oral and oropharyngeal squamous cell carcinoma [5].

The most frequently used radiopharmaceuticals for SLND are ^{99m}Tc-labelled colloidal particles. However, they are characterized by nonideal properties [6–8]; in particular, their uptake mechanism is driven by passive diffusion and show slow clearance rate from the injection site or low residence time in the SLN [9–12]. From the clinical point of view, an ideal tracer must combine persistent retention in the SLN, low distal lymph node accumulation, fast clearance rate from the injection site, safe radiation exposure level, and lack of toxicity.

New approaches based on the receptor-targeted molecular interaction have been developed with the aim to investigate specific probes for SLN. In particular, the mannose receptors expressed by lymph node macrophages became an attractive target [13,14], and multifunctional mannose-derivate ligands have been studied for the labeling with ^{99m}Tc [8,11,12]. A multifunctional ligand is commonly depicted as a molecular moiety being sufficiently large in size to accommodate a number of different chemical groups performing specific chemical and biological functions. Dextran provides a convenient macromolecular scaffold for hosting a relatively large number of functional groups and it has been recently employed to develop the ^{99m}Tc radiopharmaceutical (Lymphoseek®) for SLND [15]. The basic design of this new agent involves appending at various positions of the dextran structure a number of diethylenetriaminepentaacetic acid (DTPA) groups for the chelation of the metal together with a number of mannose residues for recognition by specific receptors on the macrophage's membrane. A strong limitation of this approach comes from the fact that DTPA is not considered an optimal chelating system for ^{99m}Tc and, as a consequence, the stability of the resulting conjugate macromolecular complex is poor. Furthermore, the technetium chemistry with DTPA is not well defined and some controversy about the nature of the complex formed with this metal exists [16]. Recently, aiming to provide more stable and chemically well-defined target-specific ^{99m}Tc complexes for SLND, ^{99m}Tc-tricarbonyl technology has been applied to label mannosylated-dextran conjugates in combination with pyrazolyldiamine chelator that selectively react with the fac-$[^{99m}Tc(CO)_3(H_2O)_3]^+$ metal fragment [11]. According to the mannosylated-dextran conjugates strategy, '4 + 1' mannosylated-dextran Tc(III) mixed-ligand complexes have been also reported [17].

Based on the dextran derivatives functionalized with mannose units' principle, we report in this work the design, the synthesis, and the characterization of a specific class of dextran-mannose multifunctional ligands specially designed for binding to $[^{99m}TcN]^{2+}$ group. The coordination chemistry of this metallic synthon is very well established [18–20] and can be efficiently manipulated by a careful selection of the coordinating atoms type bound to the $[^{99m}TcN]^{2+}$ group.

The compound S-methyl dithiocarbazate $[H_2N-NH-C(=S)SCH_3=HDTCZ]$ has been selected as the first chelating system to be investigated in the production of a multifunctional ligand for SLND based on ^{99m}Tc nitrido chemistry. DTCZ strongly binds to the $[^{99m}Tc\equiv N]^{2+}$ core, through the neutral thiocarbonyl sulfur atom and the deprotonated terminal amine nitrogen atom, forming both mono- and bis-substituted complexes [21,22]. Thus, the synthesis of this ligand is described in the following sections.

Another convenient chelating system for the $[^{99m}Tc\equiv N]^{2+}$ core is provided by the so-called '3 + 1' method. This approach stems from the finding that the coordination arrangement composed by a tridentate π-donor ligand, having $[S^-, N, S^-]$ as a set of donor atoms, and a monodentate π-acceptor monophosphine ligand (PR_3) usually exhibits a high stability when bound to a $[^{99m}Tc\equiv N]^{2+}$ group in a square pyramidal geometry. A very convenient tridentate $[S^-, N, S^-]$ chelating system is provided by the simple combinations of two terminal cysteine aminoacids (Cys-Cys). The schematic structure of of '3 + 1' ^{99m}Tc nitrido complexes with the Cys-Cys chelating system is illustrated in Figure 1.

In the following, the preparation and stability studies of ^{99m}Tc-radiopharmaceuticals containing mannose-dextran derivatives are described.

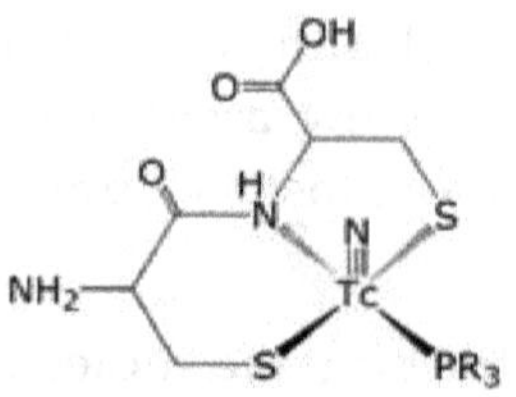

Figure 1. Structure of '3 + 1' ^{99m}Tc nitrido complexes with the Cys-Cys chelating system.

2. Results and Discussion

2.1. Design of a Dextran-Mannose Multifunctional Ligand for Coordination to the [^{99m}Tc≡N]$^{2+}$ Core

A chemical approach, usually employed for attaching different functional groups to a dextran scaffold, consists of hanging them at different positions of the polymeric chain. We used here a simplified strategy that allowed a more careful control of the number of functional groups introduced into the final macromolecule. This approach is schematically illustrated in Figure 2. As mentioned above, two functional groups are required for obtaining a new ^{99m}Tc nitrido agent for SLND, namely a suitable chelating group and a mannosyl residue. Each group was placed at one terminus of a linear chain of atoms that was also equipped with a reactive group (W) in its central position (Figure 2a). In turn, this latter group was reacted with another suitable reactive moiety, previously attached to the dextran scaffold, thus forming a stable linkage (click chemistry) (Figure 2b). Through this reaction, both functionalities remained strongly tethered to the macromolecular backbone as branched pendant arms.

(a)   (b)

Figure 2. Schematic drawing of a multifunctional fragment with a reactive group (W) (**a**) for binding to dextran (**b**).

2.2. Synthesis of Dextran-Mannosyl Multifunctional Ligands for the [^{99m}Tc≡N]$^{2+}$ Core

As mentioned above, the overall synthetic strategy employed here involved the preliminary preparation of a linear trifunctional fragment bearing a mannose residue at one terminus, a chelating group for the [^{99m}Tc≡N]$^{2+}$ core at the other terminus, and a reactive alkyne or sulfide group placed almost in the center of the linear chain (W in Figure 2a). These fragments were subsequently linked to the dextran backbone using three different procedures: (a) Thiol-ene chemistry [23]; (b) azide-alkyne Huysgen cycloaddition (click chemistry) [24], and (c) amide condensation. Specifically, the allyl-dextran (**1**), the azido-dextran (**2**), and cysteine-dextran derivative (**3**) (Figure 3) were used with thiolene condensation, click chemistry, and amide bond formation, respectively.

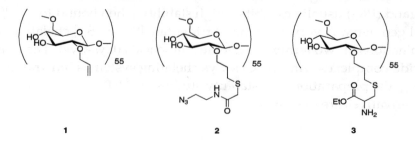

1   2   3

Figure 3. Dextran derivatives used in the synthesis of the new dextran-mannose multifunctional ligands.

2.2.1. Synthesis of Dextran Derivatives

The commercially available dextran with average molecular weight 10,000 Da was reacted with allyl bromide, sodium hydroxide, and sodium borohydride to obtain the dextran derivative **1**. The product was purified by repeated precipitation with ethanol and dried under vacuum to achieve a constant weight. The final loading of dextran polymer was achieved by comparison of ^{1}H-NMR spectra. In particular, the chemical shift and the integral value of anomeric protons (nonsubstituted and substituted dextran) at 4.96 ppm and 5.13 ppm were reported to the allylic proton at 5.96 ppm. The loading was about 18 allylic groups for every polymeric unit (18 allyl moiety for 55 monomeric sugar in the dextran); see Figure 4. As shown by the NMR spectra of allyl dextran, only one compound was reported. As suggested by Pirmettis and coworkers [12], and in agreement with our analytical data, position 2 of dextran was the most accessible, probably for steric reasons. In our experience, no other positions were touched by the alkyl group using allyl bromide and sodium hydroxide as reagents.

Figure 4. ^{1}H-NMR spectra of dextran (**left**) and allyl dextran (**right**).

Compound **1** was then treated with the azido-thioglicol amide at 50 °C in the presence of ammonium persulfate to obtain the corresponding thiol-ene adduct **2** (Figure 5). The same procedure was adopted for the reaction with the Fmoc-cysteine ethyl ester to obtain compound **1a** that was directly deprotected to obtain the free amine compound **3**.

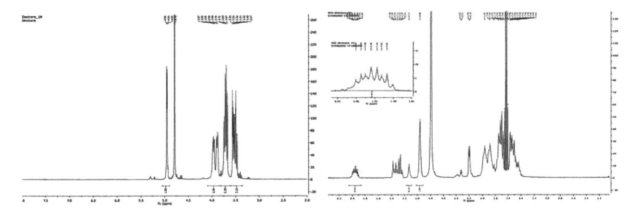

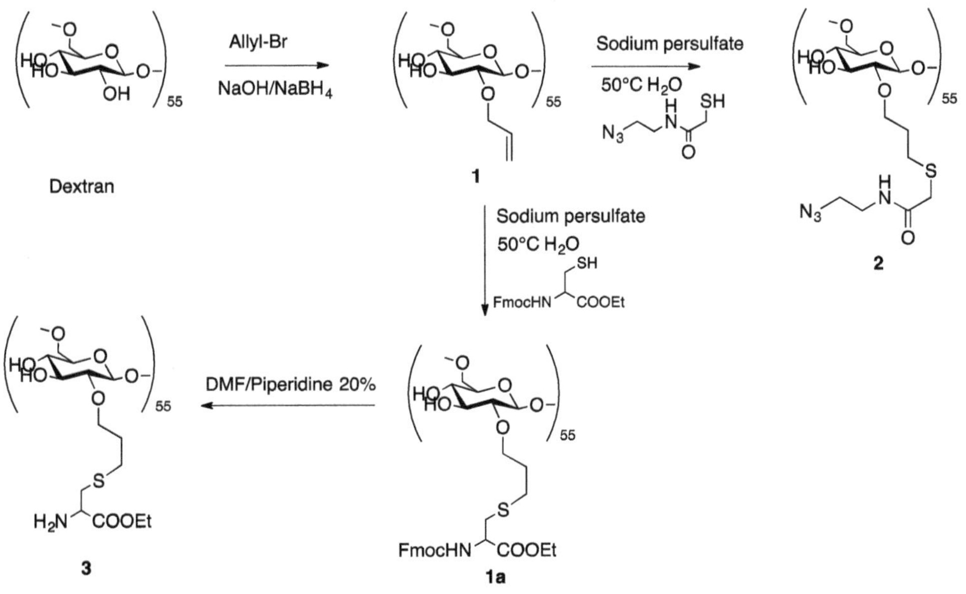

Figure 5. Synthesis of dextran derivatives.

2.2.2. Synthesis of a Dextran-DTCZ Multifunctional Ligand

A preliminary synthesis of a dextran-DTCZ derivative was carried out according to the reaction scheme depicted in Figure 6. HDTCZ was firstly functionalized with an alkyne moiety (4) and then linked to azido-dextran (2) by click chemistry. Preliminary labeling of the resulting ligand (5) was carried out in physiological solution by simple mixing with the $[^{99m}Tc\equiv N]^{2+}$ intermediate prepared by reaction of $[^{99m}Tc][TcO_4]^-$ with succinic dihydrazide (SDH) in the presence of Sn^{2+} ions. Although the labeling yield was >90%, it was found that 5 was highly unstable also in the solid state. In particular, after freeze-drying, the labelling yield dropped to 50%, thus indicating that the DTCZ group was partially removed from the dextran scaffold by the lyophilization process. Because of these difficulties, this type of dextran derivative for SLND was abandoned and the mechanism of DTCZ decomposition has not been deepened.

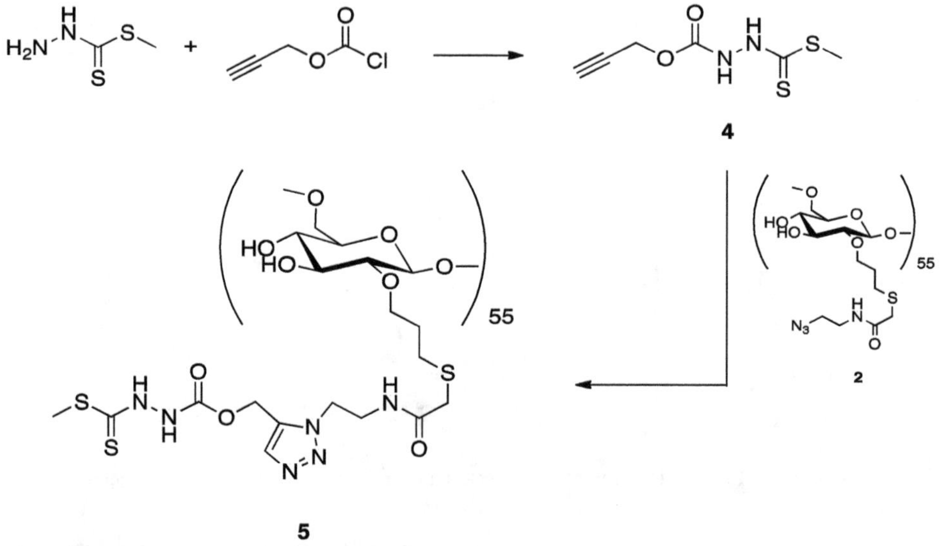

Figure 6. Schematic drawing of the synthesis of dextran-DTCZ (5).

2.3. Synthesis of 2-(2,3,4,6-tetra-O-acetyl-β-D-mannopyranosyl)-Acetic Acid

The novel 2-(2,3,4,6-tetra-O-acetyl-β-D-mannopyranosyl)-acetic acid 8 was synthesized by oxidation of the corresponding β-D-mannopyranosyl acetaldehyde 7, which in turn was prepared from the isomeric α-aldehyde 6 [25] by a previously optimized anomerization procedure [26]. It is worth noting that the challenging mannosyl derivative 8, that is a β-C-mannoside, was suitably designed to display a metabolically stable carbon–carbon anomeric linkage between the sugar moiety and the carboxylic functionality, thus preventing the corresponding glycoconjugates from chemical and enzymatic degradation (deglycosylation) in vivo [27]. Accordingly, the α-mannosyl acetaldehyde 6 was dissolved in MeOH and treated with L-proline organocatalyst (30 mol%), which promoted the anomeric process to the corresponding β-aldehyde 7 with the aid of microwave (MW) dielectric heating (constant power at 13 W for 3 h). The target β-mannosyl aldehyde 2 (thermodynamic product) was duly isolated in pure form by column chromatography (75% yield) and then subjected to a standard oxidation procedure with sodium chlorite [28] to give the corresponding acid 8 in almost quantitative yield (Figure 7).

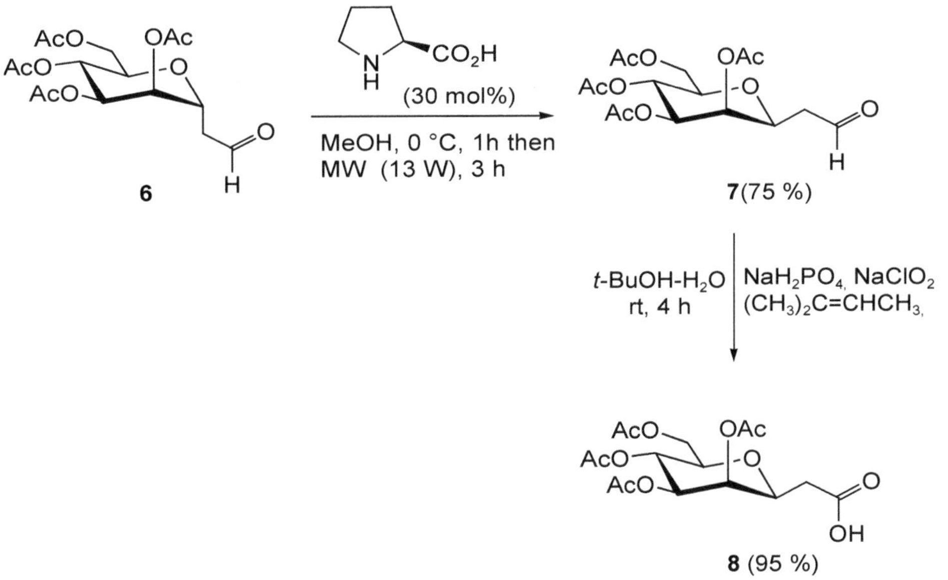

Figure 7. Synthesis of 2-(2,3,4,6-tetra-*O*-acetyl-β-D-mannopyranosyl)-acetic acid **8**.

2.4. Synthesis of a Dextran-Mannose-CysCys Multifunctional Ligand

A pair of multifunctional mannosylated CysCys ligands **9** and **10**, (Figure 8a) suitable for the labeling through the 3 + 1 method, was obtained using the reactions depicted in Figure 8b.

As a first step, the two linear pseudopeptides **9** and **10** were produced following the procedures illustrated in Figure 8b. Essentially, these compounds have the same basic structural features given by a terminal mannose group and a terminal combination of two cysteine aminoacids, but differ from the reactive group positioned approximately at the center of the linear pseudopeptide chain. In particular, **9** carries an alkyne group that is replaced by a carboxylic group in **10**. Pseudopeptide **9** was then linked to the dextran derivatives **2** through click chemistry reaction. Instead, pseudopeptide **10** was appended to the dextran derivative **3** via amide condensation (Figure 9).

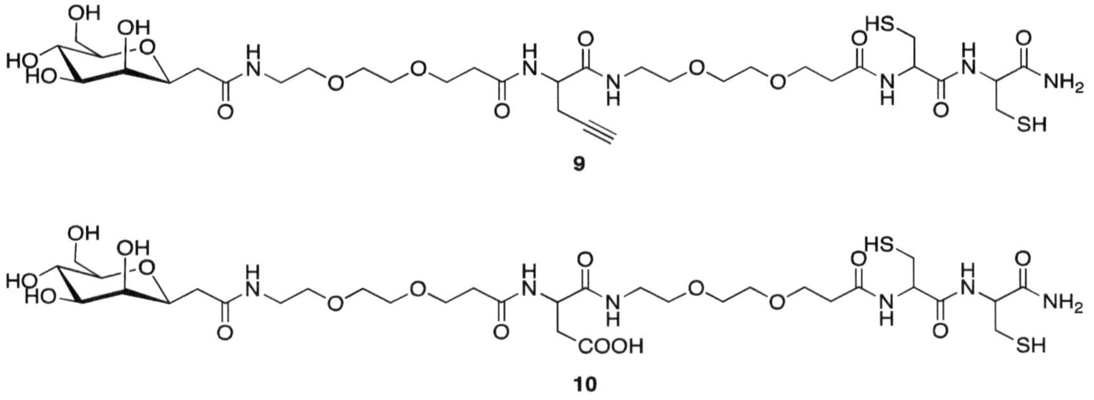

(a)

Figure 8. *Cont.*

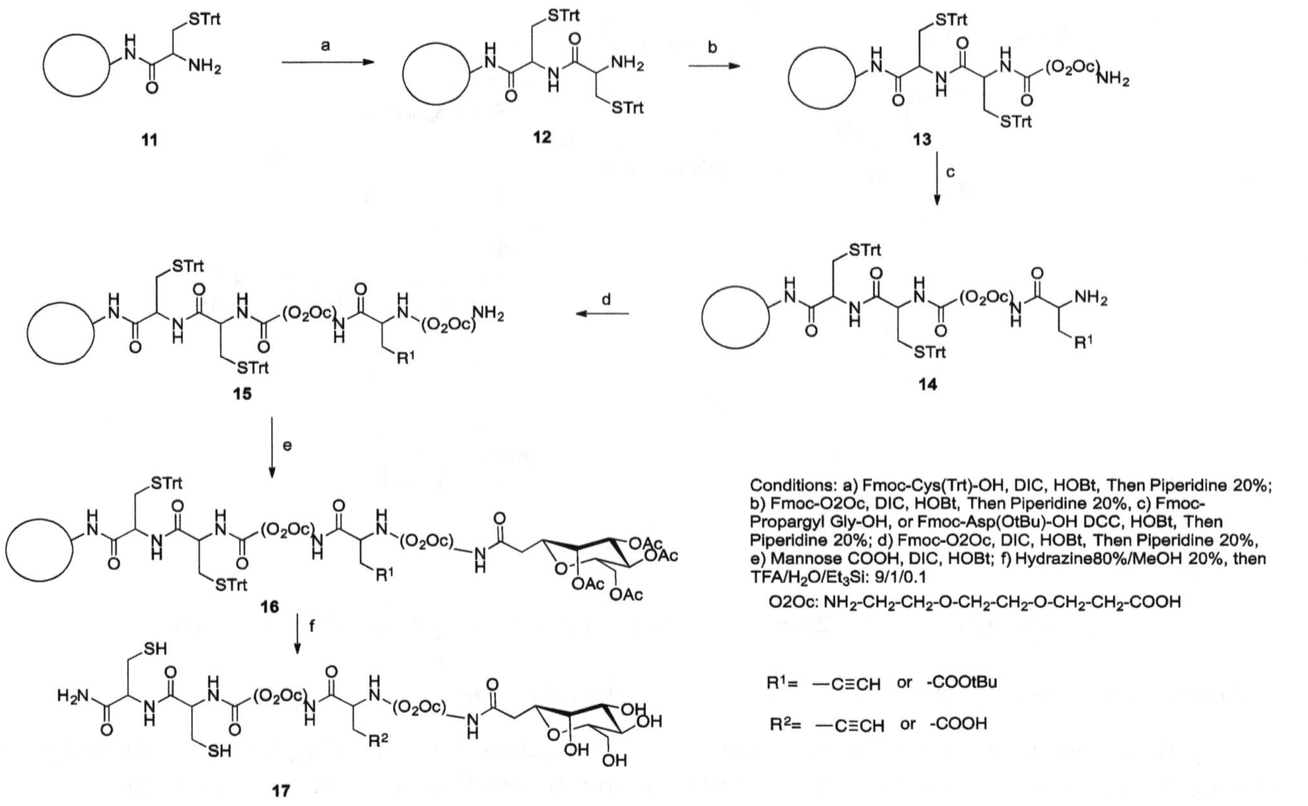

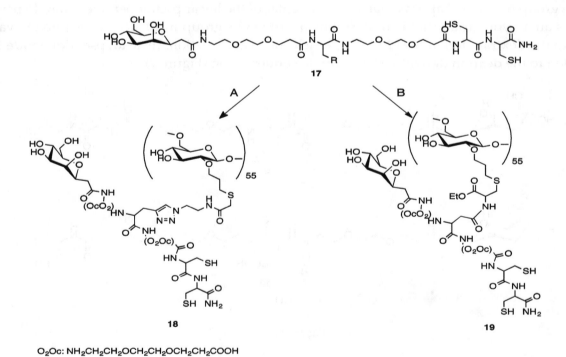

Figure 8. Structure (a) and synthesis (b) of mannosyl-CysCys ligands.

Figure 9. Synthesis and structure of dextran-mannosyl-CysCys ligands 18 and 19.

2.5. Preparation of ^{99m}TcN-"3 + 1" Labeled Dextran-Mannose Derivates

The resulting multifunctional ligands **18** and **19** (Figure 9) were labeled with the $[^{99m}Tc\equiv N]^{2+}$ core by applying the 3 + 1 approach, as shown in Figure 10. The monophosphine PCN (tris-cyanoethyl phosphane) was employed as ancillary ligand. Labeling yields were >95% (Figure 11a,b), and the resulting complexes exhibited a prolonged stability (>6 h) in physiological solution.

The formulation developed to prepare the ^{99m}TcN-"3+1" labeled dextran-mannose compound contains 0.1 mg of dextran-derivate, about half of that involved in the Lymphoseek® formulation (0.250 mg). Therefore, even if this dextran-derivate could have hypersensitivity effect, still to be verified, it is reasonable to assume that the reactions by patients to dextran in our formulation could be smaller than with Lymphoseek®. Further studies must be performed on this topic.

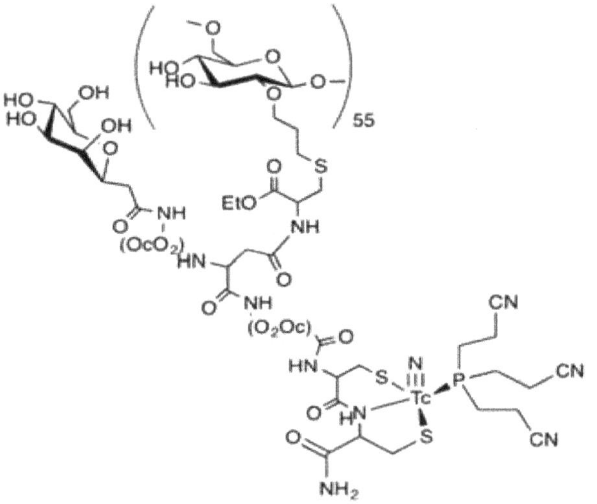

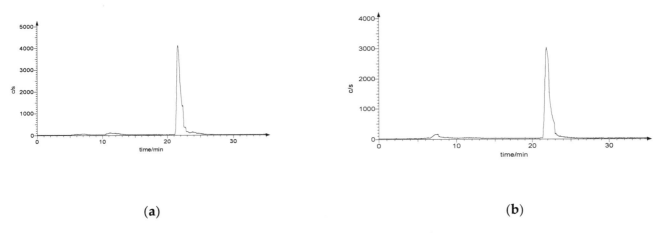

Figure 10. Representative labeling of the dextran-mannosyl-CysCys ligand **19** with the $[^{99m}Tc\equiv N]^{2+}$ core.

Figure 11. HPLC chromatograms of $[^{99m}Tc\equiv N(\textbf{18})PCN]$ (**a**) and $[^{99m}Tc\equiv N(\textbf{19})PCN]$ (**b**) complexes.

2.5.1. Stability Studies

The in vitro stability of ^{99m}Tc-complexes was evaluated by monitoring radiochemical purity (RCP) at different time points (15, 30, 60, 120 min) by high-performance liquid chromatography (HPLC). After preparation, 100 µL of the selected radioactive compound were incubated at 37 °C with 900 µL of saline or, alternatively, rat serum. No significant variation of RCP was observed in both conditions.

2.5.2. Cysteine and Glutathione (GSH) Challenge

An aliquot of freshly prepared aqueous solution of L-cysteine or GSH (50 μL, 10.0 mM) was placed in a test tube containing phosphate buffer (250 μL, 0.2 M, pH = 7.4), water (100 μL), and the appropriate ^{99m}Tc-complex (100 μL). The mixture was incubated at 37 °C for 2 h. A blank experiment was carried out using an equal volume of saline. Aliquots of the resulting solutions were withdrawn at 15, 30, 60, 120 min after incubation and analyzed by HPLC chromatography. The complexes were found to be inert toward transchelation by cysteine and GSH.

3. Materials and Methods

3.1. General

Dextran with average molecular weight 10,000 Da, succinic dihydrazide [SDH=H$_2$N–NH–(O=)C–(CH$_2$)$_2$–C(=O)–NH–NH$_2$], sodium dihydrogen phosphate monohydrate (NaH$_2$PO$_4$·H$_2$O), disodium hydrogen phosphate heptahydrate (Na$_2$HPO$_4$·7H$_2$O), SnCl$_2$·2H$_2$O, tris(2-cyanoethyl)phosphine [PCN=P(CH$_2$CH$_2$CN)$_3$], γ-hydroxypropylcyclodextrin, L-cysteine, and glutathione (GSH) were obtained from Sigma Aldrich, Milan, Italy.

Technetium-99m, as Na[^{99m}TcO$_4$] in physiological solution, was obtained from a Drytec™ ^{99}Mo/^{99m}Tc generator (GE Healthcare, Belfast, UK).

The infrared spectra (IR) (PerkinElmer, Waltham, Massachusetts, US) were recorded with FT-Perkin Elmer Spectrum 100 using a universal ATR crystal Zr/Se Diamond Bounces 1, serial number 14031; 1H-NMR spectra were recorded on a Varian 400 NMR instrument (Varian Inc., Palo Alto, CA, USA); the chemical shift (δ) is expressed in ppm.

3.1.1. Synthesis of 1

Sodium hydroxide (NaOH, 0.5 g, 12.5 mmol) and sodium borohydride (NaBH$_4$, 20.0 mg, 0.53 mmol) were added to a stirred solution of dextran (average molecular weight = 10,000 Daltons) (2.0 g, 0.2 mmol) in water. Allyl bromide (BrCH$_2$CH=CH$_2$, 3.5 g, 30 mmol) was then added to this solution at 40 °C. The mixture was stirred at 60 °C for 3 h and then neutralized with acetic acid. The product was purified by repeated precipitation with ethanol and dried under vacuum to achieve a constant weight. The final loading of dextran polymer was achieved by comparison of ^{1}H-NMR spectra. In particular, the chemical shift and the integral value of anomeric protons (nonsubstituted and substituted dextran) at 4.96 ppm and 5.13 ppm were reported to the allylic proton at 5.96 ppm. The loading was about 18 allylic groups for every polymeric unit (18 allyl moiety for 55 monomeric sugar in the dextran).

3.1.2. Synthesis of Thioglycol Amide

Sodium azide (NaN$_3$, 3.34 g, 51.38 mmol) was added to a stirred solution of 2-chloro-ethylamine hydrochloride (H$_2$NCH$_2$CH$_2$Cl, 2.0 g, 17.39 mmol) in water, and the reaction solution was heated at 80 °C for 15 h. After cooling the reaction at 0 °C, KOH pellets were added until pH = 14. The aqueous solution was extracted 3 times with diethyl ether (30 mL each), and the resulting organic phase was separated, dried, and concentrated under vacuum to obtain the corresponding amino-azide compound H$_2$NCH$_2$CH$_2$N$_3$ (caution: explosive compound).

This compound was successively used to prepare the corresponding thioazide using the following procedure. The amino-azide (H$_2$NCH$_2$CH$_2$N$_3$, 0.33 g, 3.8 mmol), WSC (0.42 g, 2.19 mmol), and HOBt (0.18 g, 2.19 mmol) were added to a stirred solution of thioglicolic acid (0.33 g, 1.99 mmol) in DMF at 0 °C. The reaction mixture was stirred at room temperature for 24 h and then concentrated under vacuum and diluted with ethyl acetate. The organic phase was washed with a citric acid solution (10% in water, 30 mL), NaHCO$_3$ (5% in water, 30 mL), and Brine (30 mL). The organic phase was dried and concentrated to dryness to obtain the thiozide.

^{1}H NMR (400 MHz, Chloroform-d) δ 6.64 (bs, 1H), 3.59–3.54 (m, 1H), 3.36–3.31 (m, 4H), 3.29–3.23 (m, 2H).

^{13}C NMR (100 MHz, Chloroform-d) δ 171.60, 49.84, 41.37, 32.75.

The allyl dextran (**1**) (80.0 mg) and the thioazide HSCH$_2$C(=O)NHCH$_2$CH$_2$N$_3$ (86.0 mg, 0.53 mmol) were dissolved in a mixture of water and THF(1:1). Ammonium persulfate (80.0 mg, 0.35 mmol) was added in one pot and the mixture was then heated at 50 °C for 2 h. After evaporation of the solvent under vacuum, the resulting product (**2**) was purified by gel filtration using a Sephadex G25 PD 10 column using water as eluent.

As depicted in Figure 12, the infrared spectra of azido dextran showed the classical absorption peak at 2101 cm^{-1}.

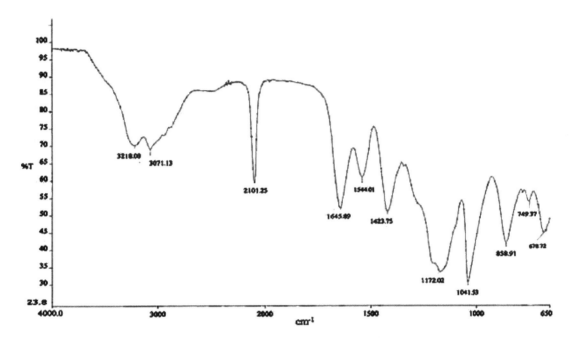

Figure 12. IR spectra of azido dextran after purification procedure.

3.1.3. Synthesis of **3**

The dextran moiety **3** was prepared according to literature methods [29]. The Fmoc-Cys-OEt group was attached to the allyl moiety using ammonium persulfate in water. In order to evaluate the derivatization loading of allyl-dextrane, we performed, in a small part of the product, a Fmoc deprotection and titration [30]; this analysis allowed us to determine the final loading of dextran in 0.20 mmol/g. The deprotection of Fmoc residue from the cysteine with DMF/20% piperidine yielded the free amine product **3**.

3.1.4. Synthesis of **4**

To a stirred solution of HDTCZ (2.0 g, 14.68 mmol) in anhydrous THF (60 mL), DIPEA (2.84 g, 22.02 mmol) and propargyl chloroformate (2.61 g, 22.02 mmol) were added at 0 °C. The reaction was stirred at room temperature for 4 h and then quenched with a saturated solution of ammonium chloride to afford compound **4**.

^{1}H NMR (400 MHz, Chloroform-d) δ 8.01 (bs, 1H), 4.85 (s, 2H), 2.61 (m, 4H).

3.1.5. Synthesis of **5**

Compound **4** (5.3 mg, 3.69 × 10^{-4} mmol), sodium ascorbate (0.8 mg, 4.059 × 10^{-5} mmol), and CuSO$_4$ (0.01 mg, 4.059 × 10^{-6} mmol) were added to a stirred solution of compound **2** (5.69 mg, approximately 4.06×10^{-4} mmol) in water (3.0 mL). The solution was stirred at room temperature for 12 h and then concentrated under vacuum to yield compound **5**.

3.1.6. Synthesis of 2-(2,3,4,6-Tetra-*O*-acetyl-β-D-Mannopyranosyl)-Acetaldehyde (7)

A 0.5–2.0 mL process vial was filled with the α-mannosyl aldehyde **6** (150 mg, 0.40 mmol) and MeOH (1.5 mL). The resulting solution was cooled to 0 °C, and then L-proline (14 mg, 0.12 mmol) was added in one portion. The vial was sealed with the Teflon septum and aluminium crimp by using an appropriate crimping tool. The mixture was then vigorously stirred at 0 °C for 1 h, then the vial was placed in its correct position in the Biotage Initiator cavity where irradiation at constant power (13 W) was performed for 3 h with simultaneous cooling of the vial (internal temperature $\approx$60 °C) by means of pressurized air (4 bar). After the full irradiation sequence was completed, the vial was cooled to room temperature and then opened. The mixture was diluted with AcOEt (80 mL) and washed with saturated $NaHCO_3$ (2 × 15 mL) and brine (2 × 5 mL). The organic phase was dried (Na_2SO_4), filtered, and concentrated to give crude β-mannosyl aldehyde **7** (β/α ratio 10:1). Flash column chromatography with 1:1 cyclohexane-AcOEt (containing 20% of CH_2Cl_2 and 1% of MeOH) afforded pure **7** (112 mg, 75%) as a white amorphous solid. ^1H NMR: δ = 9.75 (dd, 1 H, J = 0.5 Hz, J = 1.5 Hz, CHO), 5.36 (dd, 1 H, J = 0.5 Hz, J = 3.0 Hz, H-2′), 5.24 (dd, 1 H, J = 9.0 Hz, J = 9.2 Hz, H-4′), 5.12 (dd, 1 H, J = 3.0 Hz, J = 9.2 Hz, H-3′), 4.30–4.20 and 4.18–4.06 (2 m, 3 H, H-1′, 2 h-6′), 3.72 (ddd, 1 H, J = 2.5 Hz, J = 6.0 Hz, J = 9.0 Hz, H-5′), 2.77 (ddd, 1 H, J = 1.5 Hz, J = 7.5 Hz, J = 17.0 Hz, H-2a), 2.54 (ddd, 1 h, J = 0.5 Hz, J = 4.5 Hz, J = 17.0 Hz, H-2b), 2.20, 2.10, 2.05, and 1.98 (4 s, 12 H, 4 Me). ESI MS (374): 397 (M + Na^+).

3.1.7. Synthesis of 2-(2,3,4,6-Tetra-*O*-Acetyl-β-D-Mannopyranosyl)-Acetic Acid (8)

A mixture of β-aldehyde **7** (112 mg, 0.30 mmol), sodium chlorite (271 mg, 3.00 mmol), sodium dihydrogen phosphate monohydrate (311 mg, 2.25 mmol), 2-methyl-2-butene (1.2 mL), *t*-BuOH (5.5 mL), and H_2O (2.1 mL) was stirred at room temperature for 4 h and then diluted with CH_2Cl_2 (15 mL) and H_2O (5 mL). The organic layer was separated and the aqueous layer was extracted with CH_2Cl_2 (3 × 10 mL) then acidified (pH 2) with 5% HCl and extracted again with CH_2Cl_2 (3 × 10 mL). The combined organic phases were dried (Na_2SO_4), filtered, and concentrated to give the β-mannosyl acetic acid **8** (111 mg, 95%) at least 95% pure as established by ^1H NMR analysis. ^1H NMR: δ = 5.40 (dd, 1 h, J = 0.5 Hz, J = 3.0 Hz, H-2′), 5.24 (dd, 1 H, J = 9.0 Hz, J = 9.2 Hz, H-4′), 5.11 (dd, 1 H, J = 3.0 Hz, J = 9.2 Hz, H-3′), 4.27 (dd, 1 H, J = 5.5 Hz, J = 12.0 Hz, H-6′a), 4.14 (ddd, 1 H, J = 0.5 Hz, J = 5.0 Hz, J = 7.5 Hz, H-1′), 4.10 (dd, 1 H, J = 3.0 Hz, J = 12.0 Hz, H-6′b), 3.70 (ddd, 1 H, J = 3.0 Hz, J = 5.5 Hz, J = 9.0 Hz, H-5′), 2.68 (dd, 1 H, J = 7.5 Hz, J = 17.0 Hz, H-2a), 2.50 (dd, 1 H, J = 5.0 Hz, J = 17.0 Hz, H-2b), 2.20, 2.08, 2.04, and 1.98 (4 s, 12 H, 4 Me). ESI MS (390): 413 (M + Na^+).

3.1.8. Synthesis of Pseudopeptide 9

Fmoc-Rink amide resin (0.69 mmol/g, 0.2 g) was treated with piperidine [20% in *N,N*-dimethylformamide (DMF)] and linked with Fmoc-aa-OH (4.0 equiv) by using [*O*-(7-azabenzotriazol-1-yl)-1,1,3,3-tetramethyluronium hexafluorophosphate] (HATU, 4.0 equiv) as a coupling reagent. The coupling reaction was continued for 1 h and then piperidine (20% in DMF) was used to remove the Fmoc group at every step. The peptide resin was washed with methanol and dried in vacuum to yield the protected peptide-resin. This resin was treated with a mixture of trifluoroacetic acid (TFA)/H_2O/Et_3Si (9:0.5:0.5) for 1 h at room temperature. After filtration of the resin, the solvent was concentrated in vacuum and the residue triturated under diethyl ether. The crude linear peptide was purified by preparative reversed-phase HPLC to yield a white powder after lyophilization. Further purification was obtained by preparative reversed-phase HPLC using a Water Delta Prep 4000 system equipped with a Waters PrepLC 40-mm Assembly C18 column (30 × 4 cm, 300 A, 15 mm spherical particle size column). The column was perfused at a flow rate of 40 mL min^{-1} with solvent A (5% *v*/*v* acetonitrile in 0.1% aqueous TFA) and a linear gradient from 0 to 50% of solvent B (80% *v*/*v* acetonitrile in 0.1% aqueous TFA) over a period of 25 min. Analytical HPLC was performed on a Beckman 125 instrument fitted with an Alltech C18 column (4.6 × 150 mm, 5 mm particle size) and equipped with a Beckman 168 diode array detector. Analytical purity and retention time (t_R) of **9** were determined using the solvent system A + B as specified above, at a flow rate of 1.0 mL min^{-1}, and using a linear gradient ranging from 5 to 40% B over 25 min. Molecular weight of **9** was measured by ESI-MS analysis using a Micromass ZMD 2000 mass spectrometer.

HPLC: Rt 10.60 min; ESI MS (812): 813.3 (M + H$^+$).

3.1.9. Synthesis of Pseudopeptide **10**

Peptide **10** was obtained through a Fmoc-chemistry solid phase peptide synthesis using a Rink amide resin to elongate the peptide backbone starting from the C terminal (Cys). The pseudopeptide was cleaved from the resin using a mixture of TFA/water and triethylsilane.

HPLC: Rt 9.98 min; ESI MS (846): 847.6 (M + H$^+$).

3.1.10. Synthesis of **18**

To a stirred solution of compound **2** (5.69 mg, approximately 4.06 × 10^{-4} mmol) in water (3.0 mL) was added 9 (6.0 mg, 3.69 × 10^{-4} mmol), sodium ascorbate (0.8 mg, 4.059 × 10^{-5} mmol), and CuSO$_4$ (0.01 mg, 4.059 × 10^{-6} mmol). The solution was stirred at room temperature for 12 h and then concentrated under vacuum to yield compound **18**. As depicted in Figure 13, the IR spectra showed the disappearance of azide peak (at 2097 cm^{-1}) and the appearance of a new broad signal at 1652 cm^{-1} that could be assigned to carbonyl stretching of peptide amide moiety.

HPLC: Rt = 14.30 min.

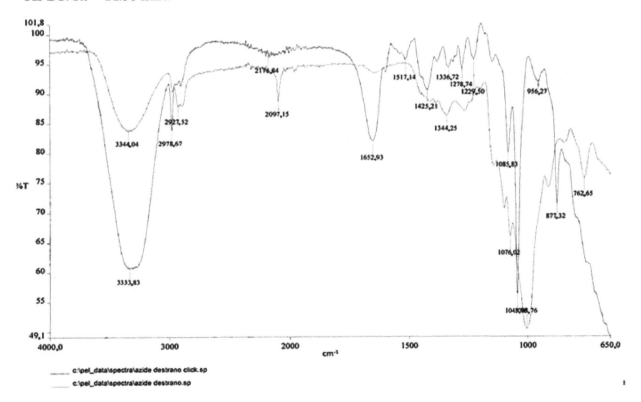

Figure 13. Comparison of IR spectra before and after click reaction.

3.1.11. Synthesis of **19**

Using a classical peptide chemistry condensation, pseudopeptide **10** (6 mg, 0.00709 mmol) was condensed with dextran moiety **3** (40 mg, loading 0.2 mmol/g, 0.00788 mmol), using as coupling agents WSC (1.5 mg, 0.007799 mmol) and HOBt (1.2 mg, 0.007799 mmol).

HPLC: Rt = 14.30 min.

3.2. Preparation of ^{99m}TcN-"3 + 1" Labeled Dextran-Mannose Derivate

Freshly generator-eluted $Na[^{99m}TcO_4]$ (100 MBq, 0.9 mL) was added to a nitrogen-purged vial containing 1.0 mg of succinic dihydrazide (SDH) and 0.1 mg of $SnCl_2$. The vial was kept at room temperature for 15 min to yield the $[^{99m}TcN]^{2+}$ group. The appropriate dextran-mannose derivate (0.1 mg dissolved in 0.5 mL of saline) and tris(2-cyanoethyl) phosphine (PCN, 0.5 mg dissolved in a saline solution containing 2.0 mg of γ-hydroxypropylcyclodextrin) were freshly prepared and then simultaneously added to the reaction vial containing the radioactive Tc-99m nitrido intermediate. The resulting mixture was heated at 80 °C for 15 min. The radiochemical yield, as determined by radio-HPLC chromatography, ranged from 95 to 98%.

3.3. Chromatography

The RCP of the final Tc-99m compounds was determined by HPLC performed on a Beckman System Gold Instrument equipped with a programmable solvent Module 126, scanning detector Module 166, and a radioisotope detector Module 170. Chromatographic analyses were carried out on a reversed-phase Agilent precolumn Zorbax 300SB-C18 (4.6 × 12.5 mm) and a reversed-phase Agilent column Zorbax 300SB-C18 (4.6 × 250 mm) using the following conditions. Mobile phase: A = water containing 0.1% TFA, B = acetonitrile containing 0.1% TFA; gradient: 0 min, B = 0%; 0–25 min, B = 100%; 25–30 min, B = 100%; 30–35 min, B = 0%; flow rate: 1.0 mL/min.

4. Conclusions

A new particular of mannosyl-dextran-derived multifunctional ligands, potentially useful for sentinel node detection, has been reported. These multifunctional ligands have been specifically designed to accommodate, in a controlled way, the same number of functional groups, each performing a specific chemical or biological function on the selected position on the dextran scaffold. Click reactions, as well as standard amide condensation, allowing the use of modular building blocks, have proven to be very efficient for building up the multifunctional ligands, containing a chelating system specifically chosen to label the $[^{99m}TcN]^{2+}$. We have found no differences between in vitro stability of the ^{99m}TcN-"3+1" labeled dextran-mannose derivate obtained through the different chemical procedures. However, further in vivo investigations should be performed to confirm our results.

Author Contributions: Conceptualization, A.D.; Formal analysis, A.F. and E.M.; Investigation, A.B., M.P., C.T., A.M. and V.Z.; Methodology, R.G.; Project administration, L.U.; Supervision, M.G.; Writing – original draft, A.B. and C.T.; Writing – review & editing, P.M.

Acknowledgments: Thanks to the Nuclear Medicine of the University Hospital of Ferrara for equipment.

References

1.   Buscombe, J.; Paganelli, G.; Burak, Z.E.; Waddington, W.; Maublant, J.; Prats, E.; Palmedo, H.; Schillaci, O.; Maffioli, L.; Lassmann, M.; et al. Sentinel node in breast cancer procedural guidelines. *Eur. J. Nucl. Med. Mol. Imaging* **2007**, *34*, 2154–2159. [CrossRef] [PubMed]
2.   Giammarile, F.; Alazraki, N.; Aarsvold, J.N.; Audisio, R.A.; Glass, E.; Grant, S.F.; Kunikowska, J.; Leidenius, M.; Moncayo, V.M.; Uren, R.F.; et al. The EANM and SNMMI practice guideline for lymphoscintigraphy and sentinel node localization in breast cancer. *Eur. J. Nucl. Med. Mol. Imaging* **2013**, *40*, 1932–1947. [CrossRef] [PubMed]
3.   Alazraki, N.; Glass, E.C.; Castronovo, F.; Olmos, R.A.; Podoloff, D. Society of Nuclear Medicine procedure guideline for lymphoscintigraphy and the use of intraoperative gamma probe for sentinel lymph node localization in melanoma of intermediate thickness. *J. Nucl. Med.* **2002**, *43*, 1414–1418. [PubMed]

4.   Wong, S.L.; Balch, C.M.; Hurley, P.; Agarwala, S.S.; Akhurst, T.J.; Cochran, A.; Cormier, J.N.; Gorman, M.; Kim, T.Y.; McMasters, K.M.; et al. Sentinel lymph node biopsy for melanoma: American Society of Clinical Oncology and Society of Surgical Oncology joint clinical practice guideline. *J. Clin. Oncol.* **2012**, *30*, 2912–2918. [CrossRef] [PubMed]

5.   Alkureishi, L.W.; Burak, Z.; Alvarez, J.A.; Ballinger, J.; Bilde, A.; Britten, A.J.; Calabrese, L.; Chiesa, C.; Chiti, A.; de Bree, R.; et al. Joint practice guidelines for radionuclide lymphoscintigraphy for sentinel node localization in oral/oropharyngeal squamous cell carcinoma. *Eur. J. Nucl. Med. Mol. Imaging* **2009**, *36*, 1915–1936. [CrossRef] [PubMed]

6.   Wilhelm, A.; Mijnhout, G.S.; Franssen, E.J.D. Radiopharmaceuticals in sentinel lymph node detection: An overview. *Eur. J. Nucl. Med.* **1999**, *26*, 36–42. [CrossRef]

7.   Eshima, D.; Fauconnier, T.; Eshima, L.; Thornback, J.R. Radiopharmaceuticals for lymphoscintigraphy: Including dosimetry and radiation considerations. *Semin. Nucl. Med.* **2000**, *1*, 25–32. [CrossRef]

8.   Hoh, C.K.; Wallace, A.M.; Vera, D.R. Preclinical studies of [99mTc] DTPA-mannosyl-dextran. *Nucl. Med. Biol.* **2003**, *30*, 457–464. [CrossRef]

9.   Sharma, R.; Wendt, J.A.; Rsmussen, J.C.; Adams, K.E.; Marshall, M.V.; Secick-Muraka, E.M. New horizons for imaging lymphatic function. *Ann. N. Y. Acad. Sci.* **2008**, *1131*, 13–36. [CrossRef] [PubMed]

10. Ravizzini, G.; Turkbey, B.; Barrett, T.; Kobayashi, H.; Choyke, P.L. Nanoparticles in sentinel lymph node mapping. *WIREs Nanomed. Nonobiotechnol.* **2009**, *1*, 610–623. [CrossRef] [PubMed]

11. Morais, M.; Subramanian, S.; Pandey, U.; Samuel, G.; Venkatesh, M.; Martins, M.; Pereira, S.; Correia, J.D.G.; Santos, I. Mannosylated dextranderivatives labeled with fac-[M(CO)3]+ (M = Tc-99m, Re) for specific targeting of sentinel lymph node. *Mol. Pharm.* **2011**, *8*, 609–620. [CrossRef] [PubMed]

12. Pirmettis, I.; Arano, Y.; Tsotakos, T.; Okada, K.; Yamaguchi, A.; Uehara, T.; Morais, M.; Correia, J.D.G.; Santos, I.; Martins, M.; et al. New Tc-99m (CO)3 mannosilated dextran bearing s-derivatized cysteine chelator for sentinel lymph node detection. *Mol. Pharm.* **2012**, *9*, 1681–1692. [CrossRef] [PubMed]

13. Petrova, T.V.; Makinen, T.P.; Saarela, J.; Virtanen, J.; Ferrell, R.E.; Finegold, D.N.; Kerjaschki, D.; Yla-Herttuala, S.; Alitalo, K. Lymphatic endothelial reprogramming of vascular endotelial cells by the Prox-1 homeobox transcription factor. *EMBO J.* **2002**, *21*, 4593–4599. [CrossRef] [PubMed]

14. Martilla-Ichihara, F.; Turia, R.; Miiluniemi, M.; Karikoski, M.; Maksimow, M.; Niemela, J.; Martinez-Pomares, L.; Salmi, M.; Jalkanen, S. Macrophages mannose receptor on lymphatics controls cell trafficking. *Blood* **2008**, *112*, 64–72. [CrossRef] [PubMed]

15. Wallace, A.M.; Hoh, C.K.; Limmer, K.K.; Darrah, D.D.; Schulteis, G.; Vera, D.R. Sentinel lymph node accumulation of Lymphoseek and Tc-99m-sulfur colloid using a "2-day" protocol. *Nucl. Med. Biol.* **2009**, *36*, 687–692. [CrossRef] [PubMed]

16. Liu, G.; Hnatowich, D.J. Labeling Biomolecules with Radiorhenium—A Review of the Bifunctional Chelators. *Anticancer Agents Med. Chem.* **2007**, *7*, 367–377. [CrossRef] [PubMed]

17. Giglio, J.; Fernández, S.; Jentschel, C.; Pietzsch, H.-J.; Papadopoulos, M.; Pelecanou, M.; Pirmettis, I.; Paolino, A.; Rey, A. Design and Development of 99mTc-'4+1'-Labeled Dextran-Mannose Derivatives as Potential Radiopharmaceuticals for Sentinel Lymph Node Detection. *Cancer Biother. Radiopharm.* **2013**, *28*. [CrossRef] [PubMed]

18. Boschi, A.; Cazzola, E.; Uccelli, L.; Pasquali, M.; Ferretti, V.; Bertolasi, V.; Duatti, A. Rhenium(V) and technetium(V) nitrido complexes with mixed tridentate p-donor and monodentate p-acceptor ligands. *Inorg. Chem.* **2012**, *51*, 3130–3137. [CrossRef] [PubMed]

19. Boschi, A.; Uccelli, L.; Pasquali, M.; Pasqualini, R.; Guerrini, R.; Duatti, A. Mixed tridentate p-donor and monodentate p-acceptor ligands as chelating systems for rhenium-188 and technetium-99m nitride radiopharmaceuticals. *Curr. Radiopharm.* **2013**, *6*, 137–145. [CrossRef] [PubMed]

20. Smilkov, K.; Janevik, E.; Guerrini, R.; Pasquali, M.; Boschi, A.; Uccelli, L.; Di Domenico, G.; Duatti, A. Preparation and first biological evaluation of novel Re-188/Tc-99m peptide conjugates with substance-P. *Appl. Radiat. Isot.* **2014**, *92*, 25–31. [CrossRef] [PubMed]

21. Boschi, A.; Massi, A.; Uccelli, L.; Pasquali, M.; Duatti, A. PEGylated N-methyl-S-methyl dithiocarbazate as a new reagent for the high-yield preparation of nitrido Tc-99m and Re-188 radiopharmaceuticals. *Nucl. Med. Biol.* **2010**, *37*, 927–934. [CrossRef] [PubMed]

22.   Boschi, A.; Duatti, A.; Uccelli, L. Development of Technetium-99m and Rhenium-188 Radiopharmaceuticals Containing a Terminal Metal-Nitrido Multiple Bond for Diagnosis and Theraphy. *Top. Curr. Chem.* **2005**, *252*, 85–115. [CrossRef]

23.   Holmberg, A.; Meurling, L. Preparation of Sulfhydrylborane-Dextran Conjugates for Boron Neutron Capture Therapy. *Bioconjugate Chem.* **1993**, *4*, 570–573. [CrossRef]

24.   Rostovtsev, V.V.; Green, L.G.; Fokin, V.V.; Sharpless, K.B. A Stepwise Huisgen Cycloaddition Process: Copper(I)-Catalyzed Regioselective Ligation ʃ of Azides and Terminal Alkynes. *Angew. Chem. Int. Ed. Engl.* **2002**, *41*, 2596–2599. [CrossRef]

25.   Hamzavi, R.; Dolle, F.; Tavitian, B.; Dahl, O.; Nielsen, P.E. Modulation of the Pharmacokinetic Properties of PNA: Preparation of Galactosyl, Mannosyl, Fucosyl, N-Acetylgalactosaminyl, and N-Acetylglucosaminyl Derivatives of Aminoethylglycine Peptide Nucleic Acid Monomers and Their Incorporation into PNA Oligomers. *Bioconjugate Chem.* **2003**, *14*, 941–954. [CrossRef] [PubMed]

26.   Massi, A.; Nuzzi, A.; Dondoni, A.J. Microwave-Assisted Organocatalytic Anomerization of α-C-Glycosylmethyl Aldehydes and Ketones. *Org. Chem.* **2007**, *72*, 10279–10282. [CrossRef] [PubMed]

27.   Postema, M.H.D.; Calimente, D. *Glycochemistry: Principles, Synthesis and Applications*; Wang, P.G., Bertozzi, C., Eds.; Marcel Dekker: New York, NY, USA, 2000; Chapter 4; pp. 77–131.

28.   Kosmol, R.; Hennig, L.; Welzel, P.; Findeisen, M.; Müller, D.; Markus, A.; van Heijenoort, J.J. A Moenomycin-type Structural Analogue of Lipid II some possible mechanisms of the mode of action of transglycosylase inhibitors can be discarded. *J. Prakt. Chem.* **1997**, *339*, 340–358. [CrossRef]

29.   Ossipov, D.A.; Hilborn, J. Poly(vinyl alcohol)-Based Hydrogels Formed by "Click Chemistry". *Macromolecules* **2006**, *39*, 1709–1718. [CrossRef]

30.   Gude, M.; Ryf, J.; White, P.D. An accurate method for the quantitation of Fmoc-derivatized solid phase supports. *Lett. Pept. Sci.* **2002**, *9*, 203–206. [CrossRef]

7

Evaluation of Radiolabeled Girentuximab In Vitro and In Vivo

Tais Basaco [1,2], Stefanie Pektor [3], Josue M. Bermudez [1], Niurka Meneses [1], Manfred Heller [4], José A. Galván [5], Kayluz F. Boligán [6], Stefan Schürch [1], Stephan von Gunten [6], Andreas Türler [1] and Matthias Miederer [3,*]

[1]   Department of Chemistry and Biochemistry, University of Bern, 3012 Bern, Switzerland;
      tais.basaco@dcb.unibe.ch (T.B.); josue.moreno@itg-garching.de (J.M.B.);
      niurka.meneses@dcb.unibe.ch (N.M.); stefan.schuerch@dcb.unibe.ch (S.S.);
      andreas.tuerler@dcb.unibe.ch (A.T.)
[2]   Laboratory of Radiochemistry, Paul Scherrer Institute (PSI), 5232 Villigen PSI, Switzerland
[3]   Clinic for Nuclear Medicine, University Medical Center Mainz, 55131 Mainz, Germany;
      stefanie.pektor@unimedizin-mainz.de
[4]   Department for Biomedical Research (DBMR), University of Bern, 3010 Bern, Switzerland;
      manfred.heller@dbmr.unibe.ch
[5]   Institute of Pathology, University of Bern, 3010 Bern, Switzerland; jose.galvan@pathology.unibe.ch
[6]   Institute of Pharmacology (PKI), University of Bern, 3010 Bern, Switzerland;
      kayluz.frias@pki.unibe.ch (K.F.B.); stephan.vongunten@pki.unibe.ch (S.v.G.)
*   Correspondence: matthias.miederer@unimedizin-mainz.de

Abstract: Girentuximab (cG250) targets carbonic anhydrase IX (CAIX), a protein which is expressed on the surface of most renal cancer cells (RCCs). cG250 labeled with ^{177}Lu has been used in clinical trials for radioimmunotherapy (RIT) of RCCs. In this work, an extensive characterization of the immunoconjugates allowed optimization of the labeling conditions with ^{177}Lu while maintaining immunoreactivity of cG250, which was then investigated in in vitro and in vivo experiments. cG250 was conjugated with S-2-(4-isothiocyanatobenzyl)-1,4,7,10-tetraazacyclododecane tetraacetic acid (DOTA(SCN)) by using incubation times between 30 and 90 min and characterized by mass spectrometry. Immunoconjugates with five to ten DOTA(SCN) molecules per cG250 molecule were obtained. Conjugates with ratios less than six DOTA(SCN)/cG250 had higher in vitro antigen affinity, both pre- and postlabeling with ^{177}Lu. Radiochemical stability increased, in the presence of sodium ascorbate, which prevents radiolysis. The immunoreactivity of the radiolabeled cG250 tested by specific binding to SK-RC-52 cells decreased when the DOTA content per conjugate increased. The in vivo tumor uptake was < 10% ID/g and independent of the total amount of protein in the range between 5 and 100 μg cG250 per animal. Low tumor uptake was found to be due to significant necrotic areas and heterogeneous CAIX expression. In addition, low vascularity indicated relatively poor accessibility of the CAIX target.

Keywords: carbonic anhydrase IX; girentuximab; renal cell carcinomas; ^{177}Lu-radiopharmaceuticals; radioimmunotherapy

1. Introduction

Targeted therapy with monoclonal antibodies (mAbs) carrying radioisotopes (radioimmunotherapy, RIT) has become a powerful tool in nuclear medicine, because of highly selective small molecules and targeted internal radiotherapy; it is currently being increasingly applied in the treatment of a growing number of malignant diseases [1–8]. Additionally, imaging studies with gamma emitting isotopes open the possibility of translational investigation of dosimetry [9]. The effectiveness of RIT depends on a number of factors related to the Ab such as the specificity and affinity as well as the immunoreactivity, stability and blood clearance of the resulting radioimmunoconjugate [10,11]. Three radiolabeled mAbs—two murine, ^{90}Y-ibritumomab tiuxetan (Zevalin; Biogen Idec) and ^{131}I-tositumomab (Bexxar; Corixa/GSK), and one chimeric, ^{131}I-ch-TNT (Shanghai Medipharm Biotech)—have been approved for non-Hodgkin's lymphoma (NHL) or lung cancer, but only a minority of anticancer mAbs currently in the clinics, are radioimmunoconjugates [12]. A suitable therapeutic window exists, only when RIT leads to a sufficient deposition of radioactivity in the tumor and, at the same time, acceptably low doses to healthy organs and tissues. Clinical studies revealed the limitations of radioimmunoconjugates as cancer therapeutics (for example, mAbs did not deliver effective radiation doses, especially to solid tumor sites [13], complex chemistry was often required for conjugation, and there were potentially toxic effects on normal tissues). In addition, in solid large tumors, accumulation of radioactivity by RIT is negatively influenced by slow diffusion properties of large molecules when interstitial fluid pressure is high and perfusion and vascular permeability are heterogeneous [10,14]. Furthermore, antigen expression can be reduced due to the presence of necrotic areas in those tumors, leading to a reduction of the radionuclide uptake.

Reaching cancer cells within solid tumors by mAbs, follows slower kinetics, compared to small molecules, such as peptides. Thus, long circulation times require therapeutic radionuclides with relatively long half-lives and with high stability of the radioimmune-conjugation. The released energy from the radiometal can also induce radiolysis and degradation of the protein, and thus loss of specificity. The formation of free radicals can be attenuated with the addition of quenching reagents like human serum albumin (HSA), gentisic acid, ascorbic acid, and other antiradicals [15]. β^- emitting radionuclides are currently prevalent in RIT since they have shown particular efficacy against a larger number of diseases. Radionuclides such as ^{131}I, ^{90}Y, ^{188}Re, and ^{177}Lu have been used extensively for the RIT of neoplastic lesions [3,16–18]. ^{177}Lu is increasingly being used as a potent radionuclide for use in in vivo therapy because of its favorable decay characteristics. It decays by the emission of beta particles with maximum energies of 497 keV (78.6%), 384 keV (9.1%), and 176 keV (12.2%) to stable ^{177}Hf [19] allowing delivery of therapeutic doses to the tumor and minimal doses to healthy tissues (i.e., low renal toxicity). The β-emission energy of ^{177}Lu (β_{mean} = 166 keV) is lower than for other radionuclides commonly used for therapy such as ^{131}I (β_{mean} = 191 keV), ^{90}Y (β_{mean} = 699 keV), or ^{188}Re (β_{mean} = 770 KeV). In addition, the emission of gamma rays of 113 keV (6.4%) and 208 keV (11%) with relatively low abundances, provides advantages that allow simultaneous scintigraphic studies, which help to monitor proper in vivo localization of the injected radiopharmaceutical and to perform dosimetric evaluations. Another important aspect for consideration is the relatively long $t_{1/2}$ of ^{177}Lu (6.73 days), which provides logistical advantages that facilitate its supply to locations far from reactors. The relatively long $t_{1/2}$ also favors this nuclide for use in RIT [20].

An essential criterion for successful targeted radiotherapy with ^{177}Lu depends on the choice of the proper bifunctional chelator (BFC). ^{177}Lu is a bone-seeking element [14], its premature release and accumulation in the bone can lead to dose-limiting bone marrow toxicity. A number of acyclic and cyclic ligand systems have already been investigated for the labeling of mAb (full-length and fragments) with ^{177}Lu [21–23]. Macrocyclic BFCs such as 1,4,7,10-tetraazacyclododecane-1,4,7,10-tetraacetic acid (DOTA) are of particular interest for the use of lanthanides in RIT because they are very well organized structures, enabling the formation of metal complexes, with a high thermodynamic stability and slow decomposition kinetics [22,24–26].

During the preparation of conjugated mAbs and the radiolabeling process, the protein might suffer some modifications, resulting in the loss of target recognition [27–29]. First, binding affinity to target and nontarget tissue might be affected during the immunoconjugation step, because the amino acids or peptides involved in the recognition of the antigen can be occupied by the BFC [11]. Amino acids with side chains amenable to modifications are found in all regions of Abs. Therefore, modification methods are not site-specific and there is no control over which amino acids are modified.

First, immunoconjugates with modifications in the binding structures result in decreased efficacy of the targeting system [30–32]. Second, the sensitivity of Abs to heating and extreme pH values during the labeling process. The labeling reaction with DOTA and its analogues is very slow and largely depends on the conditions at which it is performed, which includes DOTA-mAb concentration, reaction temperature, time, pH, buffer used and its concentration, and the presence of metal ions such as Zn^{2+} and Fe^{3+}. In order to achieve a good radiolabeling yield it is necessary to increase the temperature (>50 °C). The released energy from the radiometal might induce radiolysis and degradation of the protein, and thus loss of the specificity of the mAb to reach the target. The formed free radicals during the labeling can be attenuated with the addition of quenching reagents like HSA, gentisic acid, ascorbic acid, and others antiradicals [15].

Girentuximab (cG250) is a chimeric mAb reactive to the protein carbonic anhydrase IX (CAIX), a transmembrane glycoprotein with an intracellular enzymatic domain, which is overexpressed in hypoxic cells [33–35]. This antigen CAIX is also expressed on a variety of other solid tumors, including cervical, bladder, colon, and non-small cell lung cancer. Immunohistochemical (IHC) analysis of renal tumors showed homogeneous expression of CAIX in the vast majority (>80%) of primary renal cell carcinomas (RCCs) and about 70% of metastatic RCC lesions [36–39]. In most of the RCCs constitutive CAIX expression is common due to the presence of von Hippel Lindau mutation leading to a hypoxia inducible factor 1 alpha (HIF-1a), without expression in normal kidney tissue [34,36,38–42]. Therefore, CAIX is a promising target for renal cancer and other hypoxic tumors. A clinical trial failed to show a benefit of native cG250 in adjuvant treatment after surgery on the RCCs [43]. However, the patient collective showed a better overall prognosis than expected, which points to a lack of tumor cells that were available for targeting. Safety and tolerability of the antibody was demonstrated. Clinical and preclinical attempts have been made to use cG250 as carrier molecules for radioisotopes [44,45]. Therefore, there are many ongoing experiments in the therapeutic area. The first clinical trial for therapy was carried out with [^{131}I]-girentuximab but the results were not as positive as expected. The widely used beta emitting isotope ^{177}Lu ($t_{1/2}$ = 6.7 days, 497 keV end-point energy) has also been investigated in preclinical and clinical studies treating metastasized RCCs [2,46–48].

Here, a detailed evaluation of the parameters affecting conjugation of S-2-(4-isothiocyanatobenzyl)-1,4,7,10-tetraazacyclododecane tetraacetic acid (p-SCN-Bn-DOTA) to girentuximab by the isothiocyanate group was conducted [49]. In order to characterize the conjugated cG250 the modification sites and the number of BFC modifications per mAb were determined by mass spectrometry. The loss of immunoreactivity post conjugation was evaluated in cells and tumor tissues. DOTA(SCN)-girentuximab conjugates with different BFC/mAb ratios were labeled with ^{177}Lu and the influence of sodium ascorbate on the radiostability was studied. A comparison between the one-step labeling method and the two-step labeling method was another variable to consider, in regards to the preparation of the radioconstructs. In addition, the dependence of the in vitro binding of the radioconjugates, in vivo pharmacokinetics, tumor uptake on the mAb protein dose, and the heterogeneity of CAIX expression was studied in xenograft mice.

2. Results

2.1. Conjugation of p-SCN-βn-DOTA to cG250

DOTA(SCN)-cG250 immunoconjugates with a range of BFC/mAb loading ratios were prepared and purified by modulating the duration of the bioconjugation reaction times between 30 and 90 min. Immunoconjugates were classified by their molecular weight (MW) after conjugation with DOTA(SCN): C2 (90 min reaction time) > C3 (60 min reaction time) > C7 (30 min reaction time) detectable by size exclusion-high performance liquid chromatography (SE-HPLC/UV) and sodium dodecyl sulfate polyacrylamide gel electrophoresis (SDS-PAGE) (Figure 1). For example, conjugate C2 obtained after 90 min of incubation time showed a retention time of 12.24 min compared to 15.1 min for the native mAb; a shift of 3 min on the SE chromatograms. Likewise, conjugates C3 (12.72 min elution time) and C7 (13.66 min elution time) were incubated for 60 and 30 min, respectively, which correlated with the expected increment of the MW of the conjugates after the protein conjugation with the BFC was indicated by the left shifting of the peak on the SE-HPLC chromatogram, compared to the native cG250 (Figure 1a). The completeness of the protein purification by filtration–centrifugation in the conjugates was corroborated by monitoring the signal intensity within the 30 min region on the SE-HPLC chromatogram, which corresponded to the elution time of the free BFC. The complete removal of BFC in the purified conjugate is a critical parameter to ensure high radiochemical purity.

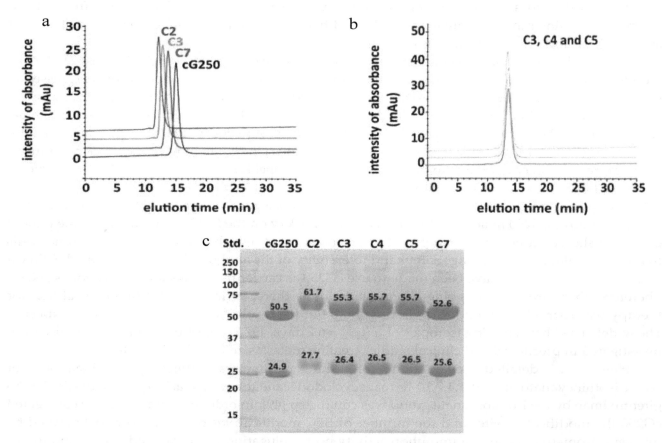

Figure 1. Conjugation of cG250 with DOTA via benzylthiocyano group: **(a)** Size exclusion-high performance liquid chromatography (SE-HPLC) chromatograms of different selected DOTA(SCN)-cG250 conjugates compared to the native cG250; **(b)** size exclusion-high performance liquid chromatography/ultraviolet (SE-HPLC/UV) chromatograms of DOTA(SCN)-cG250 conjugates prepared from the same batch; and **(c)** SDS-PAGE chromatograms of cG250-conjugates in reduced conditions.

As expected for a denaturing analytical technique, SDS-PAGE chromatogram of the DOTA(SCN)-cG250 conjugates C2, C3, C4, C5, and C7 showed easily distinguishable bands corresponding to the light (LC) and heavy chain (HC) of the Abs. The conjugated protein bands of the LC and HC were, as expected, broader and shifted to higher molecular weights, when compared to the LC and HC bands of the native mAb (Figure 1c). Using a standard (Precision Plus™ Protein Unstained, 10–25 kDa, BioRad) the MW of the HC and LC bands of cG250 could be estimated. The results correspond to the same order of MW (C2 (90 min) > C3 (60 min) > C7 (30 min)) obtained by SEC chromatography.

For large-scale clinical production of immunoconjugates the reproducibility of the conjugation process is relevant. Consistency of the conjugation process was explored by undertaking the conjugation process in triplicate. Three conjugates (C3, C4, and C5) were prepared and purified by using a 60 min incubation time. The retention times of conjugates C3, C4, and C5 by SE-HPLC were similar, and the retention times of the conjugates varied by 12.64 ± 0.08% with less than 7% uncertainty

(Figure 1b). In the case of the SDS-PAGE, the reproducibility obtained was less than 1% of uncertainty of the MW of the HC and LC (Figure 1c). Based on the SE-HPLC and SDS-PAGE results, the conjugates C3, C4, and C5 could be classified within the same group. The ratio of DOTA molecules per molecule of mAb, was calculated by the difference of the MW between the conjugated and the native mAb. The average ratio ranged from 1 to 6 in LC and from 4 to 23 in the HC based on the information from the SDS-PAGE chromatograms; using an uncertainty of 10% of the MW estimation by SDS-PAGE (Supplementary Table S1). Another important aspect that might influence the accuracy of the MW determination by SDS-PAGE is the preservation of the separation conditions. Different conditions such as the gel concentration and voltage during the protein separation would influence the migration of proteins in the tested sample, when compared to the standard sample, changing the standard mass calibration procedure as a consequence. In order to measure the MW with better accuracy, another analytical tool like mass spectrometry is required.

For SE-HPLC/UV, the stability of the conjugates was evaluated based on the shift between the retention times of the conjugates compared to the native mAb. This way, the variability of the retention time measurements at different days was excluded. These variations of retention time signals were observed due to the interactions of the stationary phase with the mobile phase (eluent or sample) components. After 24 months the difference between the retention times of the conjugates and the native monoclonal antibody were 2.91 ± 0.03, 2.51 ± 0.01, and 1.48 ± 0.03 for conjugates C2, C3, and C7, respectively. The intensity of the peak was the same using 0.05 mg/mL as protein concentration. The chromatogram of the conjugates showed no significant changes to peak positions or bands in SE-HPLC chromatograms or SDS-PAGE, respectively.

2.2. Identification of DOTA Modification Sites

The conjugates were analyzed through peptide-mass mapping using tandem liquid chromatography–mass spectrometry (LC–MS/MS). The modification sites by DOTA, were identified by comparing the peptide-mass mapping of the conjugates with the data base of peptide masses of the native cG250 after the digestion processes were completed with trypsin. The native cG250 sequence coverage LC–MS/MS was 96% and 88% for LC and HC, respectively. The data obtained was used as a control to identify the modified peptides in the conjugated protein and to calculate the occupancy by DOTA molecules on the amino acid sequence. The peptide mapping of the DOTA(SCN)-cG250 conjugates resulted in sequence coverages from 71% to 87% for HC and from 73% to 95% for LC, respectively. The lower coverage values were obtained in the conjugates with higher ratio DOTA(SCN) per molecule of mAb ratios. The higher the BFC/cG250 ratios led to a higher heterogeneity of the conjugated peptides, which resulted in decreased digestion efficiency of trypsin due to blocked trypsin cleavage sites, resulting in longer peptide sequences and consequently reduced extraction efficiency from the gel matrix. In order to increase the peptide sequence coverage, a second digestion process with chymotrypsin was performed for the conjugate C2. The combined data of two different digests resulted in almost 100% sequence coverage of both mAb subunits, HC (98.4%) and LC (98.6%). The combination of trypsin and chymotrypsin digests successfully increased the sequence coverage of the conjugates to 97.6% for the HC, and 92.5% for the LC. Short peptides could not be identified, which was due to chromatographic and data analysis/processing limitations.

Figure 2 shows that the DOTA(SCN)-modified peptides sites were, as expected, mostly through lysine amino acid residues (K and Lys), as previously described [25]. Also, DOTA modifications were not consistently allocated to the same K residues across all replicates on the HC and LC as shown by Figure 2a. The occupancy of K residues with DOTA(SCN) modification was calculated by MaxQuant, using peptide intensities and search parameter settings as previously for EasyProt. DOTA conjugated peptides were eluted at different retention times from the reversed phase chromatography column and detected with higher charge states than the nonconjugated peptides, as expected. DOTA(SCN)-labeled peptides eluted at different retention times from the reversed phase column than the native peptides, due to different matrix effects at the time of elution and possibly different ionization efficacies of native and conjugated peptide forms. The latter is supported by the observation that DOTA-labeled peptides were usually detected with a higher charge state than the nonlabeled peptides. We assumed that higher ratios represent a better accessibility of DOTA to the corresponding K residue.

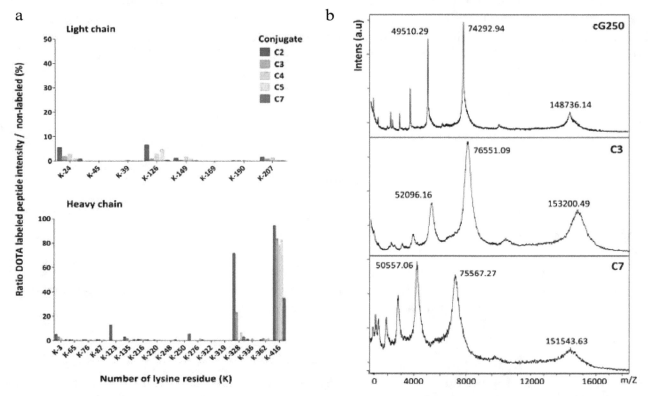

Figure 2. Characterization of the DOTA(SCN)-cG250 conjugates by mass spectrometry: (**a**) Lysine occupancy in the LC (top) and HC of DOTA(SCN)-cG250 post trypsin in-gel digestion of the proteins (n = 3) in conjugate C2 (90 min), C3, C4, C5 (60 min), and C7 (30 min) and (**b**) mass measurements by MALDI-TOF MS of native cG250 and conjugates C3 and C7.

K-416 of the HC appears to be almost quantitatively labeled, meaning that the probability of the conjugation of the K-416 is higher compared to the other K residues. Based on the incomplete sequence coverage achieved by in-gel digestion LC–MS/MS using trypsin enzyme, we also have to assume that there are K residues on peptides modified by DOTA(SCN), which could not be extracted from the gel matrix. Furthermore, DOTA(SCN) labeling renders peptides more hydrophobic, thus making it more difficult to extract them from the gel matrix. Therefore, nonlabeled peptides were extracted more efficiently than labeled ones, leading to an over-representation of the nonlabeled forms. It is well known and has been described that K is the most nucleophilic amine in proteins; however, K-416 has an additional input because it is the C-terminus of the HC of native cG250 [50,51]. The reaction that takes place does not have steric hindrance compared with the other K residues rendering the substitution reaction more efficient. In general, the reactivity of the N-terminal amino group is higher because its pKa value is lower than the K. Thus, DOTA(SCN) modifications were also observed at the amino terminus through aspartic acid amino residues (D, Asp) in the HC and LC.

2.3. Ratio of DOTA Molecules Per Molecule of Antibody

In general, when the average number of BFCs per protein (N) increases the immunoreactivity of the obtained product decreases. It is possible to determine "N" by calculating the difference in mass between the mass of the conjugates and the native mAb [52,53]. The mass of the conjugates was measured by matrix-assisted laser desorption/ionization time-of-flight mass spectrometry (MALDI-TOF MS) (Figure 2b) and the average number of DOTA(SCN) molecules per molecule of cG250 was then calculated. The native cG250 shows the presence of three major peaks corresponding to the MW of 148,736.14 Da (monocharged and unconjugated mAb, $[M+H]^+$), 74,292.94 Da (doubly charged unconjugated mAb, $[M+2H]^{2+}$), and 49,510.29 Da (triply charged unconjugated mAb, $[M+3H]^{3+}$). Furthermore, the MALDI-TOF mass spectra of the DOTA(SCN)-cG250 conjugates also showed three peaks corresponding to the mono, doubly and triply charged conjugates species. Compared to the spectrum of the native cG250 mAb, these spectra show a broadening of the peaks, which indicates heterogeneity in the number and location of DOTA(SCN) molecules conjugated to the Abs, thus confirming the results of the LC–MS analysis. The MW of the peak $[M+H]^+$ (151,543.63 Da) is lower for the conjugate C7 than for conjugate C3, corresponding to the results obtained by SE-HPLC/UV and SDS-PAGE (Figure 1). The MW of the conjugates C4 and C5 were also measured. The uncertainty of the MW by MALDI-TOF was also less than 1% in the three major peaks of conjugates C3, C4, and C5, which were prepared in the same conditions (data not shown). These results show a similar MW and, therefore, similar ranges of BFC/mAb ratios. The average number of DOTA(SCN) molecules per molecule of cG250 calculated for the conjugates are summarized in Table 1. Similar BFC per Ab ratios were obtained, by using the same conjugation method and incubation time but different mAbs [3,49].

Table 1. Average of DOTA(SCN) molecules per molecule of cG250 by mass spectrometry.

Conjugate	MW (Da)	Ratio Non Reduced	Ratio Reduced	
			HC	LC
C2 (90 min)	-	-	12–23 [1]	6–7 [1]
C3 (60 min)	154,187.07	8–10	3–4	1–2
C7 (30 min)	151,543.63	5–6	1–2	1–2

[1] Values obtained by intact mass.

In order to know the number of conjugated molecules of BFC in the HC and LC of the mAb, the native cG250 and conjugates were incubated with dithiothreitol (DTT) (40 mM) for 1 h before injecting the test sample in the MALDI-TOF spectrometer. The mass spectrum of the native cG250 showed peaks which corresponded to LC and HC. The mass spectrum of the reduced conjugate C3 also showed two main peaks at 51,546.27 Da and 24,151.98 Da, which corresponded to the MW of the HC and LC of the conjugated cG250, respectively. Those peaks were also broader compared to the spectrum of the reduced native cG250 (Supplementary Figure S1). The average of DOTA(SCN) moieties was found to be 1–2 and 3–4 in the LC and the HC of conjugate C3, respectively (Table 1). The ratios were obtained per chain and were multiplied by two based on the antibody structure matched well with the ratios obtained for the nonreduced conjugate.

It was not possible to determine the ratio of BFC molecules in the HC and LC of conjugate C2 because it was not possible to measure the MW by MALDI-TOF, presumably due to the high heterogeneity of the conjugate. However, it was possible to determine the ratio of BFC molecules in the LC by intact mass using a QExactive mass spectrometer (ThermoFisher, Bremen, Germany) via a nanospray electrospray ionization (ESI) source. The samples (the native and the conjugated cG250) were treated with DTT to cleave the LC and HC. Very clean signals could be measured for the native LC and HC as well as the conjugated LC, while the conjugated HC spectrum was extremely complex and deconvolution resulted in several signals with an inherent uncertainty of being correct (data not shown). From the LC of conjugate C2, accurate mass determination was possible, however the HC presented challenges. The software was able to extract a few masses in the HC of the conjugate C2, but they were less certain than in all other measurements (95% vs. 99%). Using the obtained MWs of the native and the conjugate divided by the MW of the BFC (552.6 Da), the DOTA(SCN)/cG250 mAb ratio ranged from 5 to 6 in the LC. For the higher intensity MW peaks (50,682.105 Da and 50,519.625 Da) the average number of BFC ranged from 12 to 23 per mAb. Therefore, those results are not reliable because of the intensity of the rest of the peaks (background) on the chromatogram. The range of values corresponded to the ones obtained by SDS-PAGE with the range of the total MW of C2 obtained by MALDI-TOF (Table 1).

2.4. In Vitro Characterization of the Conjugates

Immunoreactivity of the conjugates was evaluated by flow cytometric and IHC analyses before labeling the cG250 with ^{177}Lu. An increasing extent of conjugation of the cG250 with DOTA(SCN) moieties, correlates with a reduction in binding to CAIX on the SK-RC-52 cells compared to the native cG250 by flow cytometry and IHC (Figure 3). Staining of the cell lines with the native variant of cG250 showed that CAIX recognition on SK-RC-52 cell line is 20 times higher than on the SK-RC-18 cell line, which confirms the specificity of the cG250 and the suitability of these two cell lines for the remaining studies. The results were previously validated by immunocytochemistry analysis (ICC), where the SK-RC-52 cell line showed a strong staining intensity and cell membrane localization (Supplementary Figure S2). However, CAIX expression was not detected in the SK-RC-18 cell line by flow cytometry and neither by immunocytochemistry (ICC) (Supplementary Figure S2).

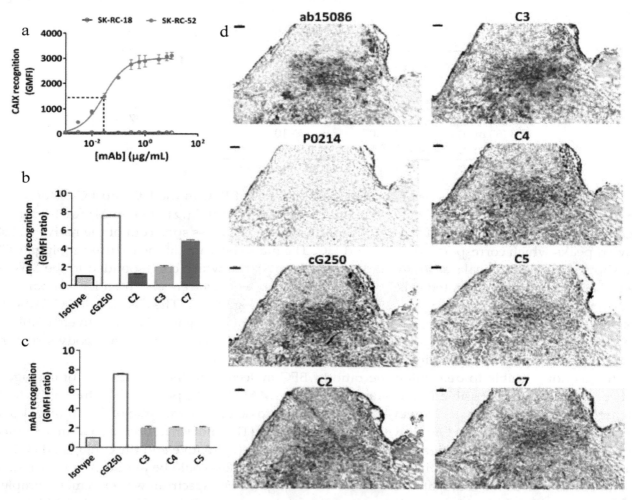

Figure 3. Immunoreactivity of DOTA(SCN)-cG250 conjugates with SK-RC-52 cells in vitro and in tumor tissue. (**a**) Concentration-dependent binding of native cG250 to SK-RC-52 cells and SK-RC-18 (control), as assessed by flow cytometry. The red dashed line corresponds to the IC50. (**b**) Flow cytometric assessment of CAIX recognition on SK-RC-52 cells of immunoconjugates C2 (90 min), C3 (60 min) and C7 (30 min). (**c**) Flow cytometric assessment of CAIX recognition on SK-RC-52 cells of immunoconjugates C3, C4, and C5 (60 min). (**d**) CAIX immunostaining in frozen SK-RC-52 tumor samples using native cG250 mAb and immunoconjugates C2, C3, C4, C5, and C7. CAIX Abcam (ab15086) as a positive control and Dako (P0214) as a negative control. 100 μm scale bar and 10X objective.

Concentration-dependent experiments demonstrated an IC50 of around 0.02 µg/mL for cG250 (Figure 3a), which was used to evaluate the effect of DOTA(SCN) on the mAb recognition in subsequent experiments. At high doses (e.g., 100 µg/mL) of protein, the geometric mean fluorescence intensity (GMFI) values increase until the cG250 saturates all the binding sites. After conjugation of the cG250 with DOTA(SCN), a reduction in the recognition of the CAIX by the conjugates on SK-RC-52 cells compared to the native variant was observed (Figure 3b). The loss of recognition was dependent on the average number of conjugated DOTA(SCN) per molecule of mAb, as C2 contains more than 12–23 DOTA, C3 contains 8–10 DOTA, and C7 contains 3–5 DOTA. In order to explore if whether or not the location of the DOTA modifications had any influence over the loss recognition by the conjugated mAb, three different conjugates (C3, C4, and C5) with the same number of BFCs located in different K residues were compared. As evidenced in Figure 3c, there were no differences ($p > 0.05$) in the recognition between the three conjugates, indicating that their biological activity was directly related to the ratio BFC/mAb rather than the location of the BFC molecules on the K residues. Those conjugates were also analyzed by IHC and no significant difference between them was observed (Figure 3d).

The recognition of the conjugates to CAIX in tumor samples was another variable that was evaluated (Figure 3d). The native cG250 was evaluated showing a staining pattern that nicely reproduced the pattern of the commercial Ab, staining the same histological areas in frozen samples. CAIX staining with the C7 conjugate (conjugated with the lowest level of DOTA) was the most specific antibody without relevant background staining. The conjugate C2 showed a high background and no specific staining, which might be due to the high number of BFCs attached to cG250. In general, all conjugates showed the same staining pattern as the native cG250. The areas that did not express CAIX by the native and conjugated cG250 were comparable and showed the same pattern as the commercial Ab (Abcam), which was used as a positive control.

To evaluate possible recognition and accumulation of the radiolabeled cG250 in subsequent animal studies, the antigen was also measured in healthy tissue which was related to the metabolism and excretion of the large proteins. In the paraffin normal tissue samples, CAIX immunostaining, showed strong intensity in the stomach and negative immunostaining in the rest of the organs (liver, gallbladder, spleen, and duodenum) by Abcam Ab. However, normal tissue frozen samples were negative for cG250 mAb and the control Abs (Supplementary Figure S3).

2.5. Radiochemical Purity and Influence of Sodium Ascorbate on the Stability In Vitro

Radioimmunoconjugates with different specific activities were obtained with >90% of radiochemical purity (RCP) by instant thin layer chromatography (ITLC) before and after the addition of DTPA. A slight excess of DTPA was added to the reaction mixture to complex any free $^{177}Lu^{3+}$ ions, which was monitored on the SE radiochromatogram. After the purification processes by SE, the typical radiochemical yield of [^{177}Lu]DOTA(SCN)-cG250 was 85% with radiochemical purity above 99%. It was possible to reach highest specific activities of 9 MBq/µg with the conjugate C3. In the case of conjugate C7 (less DOTA content), the RCP decreased when the initial activity was increased reaching as much as 5 MBq/µg. The presence of the ionic (free $^{177}Lu^{3+}$) impurities is explained by the low DOTA content in this conjugate compared to the other conjugates. The average number of ^{177}Lu atoms chelated per mAb was 1–2 for the conjugate C3 and 0–1 for the conjugates C7 postpurification. Higher initial activities of ^{177}Lu were used to increase those values of specific activities of the labeled mAb, but they resulted in lower radiochemical yields.

Stability of the radioimmunoconjugates becomes a critical issue for conjugated mAb due to their pharmacokinetics and long circulation times. In vitro stability was studied under different conditions: HSA 20%, human serum (HS) and phosphate-buffered saline (PBS) with and without the addition of sodium ascorbate (NaAsc, 50 mg/mL) postpurification. Figure 4a shows a drop in the RCP of the radioconstruct two days after labeling at 319 MBq/mL activity concentration (specific activity was > 9 MBq/µg), even in the presence of the 50 mg/mL quenching solution. We assume that the protein was damaged to a certain degree, due to the formation of radical ions by radiolysis during the labeling process. Nevertheless, radiostability of [^{177}Lu]DOTA(SCN)-cG250 at lower specific activities (<3 MBq/μg) and activity concentrations (<107 MBq/mL) was increased by the addition of NaAsc (Figure 4a). The RCP was above 90% by ITLC up to 10 d postlabeling in 20% HSA and HS for the three types of conjugates (Figure 4b).

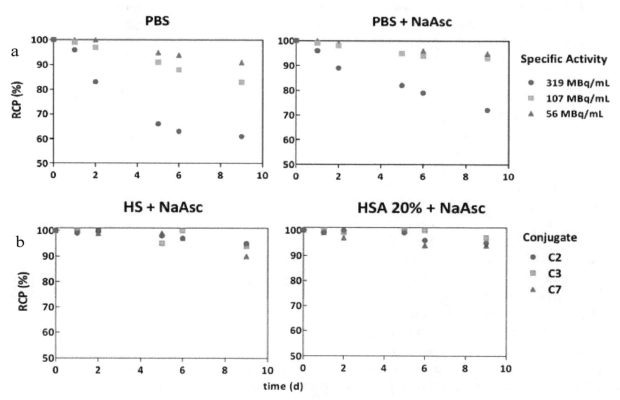

Figure 4. In vitro stability of [^{177}Lu]DOTA(SCN)-cG250 in the presence of NaAsc by TLC: **(a)** C3 radioconstructs at different activity concentrations without and with NaAsc respectively and **(b)** C2, C3, and C7 radioconstructs (2 MBq/μg) in human serum and HSA 20% in the presence of NaAsc.

2.6. In Vitro Radioimmunoreactivity of the Conjugates Labeled with ^{177}Lu

During the radiolabeling process, the biological activity of the protein may be compromised and the specificity of the biomolecule to bind to CAIX antigen may therefore be reduced. Therefore, the immunoreactivity of the radioconstructs was evaluated in vitro using the SK-RC-52 cells before in the in vivo application. First, the specific binding to SK-RC-52 cells was measured using different protein concentrations and as a result, a maximum of 60% binding was obtained (Figure 5a). After adding 5 ng of carrier antibodies to 5×10^6 cells, a decrease in the percentage of binding was observed due to the saturation of binding sites with the nonlabeled mAb. During the preparation of the radioconstructs it was not possible to separate the labeled-mAb from the nonlabeled-mAb using PD10 columns. Saturation of the binding sites was also observed by flow cytometric analysis (Figure 3a) at high protein doses. In the case of the SK-RC-18 cells (negative control) the percentage of binding and internalization was <2.0% (Figure 5a) as compared to the values for nonspecific binding using the native cG250 at the highest studied protein concentration (data not shown).

Figure 5b shows the percentage of binding and internalization of different conjugates to positive and negative CAIX cell lines (SK-RC-52 and SK-RC-18, respectively). The percentage of binding of [^{177}Lu]DOTA(SCN)-cG250 to SK-RC-52 cells ranged from 60 to 70% for conjugate C7 with a ratio of less than six DOTA(SCN) molecules per cG250. The percentage of binding to the SK-RC-52 cell line was significantly higher ($p < 0.001$) for the radioconstructs using conjugate C7 (lowest DOTA content). The percentage of internalization of the radioconstruct was >90% of the total activity bound to the SK-RC-52 cells (Figure 5b,c). In general, the percentage of binding and internalization decreased with increasing DOTA content showing the same pattern as observed in the flow cytometric analysis (Figure 3b). Figure 5c shows no significant change ($p > 0.05$) in the percentage of binding and internalization after a dilution of the radioconstructs with 20% HSA, human serum, and PBS to simulate in vivo conditions. The percentage of binding and internalization slightly decreased using higher specific activities of the radioconstructs (Figure 5d). Blocking studies with an excess of native cG250 revealed the specificity of the labeled cG250 by reducing binding and internalization to background levels. In all cases, the SK-RC-18 cells were used as a negative control to correct the percentage of binding and internalization as a nonspecific binding.

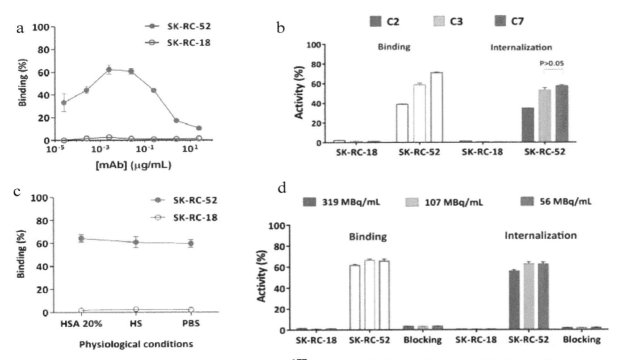

Figure 5. Radioimmunoactivity in vitro of [^{177}Lu]DOTA(SCN)-cG250 to SK-RC-52 cells ($n = 3$). (**a**) Concentration-dependent binding of [^{177}Lu]DOTA(SCN)-cG250 using the conjugate C3 (60 min). (**b**) Recognition of radioconstructs from conjugates C2 (90 min), C3 (60 min) and C7 (30 min) to SK-RC-52 cells by radioimmunoassay at 2 MBq/µg specific activity. (**c**) Radioimmunoactivity in HSA 20%, HS and PBS at 2 MBq/µg specific activity using the conjugate C3. (**d**) Radioimmunoactivity of [^{177}Lu]DOTA(SCN)-cG250 at different activity concentrations using the conjugate C3. Blocking studies were performed with 50 µg of native cG250.

2.7. Biodistribution

The biodistribution of [^{177}Lu]DOTA(SCN)-cG250 which was measured 48 h after the I.V. application of 12 MBq in BALB/c nu/nu mice across a range of Ab protein mass doses (specific activities) shows a moderate influence by the total applied protein dose (Figure 6). In vivo, blood retention increased with higher protein doses (i.e., lower specific activity) and liver uptake slightly declined with protein doses up to 60 µg/animal. In contrast, tumor accumulation was not significantly influenced ($p > 0.05$) by total protein doses between 5 and 100 µg per animal. Correspondingly, at higher protein doses blood circulation seemed prolonged and tumor uptake was highest at a relatively high amount of cG250 (30 µg) per animal (Figure 6a). In addition, a higher amount of radioactivity remained in the rest of the animal body (skin, blood, muscles, and bones) for animals with higher administered protein doses and the excretion process was low (Figure 6b). Longer circulation and the remaining activity in the rest of the animal may be correlated to the saturation of the binding sites in the target, which was observed during the blocking studies. A reduction of tumor uptake at 24 h ($p < 0.05$) was observed in the animals with a previous injection of 500 µg of native cG250 (Figure S4). The native mAb was injected shortly before the radioconjugate and CAIX receptors where partially blocked. However, a major impact by the blocking in spleen and liver was not observed.

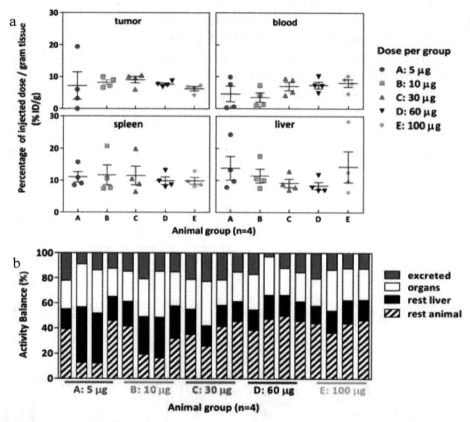

Figure 6. Biodistribution of [^{177}Lu]DOTA(SCN)-cG250 from conjugate C7 at 48 h using total protein dose adjusted between 5 and 100 µg and 12 MBq per animal ($n = 4$). (**a**) Organs: tumor, blood, spleen and liver. (**b**) Activity balance.

Tumor volume had more influence on tumor uptake when low protein doses were used (Figure 7). Interestingly, for one animal bearing a small tumor (140 µg), a positive out layer was observed in the group receiving the lowest protein dose. In case of higher doses, the %ID/g was similar across mass doses and was independent of the tumor size (Figure 7). The effect of the tumor weight on tumor retention has been studied in previous work, where an exponential decline of tumor uptake of ^{111}In-DTPA-girentuximab was demonstrated [54].

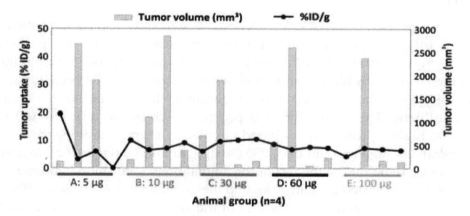

Figure 7. Relationship between tumor uptake and tumor volume per animal of the biodistribution of [^{177}Lu]DOTA(SCN)-cG250 from conjugate C7 at 48 h using total protein dose adjusted between 5 and 100 µg and 12 MBq per animal ($n = 4$).

The relationship of blood circulation values with the protein amount was also observed in the biodistribution of [177Lu]DOTA(SCN)-cG250 measured 24 h and 96 h after the I.V. application of 2 MBq (0.5 μg) and 18 MBq (5 μg) without adjusted doses (Figure 8). The animals with a 5 μg protein dose showed a slower blood clearance until 24 h. The T/B ratio of 43.25 at 96 h was almost four times higher than the ratio at 24 h in the animals with a 5 μg protein dose. Therefore, tumor uptake was higher in the animal group with lower liver uptake. The decreased %ID/g in the liver with an increased protein dose was observed independently regardless of if the protein dose was adjusted (Figures 6 and 8) [33,55].

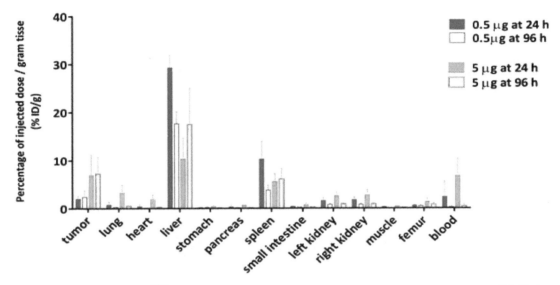

Figure 8. Biodistribution of [177Lu]DOTA(SCN)-cG250 from conjugate C7 using a 0.5 μg (2 MBq) and a 5 μg (18 MBq) protein dose per animal ($n = 4$).

In order to determine the availability of the radioconstruct in blood and in vivo stability, a metabolism analysis was performed by protein precipitation (data not shown). The percentage of the activity was >50% in plasma showing a low complexation with blood cells. Another important parameter is the percentage of free 177Lu activity in blood plasma relative to the intact labeled radioconstruct. The percentage of free 177Lu was <5% at 24 h and increased to 10% at 96 h from the release of the radiometal. Indeed, the tumor/blood (T/B) ratio increased at 96 h (0.5 μg) to 10.16 (Figure 8a) when the specific activity was <3 MBq/μg. This could indicate the importance of the radiostability of the radioconstructs in vivo. Therefore, tumor uptake was low but in line with the values obtained by Muselaers, C. H. (escalating doses of 111In-DTPA-G250) comparing the lower protein dose (<5 μg) [56].

2.8. Effect of Tumor Volume, Hypoxia, and Necrosis on cG250 Tumor Retention

The accumulation of the radioactivity in the tumor is also related to the properties of the target such as the location, size, antigen expression, and others. To study the target influence in the radiopharmaceutical uptake and diffusion, tumor properties such as CAIX expression and the vascularity were studied in different-sized tumors. IHC analysis of SK-RC-52 tumors ($n = 20$) showed a CAIX expression depending on the tumor size and tumor growth. In general, it resulted in decreased availability of the antigen when the tumor volume was increased. Tumors smaller than 20 mm^3 (Figure 9a) and tumors larger than 200 mm^3 (Figure 9c,d) usually developed necrosis after 6 weeks of tumor growth. The extent of necrosis consequently reduces the expression of CAIX. Large tumors (544 mm^3) showed 80% necrosis (as observed by H&E stain) (Figure 9c). However, tumor volumes smaller (161 mm^3) showed mostly homogeneous patterns and a strong intensity of CAIX localized in cell membranes of the SK-RC-52 tumors and no necrosis (Figure 9b).

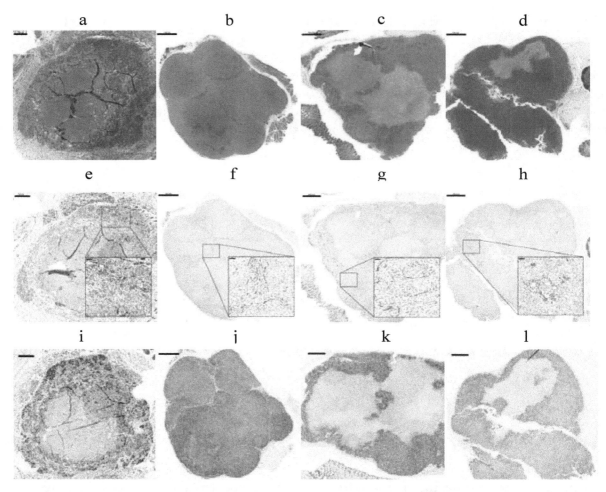

Figure 9. Evaluation of vascular density and hypoxia in FFPE from four different SK-RC-52 tumors: (**a–d**) (H&E) staining; (**e–h**) CD31 immunostaining; and (**i–l**) HIF1α staining. (**a**) 200 μm scale bar, 5x objective. (**b–d**) 1000 μm scale bar, 1.5x objective; (inset) 50 μm scale bar, 20x objective.

The vascular density was determined by CD31 (a marker of endothelial cells) (Figure 9e–h). Additionally, CD31 staining showed an average percentage of vascular density of 2.5 ± 0.5% in the tumors, which was also independent of the tumor size and the CAIX expression. Results are in line with the values obtained by Oosterwijk-Wakka, J.C. in 2015 [57]. Hypoxia-inducible factor 1 (HIF-1) marker, which is a key mediator of tumor survival and adaptation to a hypoxic environment, was evaluated by IHC [58]. IHC analysis of the SK-RC-52 tumors with different size showed the presence of HIF1α in all nuclei from tumor cells (Figure 9i–l) but also reflects necrosis and a high heterogeneity of CAIX expression across the tumor. These effects have a direct influence on the targeting of the mAb and resulting radiation dose accumulation to the tumor [59].

3. Discussion

In the present study we evaluated some variables that might affect the immunoreactivity of the cG250 during the conjugation and radiolabeling processes in comparison with the initial properties of the native cG250. DOTA isothiocyanate modifications occurred via K residues with the formation of a stable and strong thiourea bond (SC(NH$_2$)$_2$). The precision of the isothiocyanate conjugation to mAbs via lysine residues allows for higher selectivity and control compared to the iodination reaction. Higher levels of modification can still lead to impaired binding, and, therefore, loss of efficacy. However, the extent of Ab modifications via BFC/mAb ratio can be controlled during the bioconjugation reaction. The absence of DOTA(SCN) labeling in the CDR is an additional advantage of the labeling of mAb with radiometals compared to previous studies with [131]I [55]. The radioiodination of cG250 using the standard method Chloramine–T is performed through tyrosine amino residues (Y, Tyr), which are part of the complementarity determining regions (CDRs) of the cG250. In in vivo studies the bond ^{131}I-Y amino residues might be affected due to the action mechanism of the mAb during the internalization process into the cancer cells [60]. The use of the radiometals is a tool more suitable for RIT of RCC [2]. However, the occupancy of the K in the neighborhood of the CDRs can compromise the biological activity of conjugates and limit the effectiveness of the therapy. The higher the number of DOTA(SCN) attached to K residues in the mAb sequence, the more heterogeneity the conjugate has and the more difficult it is to characterize. For example, conjugate C2 (90 min) was impossible to measure the MW and calculate then the BFC/mAb ratio by mass spectrometry.

The effectiveness of RIT depends on a number of factors and processes. Some factors relate to the specificity, affinity, and immunoreactivity of the mAb postconjugation and post-radiolabeling. The in vitro evaluation of the immunoreactivity of the conjugates showed that the conjugates with the lowest DOTA content have a better recognition of the CAIX compared to conjugates with higher DOTA content using the native cG250 as a reference. Meanwhile, conjugates with the same BFC/mAb ratio showed similar percentage of binding to the CAIX antigen in SK-RC-52 cells and tumor samples, which was observed by flow cytometry and immunohistochemistry. The immunoreactivity of the DOTA(SCN)-cG250 conjugates seemed mainly determined by the average number of the BFC attached to the mAb. Also, the introduction of multiple BFC modifications might enhance blood clearance and thus the deterioration of pharmacokinetic properties occurred [29]. Another critical point for the use of radiolabeled mAbs is stability and immunoreactivity after the labeling or chelation with the radiometal. The radiochemical yield of DOTA(SCN) conjugates at room temperature in general, is very low; but offers advantages over heating most importantly, such as the preservation of the protein. To complete the radiolabeling (RCP > 90%) without loss of immunoreactivity of the radiolabeled Abs, longer reaction times (90 min) and elevated temperatures (below 42 °C) were used. We were able to label DOTA(SCN)-cG250 conjugates with ^{177}Lu obtaining RCP > 95% for each conjugate (different BFC/mAb ratios). Compared to a two-step method the ratio of ^{177}Lu to mAb was orders of magnitude higher. As the effectiveness of the RIT also depends on the accumulation of radioactivity at the tumor site, the specific activity of the radioconstruct might play a determining role in accessible tumor sites such as circulating tumor cells and tumor cell clusters. With prevention of radiolysis it was possible to keep the stability in vitro in physiological conditions for specific activities < 3 MBq/µg (<107 MBq/mL) by adding sodium ascorbate to the formulation after labeling. In general, the immunoreactivity of the radiolabeled cG250 to the specific binding of SK-RC-52 cells decreased when the DOTA content per conjugates was high. The internalization and accumulation of the radionuclide into the target is an important parameter in RIT [24], and does not seem significantly influenced by the increment of DOTA modifications. However, the percentage of internalization to the SK-RC-52 cells was not significantly different ($p > 0.05$) between conjugate C3 (8–10 BFCs/mAb ratio) and conjugate C7 (5–6 BFCs/mAb ratio).

The biodistribution of [^{177}Lu]DOTA(SCN)-cG250 in Balb/c nu/nu mice with subcutaneous SK-RC-52 showed more than 20% ID/g in the liver and less than 10% ID/g in the tumor, independent of the protein dose which ranged from 5 to 100 µg. Both lower as well as higher tumor uptakes were observed when increasing the protein dose. The blood clearance appeared generally slightly faster with lower amounts of protein. Typically, the therapeutic index between the tumor effect and systemic toxicity is determined by accumulation and retention within tumor tissue on one side and blood circulation on the other. Due to the possibility of slow accumulation and further internalization into the tumor tissue, long blood circulation might enhance both tumor accumulation and systemic toxicity. Thus, a complex in vivo interaction between pharmacokinetic (PK) properties of the radioconstruct and tissue properties of the tumor exist. For smaller molecules like ^{99m}Tc-(HE)3-ZCAIX:1 the influence on PK on tumor uptake is generally less pronounced [61]. At very low protein amounts (0.5 µg girentuximab/animal) rapid clearing from blood was observed, which results in a shorter time of availability of the radioimmunoconjugate for internalization into the tumors and correspondingly very low tumor uptake. At high mAb doses oversaturation of binding sites occurs and tumor uptake is obviously maximized mainly by the possibility of long diffusion into the tumor and by resaturation of recycled antigens after internalization. Although higher specific activities are very feasible, the lowest amount of cG250 showing acceptable PK was 5 to 30 µg/animal. This resulted in typical tumor accumulation of 10% ID/g in tumors with higher uptake in small and homogenous tumors. This compares well to tumor uptake of F(ab')2 fragments in head and neck squamous cell carcinomas (HNSCC) xenografts of 1 to 4% ID/g [45]. Nevertheless, tumor accumulation is highly influenced by the heterogeneity of tumor microstructure. However, at much lower protein doses, the PK might be an obstacle when the radiolabeled Ab is rapidly cleared from the blood and distributed to organs like the liver and spleen. Thus, PK of [^{177}Lu]DOTA(SCN)-cG250 (3 MBq/µg) was influenced by the applied total protein dose, whereby at low amounts of mAb rapid clearance from blood by to liver and spleen occurred.

For disseminated small tumors, including single cancer cells, diffusion is less important than saturation of antigens. This is particularly true for systemic disease-spreads where tumor cells and tumor cell clusters are distributed through the body. Here, a high ratio between radioactivity and the amount of protein carrier mAbs might be beneficial. When binding occurs in relation to the circulation time, it is plausible to measure a relationship between tumor accumulation and tumor size. However, if oversaturation occurs, such a relationship declines when binding sites stay saturated over the blood clearance time. Subsequently, the expected inverse relationship between tumor size and tumor uptake was not observed at protein doses of 60 and 100 µg per mouse. This indicates that protein amounts above 60 µg will not be optimal for binding, in particular, for small tumors and single cells. To target subclinical tumor manifestations—either single cells or small tumor cell clusters—replacement of a beta emitting isotope by long lived alpha emitting isotopes might be promising [4,5,62,63]. Furthermore, the effect of longer blood circulation with a higher protein amount is evident with a higher inverse relationship between the tumor size and tumor targeting for animals receiving 5 µg, over animals receiving only 0.5 µg cG250 without adjusting for specific activity. Therefore, future development of targeting smaller tumor clusters without the observed tendency to necrosis and heterogeneity might include alpha emitting isotopes like Actinium-225.

Other factors related to the target or antigen such as density, location, and heterogeneity of expression of tumor-associated antigen within tumors will affect the therapeutic efficacy of RIT, as will physiological factors such as the tumor vascularity, blood flow, and permeability [10,59]. Consistent with decreased vessel density, elevated intratumoral pressure, and the presence of necrotic areas, large tumors only display a very low uptake. A minimum value of tumor–antigen density is a prerequisite for mAb/ADC efficacy [11]. In view of tumor properties influencing radiopharmaceutical uptake and diffusion, great heterogeneity with regards to the occurrence of necrosis and expression of CAIX was detected. Those properties were studied in different sized-tumors and resulted in decreased availability of the antigen when the tumor volume was large. In addition, the poor vascularization could influence the reachability of the target and thus the tumor uptake.

We show that, the transportation of therapeutic activities to the tumor tissue by cG250 was influenced by several factors. Thus, an optimization of the radiolabeling and BFC/mAb ratio along with an optimized protein dose is important to be able to preferentially target small and homogeneous CAIX expressing tumors. An inverse relationship between the tumor volume and tumor uptake was found. Tumors smaller than 20 mm^3 and larger than 200 mm^3 mostly developed necrosis after six weeks of tumor growth. In addition, after four weeks of tumor growth variation in the tumor volume increased because the growth of the tumor size among the animals was very different. This resulted in dispersed %ID/g values in the animal experiments and resulted in the interpretation of the results being difficult. Heterogeneous expression of the CAIX antigen and necrosis resulted in lower tumor uptake. In particular, large tumor sizes are not ideal targets. However, investigations targeting small tumor cell clusters are typically not directly possible, due to the difficulties of detection within the organism. Therefore, we conclude that specific activities of 2–10 MBq/ug and antibody amounts of 5–30 µg per mouse are optimal to investigate [^{177}Lu]cG250-mediated therapies regarding differently accessible target cells and to optimize repeated application schemes.

4. Materials and Methods

4.1. Preparation of cG250 Conjugates

cG250 was provided by the company Wilex (Munich, Germany). Isothiocyanate-benzyl-DOTA (p-SCN-βn-DOTA) was purchased from Macrocyclics (Dallas, TX). cG250 (5 mg) was mixed with p-SCN-Bn-DOTA (2.5 mg) in 50 µL of sodium bicarbonate buffer (1 M NaHCO$_3$) following the previously described protocol [49]. The mixture was incubated at 37 °C for 30, 60, and 90 min using a thermomixer to obtain conjugates with different BFC molar ratios per molecule of mAb. The mixture was purified by filtration–centrifugation using a Millipore centrifugal device YM-10 (10,000 MW cut off, Millipore). The sample was centrifuged (4000 g × 5 min) at 4 °C to remove the unreacted BFC and buffer exchange the conjugation into a saline solution (NaCl 0.9%) using five volumes of NaCl 0.9%. Postpurification, the samples were transferred to Eppendorf vials (2 mL) previously weighted and labeled C2 (90 min), C3–C5 (60 min), and C7 (30 min). The concentration of the conjugates were determined by ultraviolet spectroscopy (UV) using 1.4 mL/mg/cm as extinction coefficient (Nanovue-GE Healthcare Life Sciences).

The purified fraction was analyzed by SE-HPLC/UV using a G3000 column (7.5 × 300 mm, 10 µm, Waters). The samples were prepared in triplicate for each of the conjugates (0.05 µg/mL) and measured at 280 nm with a flow rate of 0.5 mL/L of 0.9% NaCl (Dionex, P680 HPLC pump, UVD1704 detector). The spectra were evaluated by the software Chromeleon from Dionex (Chromeleon 6.8 SR13 Build 3967 Version). The native cG250 was used as a reference in all cases. The elution time of the peaks of the conjugate were compared with the native cG250.

The conjugates were also analyzed by electrophoresis SDS-PAGE using 10% gel. The native cG250 and conjugated samples were incubated with a sample buffer (0.125 M Tris-HCl pH 6.8, 4% (w/v) SDS, 10% (v/v) glycerol, 0.01% bromophenol blue, 40 mM DTT) and heated at 95 °C for 5 min following the protocol by Laemmli [64]. The electrophoresis was run at a constant voltage of 100 mV (Hoefer SE250 Mini-Vertical gel Electrophoresis unit, USA). The visualization of the light chain (LC) and heavy chain (HC) bands were performed by Coomassie blue G-250 al 0.05% (Merck) blue-stained [65] and analyzed with ChemiDoc XL Imager (Bio Rad) by Image Lab Software 5.2.1 (Bio Rad). Precision Plus™ Protein Unstained (10–25 kDa, BioRad) was used as a MW marker.

4.2. Characterization by Mass Spectrometry

Prior to the mass spectrometric identification by LC–MS/MS, HC, and LC bands were excised and in-gel digested to generate the peptides as previously described [66]. Extracted peptides were loaded onto a precolumn (PepMap C18, 5 µm, 300 A, 300 µm × 15 mm length) at a flow rate of 20 µL/min with solvent A (0.1% formic acid in water/acetonitrile 98:2) with an Ultimate-3000 (ThermoFisher, Reinach, Switzerland), thereafter eluted in back flush mode onto the analytical nanocolumn (C18, 5 µm, 300A, 0.075 mm i.d., × 150 mm length) using an acetonitrile gradient of 5 to 40% of solvent B (0.1% formic acid in water/acetonitrile 4.9:95) in 40 min at a flow rate of 400 nL/min. The column effluent was directly coupled to a Fusion LUMOS mass spectrometer (ThermoFischer, Bremen; Germany) via a nanospray ESI source. Data was acquired in data-dependent mode with precursor ion scans recorded in the Orbitrap at a resolution of 120,000 (at $m/z = 250$), which is parallel to the top speed of the fragment spectra of the most intense precursor ions in the linear trap, for a maximum cycle time of 3 s. Peptides were fragmented in parallel by high-energy collision and electron transfer.

The fragment spectra acquired by LC–MS/MS were converted to a mascot generic file format (mgf) by ProteomeDiscoverer 2.0 (ThermoFisher Scientific) and interpreted with Easyprot (version 2.3) searching against the SwissProt human protein sequence database (version 2014_01) including the sequence of native cG250 using fixed modification of carbamidomethylation on cysteine

(Cys, C), variable modifications of oxidation on methionine (Met, M), deamidation on glutamine (Gln, Q)/asparagine(Asn, N), and DOTA on K residues and on protein N-Terminus, respectively. A forward + reversed sequence database search was used to estimate the false discovery rate. Parent and fragment mass tolerances were set to 10 ppm and 0.4 Da, respectively. Protein identifications were only accepted, when two unique peptides fulfilling the 1% false discovery rate (FDR) criteria were identified. Furthermore, the occupancy of K residues with DOTA modification were calculated by MaxQuant (version 1.5.0.0) using peptide intensities and the search parameter settings as used for EasyProt. Mass spectrometry sequencing data was acquired at the Proteomics and Mass Spectrometry Core Facility, Department for Biomedical Research (DBMR), University of Bern, Switzerland.

The determination of the MW and the average number of BFC groups attached to each mAb molecule was performed by MALDI-TOF-MS. Samples were injected on an Autoflex III Smartbeam instrument (Bruker Daltonics, Bremen, Germany). An analysis was performed in the linear mode with a positive polarity, and a mass range of 200 kDa. Conjugated cG250 solution was diluted (1:10) with saturated α-cyano-4-hydroxycinnamic acid (CHCA, MW 189.04 Da) solution. Data acquisition and processing was performed by flexAnalysis software (Built 75, version 3.3). MALDI-TOF mass spectra data was obtained at the mass spectrometry group, Department of Chemistry and Biochemistry, University of Bern, Switzerland.

4.3. Cell Culture

The human kidney carcinoma cell lines, SK-RC-52 and SK-RC-18, were kindly provided by Dr. Weis-Garcia from Memorial Sloan Kettering Cancer Centre (MSKCC, New York, USA). SK-RC-52 is a CAIX-expressing human RCC cell line derived from mediastinum and SK-RC-18 is derived from lymph node cells, negative for CAIX [39]. The cells were cultured in RPMI medium (Life Technologies) supplemented with 10% fetal calf serum (FCS), 100 IU/ml of penicillin and 100 μg/ mL of streptomycin at 37 °C in a humidified atmosphere with 5% CO_2.

4.4. Flow Cytometric Analysis

The Abs were briefly diluted in 100 μL of fluorescence-activated cell sorting (FACS) buffer (Dulbecco's phosphate buffered saline with 0.2% bovine serum albumin, BSA) in concentrations ranging from 3 ng/mL to 100 μg/mL, or as otherwise indicated. The mAb dilutions were mixed with 10^5 cells and incubated for 60 min at 37 °C. Subsequently, the cells were washed three times with a FACS buffer and incubated with a R-Phycoerythrin AffiniPure F(ab')$_2$ Fragment Goat Anti-Human IgG + IgM (H + L) (Jackson Immunoresearch) for 30 min at 4 °C in the dark. Next, the samples were washed and resuspended in the FACS buffer for analysis. An IgG1 from myeloma (Sigma) was used as an isotype control to define the threshold of the background staining. The analysis was carried out on a FACSVerse (BD Biosciences, San Jose, CA, USA). The data was analyzed by FlowJo (Tree Star, Ashland, OR, USA). The flow cytometry analysis was performed at the Institute of Pharmacology (PKI), University of Bern, Switzerland.

4.5. Radiolabeling, Quality Control, and Radiostability

DOTA(SCN)-cG250 conjugates were labeled with ^{177}Lu (>500 GBq/mg, IDB Holland) in an ammonium acetate buffer, pH 5.5–6.5, at 37 °C for 90 min as described previously [49]. All solutions used for the labeling were prepared with metal-free water and filtered using 0.22 μm filters (Millipore). Conjugates with different specific activities were obtained by labeling 100 μg of protein with ^{177}Lu activities (0.05 M HCl) from 0.1 to 3 GBq. The reaction was stopped after 90 minutes by adding diethylene triamine pentaacetic acid (DTPA, 10 mM) and incubation at 37 °C for another 30 min. The radioconstructs were purified by size exclusion (SE) using a PD 10 column and 1% HSA in PBS. ITLC was performed using a silica gel (SG 1.5 × 10 cm, Varian) as stationary phase and 20 mM of DTPA as a mobile phase (Raytest, MiniGita Firm, ver. 1.10). The chromatograms were evaluated by Gina Star TLC software (ver. 5.0.1 Rel 2). Purified radioconstructs were diluted with human serum,

20% of HSA and PBS in order to simulate in vivo conditions. The stability of the radioconstructs at different specific activities was studied in the presence or absence of sodium ascorbate at 37 °C.

4.6. Radioactivity Binding Assay

The binding assay was performed in triplicate using 200 µL of SK-RC-52 and SK-RC-18 cells. As a control, nonspecific binding was carried out incubating 500 µg of the native cG250 with the SK-RC-52 cell for 5 min before the addition of the radioconstruct. The radiocontructs were diluted in HSA/PBS to 5×10^{-2} µg/mL and 10 µL of the radiolabeled mAb was added to the cells and incubated at 37 °C for 1 h. After incubation, the cell pellets were washed twice with 1% HSA/PBS, centrifuged ($400 \times g$, 5 min) and measured by an automatic gamma counter (WIZARD2, PerkinElmer). The pellets were then treated with a stripping buffer (0.1 M CH_3COOH, 0.15 M NaCl, PBS, pH = 3) to determine the percentage of internalization.

4.7. Animals

3×10^6 SK-RC-52 cells in 100 µL PBS were injected subcutaneously into the right flank of 6–8 week old male BALB/c nu/nu mice (Janvier, le Genest-Saint-Isle, FR). Two different dimensions (length and width) of tumor size were measured at least twice a week with a caliper. The tumor volume was calculated using the equation: $V = (\pi/6)*(\text{higher diameter})*(\text{lower diameter})^2$. All animal experiments were performed in accordance with German law and guidelines for care and use of laboratory animals. The experiments were approved by the competent authority (Landesuntersuchungsamt Rheinland-Pfalz, Germany; according to §8 Abs. 1 Tierschutzgesetz; permission no. 23177-07/G15-1-033).

4.8. Immunohistochemical Analysis (IHC)

Tissue samples of the stomach, liver, gallbladder, spleen, and tumor were collected and divided into two parts. One part of the tissue sample was fixed in a formaldehyde solution at 4% and embedded in paraffin (FFPE). The other remaining tissue sample was embedded in OCT (Tissue-Tek®) and frozen at −80 °C. The samples were transported to the Translational Research Unit (TRU) at the Pathology Institute, University of Bern, Switzerland to perform the immunohistochemical analysis (IHC). The samples were cut to 3 µm thickness and IHC analysis was carried out in the automated system BOND RX (Leica Biosystems, Newcastle, UK). FFPE sections were deparaffinized and rehydrated in a dewax solution (Leica Biosystems) and the antigen was retrieved by heating in a citrate buffer solution (pH = 6.5) at 95 °C for 20 min. Endogenous peroxidase activity was blocked with a H_2O_2 solution for 4 min. Carbonic anhydrase rabbit polyclonal Ab (Abcam, ab15086) was incubated at 1:1500 dilution for 30 min at room temperature. This Ab was used to validate the native and conjugated cG250. Hypoxia-inducible factor 1 (HIF-1) rabbit polyclonal Ab (Genetex, GTX127309) was diluted at 1:1000 and incubated for 30 min to confirm the hypoxia conditions into the tumor. The CD31 rabbit polyclonal Ab, (Abcam, ab28364) was diluted at a 1:30 dilution and incubated for 2 h to detect the endothelial cells from blood vessels to show extent of vascularization of the tumors. The frozen samples were fixed in acetone for 15 min at −20 °C and then air-dried. The samples were incubated with native and conjugated cG250 at a 1:1000 dilution for 30 min and subsequently the secondary rabbit anti-human Ab (Dako, P0214) was used at a 1:400 dilution for 15 min. As a negative control, the same tissue samples were incubated in parallel with only a secondary rabbit anti-human Ab.

All the samples were visualized with the Bond Polymer Refine Kit with 3-3′-Diaminobenzidine-DAB as the chromogen (Leica Biosystems). The samples were then counterstained with hematoxylin and mounted in Aquatex (Merck, Darmstadt, Germany). Finally, all slides were scanned and photographed in a Pannoramic P250 scanner (3DHistech, Hungary). By using ImageJ, the vascular density through CD31 expression was quantified for each tumor sample as a percentage of the CD31-positive microvessel area to the total tumor area (CD31 area/total tumor area) as previously described [67].

4.9. Biodistribution

After 4 to 6 weeks of tumor growth, groups of four mice were injected intravenously (I.V.) via the tail vein with 12 MBq of [^{177}Lu]DOTA(SCN)-cG250 with adjusted protein doses with native cG250 from 5 to 100 μg. The animals were sacrificed at 48 h post injection and the organs were collected. To determine differences in pharmacokinetics and its influence on tumor uptake at very low protein doses (n, groups of four animals were injected with 0.5 μg (2 MBq) and 5 μg (18 MBq) at a fixed specific activity of 3 MBq/μg and biodistribution was determined after 24 h and 96 h. Blood samples were collected, mixed with a 100 μL heparin solution to avoid coagulation, weighed, and the activity measured with a gamma counter. After the addition of 500 μL of PBS, the blood was centrifuged at 7500 rpm for 5 min to separate blood cells and plasma. The plasma fractions were weighed and measured with a gamma counter. Proteins were precipitated by adding 500 μL of acetonitrile and separated by centrifugation at 7500 rpm for 5 min. The supernatants were weighed followed by the determination of the activity with a gamma counter. The percentage of radioactivity in the blood cell was calculated by subtracting the activities of the supernatant from the activity of the whole blood. In all the experiments the percentage of incorporated doses (%ID/g) was calculated by the weight of the organs and the measurements by gamma counter (WIZARD2, PerkinElmer).

4.10. Statistical Analysis

All statistical analyses were performed using the program GraphPad Prism (version 6.0). The one-way ANOVA was used for the comparison between the conjugates by FACS, and radioactivity curves and blocking in vivo experiments. Two-way ANOVA was used to compare the groups at different specific activities and different stability conditions. Differences were considered to be statistically significant at a level of $p < 0.05$. The %ID/g in the biodistribution studies were presented with the average of the same group of animals and their standard deviation.

Supplementary Materials:
Figure S1: Mass measurements by MALDI-TOF MS in reduced conditions (DTT): (a) native cG250; (b) conjugates C3 (60 min); and (c) conjugate C7 (30 min); Figure S2: Validation of the CAIX expression in SK-RC-52 and SK-RC-18 cell lines: (a) Recognition of cG250 by flow cytometry. (b) CAIX immunostaining in FFPE samples using ab15086 (Abcam), 50 μm scale bar and 10× objective. Gastric mucosa was used as positive control, 100 μm scale bar and 10× objective; Figure S3: CAIX immunostaining in normal tissue: (a) FFPE samples using ab15086 (Abcam) and (b) frozen samples using cG250 (Wilex); 200 μm scale bar and 10× objective; Table S1: Average of DOTA(SCN) molecules per molecule of cG250 by SDS-PAGE; Table S2: Abbreviations.

Author Contributions: Conceptualization, T.B., S.P., J.M.B., A.T., and M.M.; Formal analysis, T.B., S.P., J.M.B., A.T., and M.M.; Methodology, N.M., M.H., J.A.G., K.F.B., S.S., and Stephan von Gunten; Supervision, S.P., J.M.B., A.T., and M.M.; Validation, T.B., S.P., J.M.B., N.M., M.H., J.A.G., K.F.B., S.S., S.v.G., and M.M.; Writing–original draft, T.B. and M.M.; Writing–review & editing, S.P., J.M.B., N.M., M.H., J.A.G., K.F.B., S.S., S.v.G., A.T., and M.M.

Acknowledgments: The authors would like to thank to Frances Weis-Garcia (MSKCC) for providing the human kidney carcinoma cell lines—SK-RC-52 and SK-RC-18—and the company Wilex for the girentuximab. Thanks to Michael Wheatcroft from Telix Pharma for his valuable comments and discussion. Also, Stephan Maus, George Otto, Natascha Buchs, Sophie Braga, and Urs Kämpfer for their help and valuable technical assistance.

Abbreviations

Ab	antibody
ADC	antibody drug conjugate
Asn, N	asparagine amino residues
BM	biomolecule
BFC	bifunctional chelator

BSA	bovine serum albumin
CAIX	carbonic anhydrase IX
cG250	monoclonal antibody anti-CAIX, girentuximab
Cys, C	cysteine amino residues
CDR	complementarity-determining regions
CHCA	hydroxycinnamic acid
CD31	cluster of differentiation 31, endotelial cells marker
DOTA	tetraxetan or 1,4,7,10-Tetraazacyclododecane-1,4,7,10-tetraacetic acid
DOTA(SCN)	p-SCN-Bn-DOTA or S-2-(4-Isothiocyanatobenzyl)-1,4,7,10-tetraazacyclododecane tetraacetic acid
DTPA	pentetic acid or diethylenetriaminepentaacetic acid
DTT	dithiothreitol
DCB	Department of Chemistry and Biochemistry, University of Bern, Switzerland
DBMR	Department for Biomedical Research, University of Bern, Switzerland
d	day
EDTA	ethylenediaminetetraacetic acid
ESI	electrospray ionization
FDR	false discovery rate
FFPE	formalin-fixed paraffin-embedded
FACS	fluorescence-activated cell sorting applied in flow cytometry
FCS	fetal calf serum
FT	Fourier transform
Fac	formic acid
Gln, Q	glutamine amino residues
HC	heavy chain of immunoglobulin
HIF-1	hypoxia-inducible factor 1
HSA	human serum albumin
HS	human serum
HNSCC	head and neck squamous cell carcinomas (HNSCC)
h	hour
HPLC	high-performance liquid chromatography
Ig	immunoglobulin
IC50	concentration of an inhibitor where the response (or binding) is reduced by half
IHC	immunohistochemistry
ICC	immunocytochemistry
ITLC	instant thin layer chromatography
ID	injected dose
i.v.	intravenously
LET	linear energy transfer
LC	light chain of immunoglobulin
LC	liquid chromatography
Lys, K	lysine amino residues
LRC	Laboratory of Radiochemistry, Paul Scherrer Institute, Villigen PSI, Switzerland
mAb	monoclonal antibody
MBq	megabecquerel
Met, M	methionine amino residues
MALDI	matrix assisted laser desorption/ionization–mass spectrometry
MS	mass spectrometry
MW	molecular weight or mass
mgf	mascot generic file format
MSKCC	Memorial Sloan Kettering Cancer Centre, New York, USA
min	minute
NaAsc	sodium ascorbate
NaCl	saline solution
NHL	non-Hodgkin's lymphoma

NHS	N-hydroxysuccinimide
OCT	optimum cutting temperature
PKM	pharmacokinetic modifying linker
PK	pharmacokinetics
PET	positron emission tomography
PBS	phosphate buffer saline
ppm	parts per million (chemical shift)
PSI	Paul Scherrer Institute, Villigen PSI, Switzerland
PKI	Institute of Pharmacology, University of Bern, Switzerland
RIT	radioimmunotherapy
RCCs	renal cell carcinomas
RCP	radiochemical purity
Rf	retardation factor
RPMI	Roswell Park Memorial Institute medium
RPM	revolutions per minute
SEC	size exclusion *chromatography*
SDS-PAGE	sodium dodecyl sulfate polyacrylamide gel electrophoresis
SCN	isothiocyanate
SG	silica gel
$t_{1/2}$	half-life
Tyr,Y	tyrosine amino residues
TOF	time of flight
TFA	trifluoroacetic acid
TRU	Translational Research Unit, University of Bern, Switzerland
Tris	hydroxymethylaminomethane
UV	ultraviolet

References

1. Fleuren, E.D.; Versleijen-Jonkers, Y.M.; Heskamp, S.; van Herpen, C.M.; Oyen, W.J.; van der Graaf, W.T.; Boerman, O.C. Theranostic applications of antibodies in oncology. *Mol. Oncol.* **2014**, *8*, 799–812. [CrossRef] [PubMed]

2. Brouwers, A.H.; van Eerd, J.E.; Frielink, C.; Oosterwijk, E.; Oyen, W.J.; Corstens, F.H.; Boerman, O.C. Optimization of radioimmunotherapy of renal cell carcinoma: Labeling of monoclonal antibody cG250 with 131I, 90Y, 177Lu, or 186Re. *J. Nucl. Med.* **2004**, *45*, 327–337. [PubMed]

3. Thakral, P.; Singla, S.; Yadav, M.P.; Vasisht, A.; Sharma, A.; Gupta, S.K.; Bal, C.S.; Malhotra, A. An approach for conjugation of (177) Lu-DOTA-SCN-Rituximab (BioSim) & its evaluation for radioimmunotherapy of relapsed & refractory B-cell non Hodgkins lymphoma patients. *Indian J. Med. Res.* **2014**, *139*, 544–554. [PubMed]

4. Kennel, S.J.; Brechbiel, M.W.; Milenic, D.E.; Schlom, J.; Mirzadeh, S. Actinium-225 conjugates of MAb CC49 and humanized delta CH2CC49. *Cancer Biother. Radiopharm.* **2002**, *17*, 219–231. [CrossRef] [PubMed]

5. Zalutsky, M.R.; Reardon, D.A.; Akabani, G.; Coleman, R.E.; Friedman, A.H.; Friedman, H.S.; McLendon, R.E.; Wong, T.Z.; Bigner, D.D. Clinical experience with alpha-particle emitting 211At: Treatment of recurrent brain tumor patients with 211At-labeled chimeric antitenascin monoclonal antibody 81C6. *J. Nucl. Med.* **2008**, *49*, 30–38. [CrossRef] [PubMed]

6. White, C.A. Rituxan immunotherapy and zevalin radioimmunotherapy in the treatment of non-Hodgkin's lymphoma. *Curr. Pharm. Biotechnol.* **2003**, *4*, 221–238. [CrossRef] [PubMed]

7. Witzig, T.E.; Wiseman, G.A.; Maurer, M.J.; Habermann, T.M.; Micallef, I.N.; Nowakowski, G.S.; Ansell, S.M.; Colgan, J.P.; Inwards, D.J.; Porrata, L.F.; et al. A phase I trial of immunostimulatory CpG 7909 oligodeoxynucleotide and 90 yttrium ibritumomab tiuxetan radioimmunotherapy for relapsed B-cell non-Hodgkin lymphoma. *Am. J. Hematol.* **2013**, *88*, 589–593. [CrossRef] [PubMed]

8. Shadman, M.; Li, H.; Rimsza, L.; Leonard, J.P.; Kaminski, M.S.; Braziel, R.M.; Spier, C.M.; Gopal, A.K.; Maloney, D.G.; Cheson, B.D.; et al. Continued Excellent Outcomes in Previously Untreated Patients With Follicular Lymphoma After Treatment With CHOP Plus Rituximab or CHOP Plus 131I-Tositumomab: Long-Term Follow-Up of Phase III Randomized Study SWOG-S0016. *J. Clin. Oncol.* **2018**, *36*, 697–703. [CrossRef] [PubMed]

9. Ray Banerejee, S.; Kumar, V.; Lisok, A.; Plyku, D.; Novakova, Z.; Wharram, B.; Brummet, M.; Barinka, C.; Hobbs, R.F.; Pomper, M.G. Evaluation of (111)In-DOTA-5D3, a Surrogate SPECT Imaging Agent for Radioimmunotherapy of Prostate-Specific Membrane Antigen. *J. Nucl. Med.* **2018**. [CrossRef] [PubMed]

10. Stillebroer, A.B.; Oosterwijk, E.; Oyen, W.J.; Mulders, P.F.; Boerman, O.C. Radiolabeled antibodies in renal cell carcinoma. *Cancer Imaging* **2007**, *7*, 179–188. [CrossRef] [PubMed]

11. Diamantis, N.; Banerji, U. Antibody-drug conjugates—An emerging class of cancer treatment. *Br. J. Cancer* **2016**, *114*, 362. Available online: https://www.nature.com/articles/bjc2015435#supplementary-information (accessed on 1 October 2018). [CrossRef] [PubMed]

12. Reichert, J.M.; Valge-Archer, V.E. Development trends for monoclonal antibody cancer therapeutics. *Nat. Rev. Drug Discov.* **2007**, *6*, 349. [CrossRef] [PubMed]

13. Sharkey, R.M.; Goldenberg, D.M. Perspectives on Cancer Therapy with Radiolabeled Monoclonal Antibodies. *J. Nucl. Med.* **2005**, *46*, 115S–127S. [PubMed]

14. Sands, H.; Jones, P.L.; Shah, S.A.; Palme, D.; Vessella, R.L.; Gallagher, B.M. Correlation of vascular permeability and blood flow with monoclonal antibody uptake by human Clouser and renal cell xenografts. *Cancer Res.* **1988**, *48*, 188–193. [PubMed]

15. Chakrabarti, M.C.; Le, N.; Paik, C.H.; De Graff, W.G.; Carrasquillo, J.A. Prevention of radiolysis of monoclonal antibody during labeling. *J. Nucl. Med.* **1996**, *37*, 1384–1388. [PubMed]

16. Macey, D.J.; Meredith, R.F. A strategy to reduce red marrow dose for intraperitoneal radioimmunotherapy. *Clin. Cancer Res.* **1999**, *5*, 3044s–3047s. [PubMed]

17. Read, E.D.; Eu, P.; Little, P.J.; Piva, T.J. The status of radioimmunotherapy in CD20+ non-Hodgkin's lymphoma. *Target Oncol.* **2014**. [CrossRef] [PubMed]

18. Wilder, R.B.; DeNardo, G.L.; DeNardo, S.J. Radioimmunotherapy: Recent results and future directions. *J. Clin. Oncol.* **1996**, *14*, 1383–1400. [CrossRef] [PubMed]

19. IAEA. *Comparative Evaluation of Therapeutic Radiopharmaceuticals*; International Atomic Energy Agency: Vienna, Austria, 2007; Available online: https://www-pub.iaea.org/MTCD/publications/PDF/TRS458_web.pdf (accessed on 28 November 2018).

20. Dash, A.; Pillai, M.R.; Knapp, F.F., Jr. Production of (177)Lu for Targeted Radionuclide Therapy: Available Options. *Nucl. Med. Mol. Imaging* **2015**, *49*, 85–107. [CrossRef] [PubMed]

21. Stimmel, J.B.; Kull, F.C. Samarium-153 and Lutetium-177 Chelation Properties of Selected Macrocyclic and Acyclic Ligands. *Nucl. Med. Biol.* **1998**, *25*, 117–125. [CrossRef]

22. Yordanov, A.T.; Hens, M.; Pegram, C.; Bigner, D.D.; Zalutsky, M.R. Antitenascin antibody 81C6 armed with 177Lu: In vivo comparison of macrocyclic and acyclic ligands. *Nucl. Med. Biol.* **2007**, *34*, 173–183. [CrossRef] [PubMed]

23. Kang, C.S.; Sun, X.; Jia, F.; Song, H.A.; Chen, Y.; Lewis, M.; Chong, H.-S. Synthesis and Preclinical Evaluation of Bifunctional Ligands for Improved Chelation Chemistry of 90Y and 177Lu for Targeted Radioimmunotherapy. *Bioconjug. Chem.* **2012**, *23*, 1775–1782. [CrossRef] [PubMed]

24. Hens, M.; Vaidyanathan, G.; Zhao, X.G.; Bigner, D.D.; Zalutsky, M.R. Anti-EGFRvIII monoclonal antibody armed with 177Lu: In vivo comparison of macrocyclic and acyclic ligands. *Nucl. Med. Biol.* **2010**, *37*, 741–750. [CrossRef] [PubMed]

25. Liu, S.; Edwards, D.S. Bifunctional chelators for therapeutic lanthanide radiopharmaceuticals. *Bioconjug. Chem.* **2001**, *12*, 7–34. [CrossRef] [PubMed]

26. Milenic, D.E.; Garmestani, K.; Chappell, L.L.; Dadachova, E.; Yordanov, A.; Ma, D.; Schlom, J.; Brechbiel, M.W. In vivo comparison of macrocyclic and acyclic ligands for radiolabeling of monoclonal antibodies with 177Lu for radioimmunotherapeutic applications. *Nucl. Med. Biol.* **2002**, *29*, 431–442. [CrossRef]

27. Liu, S. The role of coordination chemistry in the development of target-specific radiopharmaceuticals. *Chem. Soc. Rev.* **2004**, *33*, 445–461. [CrossRef] [PubMed]

28. Liu, S. Bifunctional coupling agents for radiolabeling of biomolecules and target-specific delivery of metallic radionuclides. *Adv. Drug Deliv. Rev.* **2008**, *60*, 1347–1370. [CrossRef] [PubMed]

29. Grunberg, J.; Jeger, S.; Sarko, D.; Dennler, P.; Zimmermann, K.; Mier, W.; Schibli, R. DOTA-functionalized polylysine: A high number of DOTA chelates positively influences the biodistribution of enzymatic conjugated anti-tumor antibody chCE7agl. *PLoS ONE* **2013**, *8*, e60350. [CrossRef] [PubMed]

30. Garnett, M.C. Targeted drug conjugates: Principles and progress. *Adv. Drug Deliv. Rev.* **2001**, *53*, 171–216. [CrossRef]

31. Hermanson, G.T. Chapter 3—The Reactions of Bioconjugation. In *Bioconjugate Techniques*, 3rd ed.; Academic Press: Boston, MA, USA, 2013; pp. 229–258. [CrossRef]

32. Rana, T.M.; Meares, C.F. N-terminal modification of immunoglobulin polypeptide chains tagged with isothiocyanato chelates. *Bioconjug. Chem.* **1990**, *1*, 357–362. [CrossRef] [PubMed]

33. Oosterwijk, E.; Ruiter, D.J.; Hoedemaeker, P.J.; Pauwels, E.K.; Jonas, U.; Zwartendijk, J.; Warnaar, S.O. Monoclonal antibody G 250 recognizes a determinant present in renal-cell carcinoma and absent from normal kidney. *Int. J. Cancer* **1986**, *38*, 489–494. [CrossRef] [PubMed]

34. Zatovicova, M.; Jelenska, L.; Hulikova, A.; Csaderova, L.; Ditte, Z.; Ditte, P.; Goliasova, T.; Pastorek, J.; Pastorekova, S. Carbonic anhydrase IX as an anticancer therapy target: Preclinical evaluation of internalizing monoclonal antibody directed to catalytic domain. *Curr. Pharm. Des.* **2010**, *16*, 3255–3263. [CrossRef] [PubMed]

35. Oosterwijk-Wakka, J.C.; Boerman, O.C.; Mulders, P.F.; Oosterwijk, E. Application of monoclonal antibody G250 recognizing carbonic anhydrase IX in renal cell carcinoma. *Int. J. Mol. Sci* **2013**, *14*, 11402–11423. [CrossRef] [PubMed]

36. Zatovicova, M.; Jelenska, L.; Hulikova, A.; Ditte, P.; Ditte, Z.; Csaderova, L.; Svastova, E.; Schmalix, W.; Boettger, V.; Bevan, P.; et al. Monoclonal antibody G250 targeting CA: Binding specificity, internalization and therapeutic effects in a non-renal cancer model. *Int. J. Oncol.* **2014**, *45*, 2455–2467. [CrossRef] [PubMed]

37. Oosterwijk, E.; Ruiter, D.J.; Wakka, J.C.; Huiskens-van der Meij, J.W.; Jonas, U.; Fleuren, G.J.; Zwartendijk, J.; Hoedemaeker, P.; Warnaar, S.O. Immunohistochemical analysis of monoclonal antibodies to renal antigens. Application in the diagnosis of renal cell carcinoma. *Am. J. Pathol.* **1986**, *123*, 301–309. [PubMed]

38. Ivanov, S.; Liao, S.-Y.; Ivanova, A.; Danilkovitch-Miagkova, A.; Tarasova, N.; Weirich, G.; Merrill, M.J.; Proescholdt, M.A.; Oldfield, E.H.; Lee, J.; et al. Expression of Hypoxia-Inducible Cell-Surface Transmembrane Carbonic Anhydrases in Human Cancer. *Am. J. Pathol.* **2001**, *158*, 905–919. [CrossRef]

39. Muselaers, C.H.; Boerman, O.C.; Oosterwijk, E.; Langenhuijsen, J.F.; Oyen, W.J.; Mulders, P.F. Indium-111-labeled girentuximab immunoSPECT as a diagnostic tool in clear cell renal cell carcinoma. *Eur. Urol.* **2013**, *63*, 1101–1106. [CrossRef] [PubMed]

40. Kaluz, S.; Kaluzová, M.; Liao, S.-Y.; Lerman, M.; Stanbridge, E.J. Transcriptional control of the tumor- and hypoxia-marker carbonic anhydrase 9: A one transcription factor (HIF-1) show? *Biochim. Biophys. Acta (BBA) Rev. Cancer* **2009**, *1795*, 162–172. [CrossRef] [PubMed]

41. Ivanov, S.V.; Kuzmin, I.; Wei, M.-H.; Pack, S.; Geil, L.; Johnson, B.E.; Stanbridge, E.J.; Lerman, M.I. Down-regulation of transmembrane carbonic anhydrases in renal cell carcinoma cell lines by wild-type von Hippel-Lindau transgenes. *Proc. Natl. Acad. Sci. USA* **1998**, *95*, 12596–12601. [CrossRef] [PubMed]

42. Grabmaier, K.; de Weijert, M.C.A.; Verhaegh, G.W.; Schalken, J.A.; Oosterwijk, E. Strict regulation of CAIXG250/MN by HIF-1α in clear cell renal cell carcinoma. *Oncogene* **2004**, *23*, 5624. [CrossRef] [PubMed]

43. Chamie, K.; Donin, N.M.; Klopfer, P.; Bevan, P.; Fall, B.; Wilhelm, O.; Storkel, S.; Said, J.; Gambla, M.; Hawkins, R.E.; et al. Adjuvant Weekly Girentuximab Following Nephrectomy for High-Risk Renal Cell Carcinoma: The ARISER Randomized Clinical Trial. *JAMA Oncol.* **2017**, *3*, 913–920. [CrossRef] [PubMed]

44. Cheal, S.M.; Punzalan, B.; Doran, M.G.; Evans, M.J.; Osborne, J.R.; Lewis, J.S.; Zanzonico, P.; Larson, S.M. Pairwise comparison of 89Zr- and 124I-labeled cG250 based on positron emission tomography imaging and nonlinear immunokinetic modeling: In vivo carbonic anhydrase IX receptor binding and internalization in mouse xenografts of clear-cell renal cell carcinoma. *Eur. J. Nucl. Med. Mol. Imaging* **2014**, *41*, 985–994. [CrossRef] [PubMed]

45. Huizing, F.J.; Hoeben, B.A.W.; Franssen, G.; Lok, J.; Heskamp, S.; Oosterwijk, E.; Boerman, O.C.; Bussink, J. Preclinical validation of (111)In-girentuximab-F(ab')2 as a tracer to image hypoxia related marker CAIX expression in head and neck cancer xenografts. *Radiother. Oncol.* **2017**, *124*, 521–525. [CrossRef] [PubMed]

46. Stillebroer, A.B.; Boerman, O.C.; Desar, I.M.; Boers-Sonderen, M.J.; van Herpen, C.M.; Langenhuijsen, J.F.; Smith-Jones, P.M.; Oosterwijk, E.; Oyen, W.J.; Mulders, P.F. Phase 1 radioimmunotherapy study with lutetium 177-labeled anti-carbonic anhydrase IX monoclonal antibody girentuximab in patients with advanced renal cell carcinoma. *Eur. Urol.* **2013**, *64*, 478–485. [CrossRef] [PubMed]

47. Muselaers, C.H.; Boers-Sonderen, M.J.; van Oostenbrugge, T.J.; Boerman, O.C.; Desar, I.M.; Stillebroer, A.B.; Mulder, S.F.; van Herpen, C.M.; Langenhuijsen, J.F.; Oosterwijk, E.; et al. Phase 2 Study of Lutetium 177-Labeled Anti-Carbonic Anhydrase IX Monoclonal Antibody Girentuximab in Patients with Advanced Renal Cell Carcinoma. *Eur. Urol.* **2016**, *69*, 767–770. [CrossRef] [PubMed]

48. Stillebroer, A.B.; Zegers, C.M.; Boerman, O.C.; Oosterwijk, E.; Mulders, P.F.; O'Donoghue, J.A.; Visser, E.P.; Oyen, W.J. Dosimetric analysis of 177Lu-cG250 radioimmunotherapy in renal cell carcinoma patients: Correlation with myelotoxicity and pretherapeutic absorbed dose predictions based on 111In-cG250 imaging. *J. Nucl. Med.* **2012**, *53*, 82–89. [CrossRef] [PubMed]

49. Simon, J.; King, A.G.; Moreno, B.J.M. Methods for Generating Radioimmunoconjugates. U.S. Patents 9,603,954, 3 March 2017.

50. Nakamura, T.; Kawai, Y.; Kitamoto, N.; Osawa, T.; Kato, Y. Covalent modification of lysine residues by allyl isothiocyanate in physiological conditions: Plausible transformation of isothiocyanate from thiol to amine. *Chem. Res. Toxicol.* **2009**, *22*, 536–542. [CrossRef] [PubMed]

51. Spicer, C.D.; Davis, B.G. Selective chemical protein modification. *Nat. Commun.* **2014**, *5*, 4740. [CrossRef] [PubMed]

52. Forrer, F.; Chen, J.; Fani, M.; Powell, P.; Lohri, A.; Müller-Brand, J.; Moldenhauer, G.; Maecke, H.R. In vitro characterization of 177Lu-radiolabelled chimeric anti-CD20 monoclonal antibody and a preliminary dosimetry study. *Eur. J. Nucl. Med. Mol. Imaging* **2009**, *36*, 1443–1452. [CrossRef] [PubMed]

53. Price, E.W.; Edwards, K.J.; Carnazza, K.E.; Carlin, S.D.; Zeglis, B.M.; Adam, M.J.; Orvig, C.; Lewis, J.S. A comparative evaluation of the chelators H4octapa and CHX-A"-DTPA with the therapeutic radiometal 90Y. *Nucl. Med. Biol.* **2016**, *43*, 566–576. [CrossRef] [PubMed]

54. Steffens, M.G.; Kranenborg, M.H.; Boerman, O.C.; Zegwaart-Hagemeier, N.E.; Debruyne, F.M.; Corstens, F.H.; Oosterwijk, E. Tumor retention of 186Re-MAG3, 111In-DTPA and 125I labeled monoclonal antibody G250 in nude mice with renal cell carcinoma xenografts. *Cancer Biother. Radiopharm.* **1998**, *13*, 133–139. [CrossRef] [PubMed]

55. Oosterwijk, E.; Bander, N.H.; Divgi, C.R.; Welt, S.; Wakka, J.C.; Finn, R.D.; Carswell, E.A.; Larson, S.M.; Warnaar, S.O.; Fleuren, G.J.; et al. Antibody localization in human renal cell carcinoma: A phase I study of monoclonal antibody G250. *J. Clin. Oncol.* **1993**, *11*, 738–750. [CrossRef] [PubMed]

56. Muselaers, C.H.; Oosterwijk, E.; Bos, D.L.; Oyen, W.J.; Mulders, P.F.; Boerman, O.C. Optimizing lutetium 177-anti-carbonic anhydrase IX radioimmunotherapy in an intraperitoneal clear cell renal cell carcinoma xenograft model. *Mol. Imaging* **2014**, *13*, 1–7. [CrossRef] [PubMed]

57. Oosterwijk-Wakka, J.C.; de Weijert, M.C.; Franssen, G.M.; Leenders, W.P.; van der Laak, J.A.; Boerman, O.C.; Mulders, P.F.; Oosterwijk, E. Successful combination of sunitinib and girentuximab in two renal cell carcinoma animal models: A rationale for combination treatment of patients with advanced RCC. *Neoplasia* **2015**, *17*, 215–224. [CrossRef] [PubMed]

58. Semenza, G.L. Defining the role of hypoxia-inducible factor 1 in cancer biology and therapeutics. *Oncogene* **2010**, *29*, 625–634. [CrossRef] [PubMed]

59. Lucas, A.; Price, L.; Schorzman, A.; Storrie, M.; Piscitelli, J.; Razo, J.; Zamboni, W. Factors Affecting the Pharmacology of Antibody–Drug Conjugates. *Antibodies* **2018**, *7*, 10. [CrossRef]

60. Durrbach, A.; Angevin, E.; Poncet, P.; Rouleau, M.; Chavanel, G.; Chapel, A.; Thierry, D.; Gorter, A.; Hirsch, R.; Charpentier, B.; et al. Antibody-mediated endocytosis of G250 tumor-associated antigen allows targeted gene transfer to human renal cell carcinoma in vitro. *Cancer Gene Ther.* **1999**, *6*, 564–571. [CrossRef] [PubMed]

61. Honarvar, H.; Garousi, J.; Gunneriusson, E.; Hoiden-Guthenberg, I.; Altai, M.; Widstrom, C.; Tolmachev, V.; Frejd, F.Y. Imaging of CAIX-expressing xenografts in vivo using 99mTc-HEHEHE-ZCAIX:1 affibody molecule. *Int. J. Oncol.* **2015**, *46*, 513–520. [CrossRef] [PubMed]

62. Roscher, M.; Hormann, I.; Leib, O.; Marx, S.; Moreno, J.; Miltner, E.; Friesen, C. Targeted alpha-therapy using [Bi-213]anti-CD20 as novel treatment option for radio- and chemoresistant non-Hodgkin lymphoma cells. *Oncotarget* **2013**, *4*, 218–230. [CrossRef] [PubMed]

63. Graf, F.; Fahrer, J.; Maus, S.; Morgenstern, A.; Bruchertseifer, F.; Venkatachalam, S.; Fottner, C.; Weber, M.M.; Huelsenbeck, J.; Schreckenberger, M.; et al. DNA Double Strand Breaks as Predictor of Efficacy of the Alpha-Particle Emitter Ac-225 and the Electron Emitter Lu-177 for Somatostatin Receptor Targeted Radiotherapy. *PLoS ONE* **2014**, *9*, e88239. [CrossRef] [PubMed]

64. Laemmli, U.K. Cleavage of structural proteins during the assembly of the head of bacteriophage T4. *Nature* **1970**, *227*, 680–685. [CrossRef] [PubMed]

65. Candiano, G.; Bruschi, M.; Musante, L.; Santucci, L.; Ghiggeri, G.M.; Carnemolla, B.; Orecchia, P.; Zardi, L.; Righetti, P.G. Blue silver: A very sensitive colloidal Coomassie G-250 staining for proteome analysis. *Electrophoresis* **2004**, *25*, 1327–1333. [CrossRef] [PubMed]

66. Gunasekera, K.; Wuthrich, D.; Braga-Lagache, S.; Heller, M.; Ochsenreiter, T. Proteome remodelling during development from blood to insect-form Trypanosoma brucei quantified by SILAC and mass spectrometry. *BMC Genom.* **2012**, *13*, 556. [CrossRef] [PubMed]

67. Ozerdem, U.; Wojcik, E.M.; Barkan, G.A.; Duan, X.; Ersahin, C. A practical application of quantitative vascular image analysis in breast pathology. *Pathol. Res. Pract.* **2013**, *209*, 455–458. [CrossRef] [PubMed]

8

Optimization of the Automated Synthesis of [11C]*m*HED—Administered and Apparent Molar Activities

Chrysoula Vraka [1][ID], Verena Pichler [1,*][ID], Neydher Berroterán-Infante [1][ID], Tim Wollenweber [1], Anna Pillinger [1], Maximilian Hohensinner [1], Lukas Fetty [1], Dietrich Beitzke [2], Xiang Li [1], Cecile Philippe [1], Katharina Pallitsch [3], Markus Mitterhauser [1,4][ID], Marcus Hacker [1] and Wolfgang Wadsak [1,5][ID]

[1]   Division of Nuclear Medicine, Department of Biomedical Imaging and Image-guided Therapy, Medical University of Vienna, 1090 Vienna, Austria; chrysoula.vraka@meduniwien.ac.at (C.V.); neydher.berroteraninfante@meduniwien.ac.at (N.B.-I.); tim.wollenweber@meduniwien.ac.at (T.W.); anna.pillinger@meduniwien.ac.at (A.P.); maximilian.hohensinner@meduniwien.ac.at (M.H.); lukas.fetty@meduniwien.ac.at (L.F.); xiang.li@meduniwien.ac.at (X.L.); cecile.philippe@meduniwien.ac.at (C.P.); markus.mitterhauser@meduniwien.ac.at (M.M.); marcus.hacker@meduniwien.ac.at (M.H.); wolfgang.wadsak@meduniwien.ac.at (W.W.)
[2]   Department of Biomedical Imaging and Image-guided Therapy, Division of Cardiovascular and Interventional Radiology, Medical University of Vienna, 1090 Vienna, Austria; dietrich.beitzke@meduniwien.ac.at
[3]   Institute of Organic Chemistry, University of Vienna, 1090 Vienna, Austria; katharina.pallitsch@univie.ac.at
[4]   Ludwig-Boltzmann-Institute Applied Diagnostics, 1090 Vienna, Austria
[5]   Center for Biomarker Research in Medicine, CBmed GmbH, 8010 Graz, Austria
*   Correspondence: verena.pichler@meduniwien.ac.at

Abstract: The tracer [11C]*meta*-Hydroxyephedrine ([11C]*m*HED) is one of the most applied PET tracers for cardiac imaging, whose radiosynthesis was already reported in 1990. While not stated in the literature, separation difficulties and an adequate formulation of the product are well known challenges in its production. Furthermore, the precursor (metaraminol) is also a substrate for the norepinephrine transporter, and can therefore affect the image quality. This study aims at optimizing the synthetic process of [11C]*m*HED and investigating the effect of the apparent molar activity (sum of *m*HED and metaraminol) in patients and animals. The main optimization was the improved separation through reverse phase-HPLC by a step gradient and subsequent retention of the product on a weakly-cationic ion exchange cartridge. The μPET/μCT was conducted in ten rats (ischemic model) and the apparent molar activity was correlated to the VOI- and SUV-ratio of the myocardium/intra-ventricular blood pool. Moreover, nine long-term heart transplanted and five Morbus Fabry patients underwent PET and MRI imaging for detection of changes in the sympathetic innervation. In summary, the fully-automated synthesis and optimized purification method of [11C]*m*HED is easily applicable and reproducible. Moreover, it was shown that the administered apparent molar activities had a negligible effect on the imaging quality.

Keywords: [11C]*meta*-hydroxyephedrine; radiosynthesis; separation; apparent molar activity

1. Introduction

The world health organization (WHO) estimates that almost 18 million people die of cardiovascular diseases (CVD) each year. Moreover, from the year 2000 onwards, it has been reported that CVDs have become the number one cause of death worldwide [1,2]. Therefore, there is a high demand for a reliable imaging technique enabling the investigation of CVDs. One of the most frequently used positron emission tomography (PET) tracers in this regard is [11C]*meta*-hydroxyephedrine ([11C]*m*HED), also known as 3-[(1*R*,2*S*)-1-hydroxy-2-([11C]methylamino)propyl]phenol, a false transmitter agent and a norepinephrine transporter (NET) substrate [3,4]. It has been described that [11C]*m*HED underlies the uptake-1 pathway of NET from the synaptic cleft to the cytoplasm of the sympathetic nerve terminal. Advantages of [11C]*m*HED are the metabolic resistance against the enzymes MAO (monoamine oxidase) and COMT (catechol-O-methyltransferase), and in contrast to endogenous ligands, the high selectivity towards uptake-1, the low non-specific binding to the myocardium, the fast pharmacokinetics, as well as a continuous release and re-uptake by sympathetic nerves [5,6]. Thus, the combination of these biochemical properties, together with a fast and reliable automated radiosynthesis, allows PET acquisition duration of at least one hour, despite the short half-life of carbon-11 (20 min). Additionally, flow dependent effects can be examined when combined with a [13N]NH$_3$ scan or duplex sonography [7]. In more recent studies, [11C]*m*HED has also been used to image the white-to-brown fat conversion, and it was shown that cold-induced BAT thermogenesis is controlled by the sympathetic nervous system [8,9]. Besides, [11C]*m*HED might be utilized in oncology for the diagnosis of adrenal tumors and metastasis [10,11].

The first [11C]*m*HED radiosynthesis was described in 1990 by Rosenspire et al. [4], which is still the most cited concerning radiosynthesis. Since then, only a few publications have dealt with the optimization of the radiosynthetic procedure. These studies focused mainly on automation and optimization, in terms of time efficiency and radiochemical yields. Indeed, producers of [11C]*m*HED know about the difficulties of HPLC separation and purification via solid-phase extraction, caused by the strong pH sensitivity of *m*HED. Nevertheless, this phenomenon has not been published. Furthermore, none of those investigations focused on the improvement of the molar activity or the reduction of the residual precursor concentration [3,5,12,13]. In fact, a blocking study demonstrated that the [11C]*m*HED precursor, metaraminol (*meta*-hydroxynorephedrine), can affect the image quality through displacement of the tracer itself. Consequently, the amount of residual metaraminol plays a major role in this matter. Besides the probability of triggering a pharmacological effect at high doses, both metaraminol and *m*HED are substrates for NET, and can therefore cause dose-dependent loss of image quality [14]. Thus, there is a necessity to include the sum of precursor and cold product concentrations (apparent molar activity) in the quality control criteria.

2. Results

2.1. Radiosynthesis of [11C]mHED

The radiosynthesis of [11C]*m*HED was set up on a GE Tracerlab FX C Pro and was performed fully automated. The methylation of metaraminol was highly reproducible in a mixture of DMF:DMSO as solvent, leading to a stable radiochemical yield of around 2–3 GBq. This yield was sufficient for 2–3 animals or at least 1 patient dose per production. The most common reason for a failed synthesis was the irregular reversed phase-high performance liquid chromatography (RP-HPLC) separation of metaraminol and [11C]*m*HED before radiosynthetic optimization. Changing the RP-HPLC purification to the buffer free step gradient led to a significantly more stable separation and improved reproducibility. Overall (see Table 1), 51 syntheses were performed with the reliable RP-HPLC set-up; out of these 51 syntheses 26 were used for pre-clinical and clinical studies, ten were incomplete production files or failed synthesis and were subsequently excluded. Fifteen radiosyntheses were solely performed for the purpose of experimentation with different conditions or testing the system. None of the failed syntheses was caused by separation problems.

For calculation of the molar activity, a calibration curve in the range of 0.1–5 μg/mL was prepared and the UV-Vis-signal was measured at 275 and 220 nm, respectively. For both wavelengths R^2 was >0.99, whereas the slope was steeper at 220 nm, indicating a better sensitivity.

Table 1. Overview of overall synthesis data (excluding synthesis for the purpose of condition testing and fail synthesis), as well as synthesis data for the respective pre-clinical and clinical study.

[¹¹C]mHED	Starting Activity [GBq]	Yield [GBq]	Yield [%EOB]	Molar Activity [GBq/µmol mHED]	Precursor Concentration [µg/mL]	mHED Concentration [µg/mL]
All synthesis (n = 32) Patients:	114 ± 15	3 ± 2	2.5 ± 1.5	126 ± 97	8 ± 7	3 ± 8
Morbus Fabry (n = 5)	124 ± 2	3.5 ± 0.4	2.9 ± 0.3	155 ± 85	6 ± 4	2 ± 1
HTX (n = 9)	120 ± 2	2.3 ± 1.3	2 ± 1	129 ± 148	5.5 ± 3.8	1.7 ± 2.8
Animals (n = 11)	122 ± 3	3 ± 2	2.4 ± 1.9	211 ± 152	4.6 ± 4.7	9 ± 19

2.2. μPET/μCT Imaging

The administered dose was 5 ± 8 μg/kg bodyweight for metaraminol and 2 ± 4 μg/kg for *m*HED, with an absolute mass dose of 2.3 ± 3.1 μg (sum of precursor and product), in a range of 0.1 to 9.5 μg (Table 2). No dose effects were visible in rats (Figure 1). Neither the correlation between the myocardium/intra-ventricular blood pool ratio and the molar activity, nor with the apparent molar activity or the sum of residual precursor and formed *m*HED showed any significance (*p*-value in all cases > 0.05).

Table 2. Overview on the applied mass concentrations of the precursor metaraminol and *m*HED as well as applied mass per bodyweight (BW). None of the patients received more than 0.1 μg/kg bodyweight of metaraminol and *m*HED, with a maximal administrated mass dose of 12 μg metaraminol and 4.6 μg *m*HED, respectively.

[¹¹C]*m*HED	Metaraminol		*m*HED	
Patients	[μg/applied volume]	[μg/kg BW]	[μg/applied volume]	[μg/kg BW]
Morbus Fabry (n = 5)	5.2 ± 3.3	0.06 ± 0.05	1.6 ± 1.3	0.02 ± 0.02
HTX (n = 9)	5.5 ± 3.8	0.1 ± 0.1	2.1 ± 1.5	0.02 ± 0.02
Animals (n = 11)	1.8 ± 2.9	4.9 ± 8.4	0.8 ± 1.8	1.8 ± 3.8

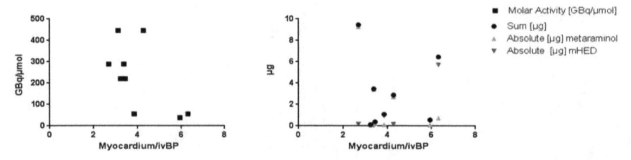

Figure 1. Correlation of the myocardium/intra-ventricular blood pool ratio and the molar activity, the mass of residual precursor and non-labelled *m*HED, as well as the sum of both.

For representative PET images see Figure 2 below. The ratios of myocardium/intra ventricular blood pool (Myo/ivBP) ranged between 3.1 and 6.3 for all animals. Infarcted areas are clearly definable within all applied masses.

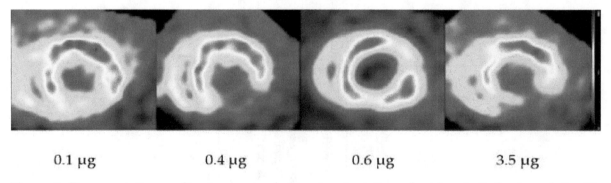

Figure 2. Representative cardiac images in short axis orientation of rat hearts (infarct model) with different applied mass doses of metaraminol and *m*HED. The sum of metaraminol and *m*HED is shown beneath the respective image.

2.3. PET/MRI Imaging

No correlation was found between the myocardium/intra-ventricular blood pool ratio and the molar activity, or the overall mass of injected metaraminol and mHED (p-values ranged from 0.1 to 1) in Morbus Fabry patients (Figure 3). The same was true for the relation between the myocardium/mediastinum ratio and the mass or molar activity of the respective compound. Even expanding the analysis to ratios based on the SUV_{mean} did not lead to any correlation (data not illustrated). Only one of the five imaged Morbus Fabry patients showed a pathological finding. Excluding this patient from the correlation causes no changes in significance.

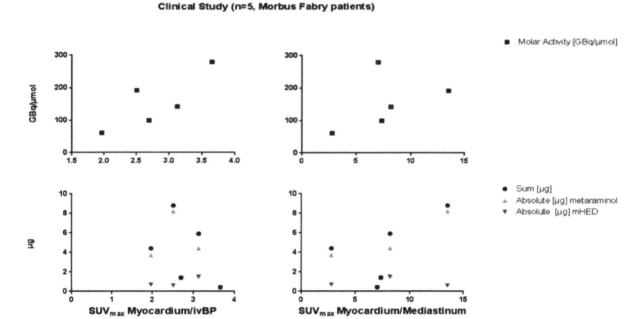

Figure 3. Correlation of the myocardium/intra-ventricular blood pool ratio (**left**) and correlation between the myocardium/mediastinum ratio (**right**) and the molar activity, the mass of residual precursor and non-labelled mHED, as well as the sum of both (Morbus Fabry patients).

The ratio of myocardium/intra ventricular blood pool (Myo/ivBP), calculated from SUV_{mean} values, were in all cases 4 (ratio range for SUV_{max}: 3 to 4). The myocardium/mediastinum ratio (Myo/Med) varies between 7 and 13 for the calculation, with SUV_{max} and SUV_{mean} (Figure 4).

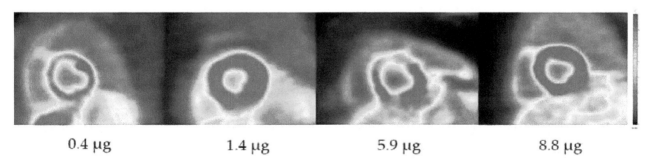

Figure 4. Cardiac images (short axis orientation) of Morbus Fabry patients with different applied mass doses of metaraminol and mHED. The sum of metaraminol and mHED is shown beneath the respective image. The patient with abnormality of sympathetic innervation was excluded in the figure, showing a Myo/Med ratio of <4 with an applied mass dose of 4.5 µg.

The correlations using the SUV_{mean} for the heart transplantation patients (HTX) showed again no significance for the Myo/ivBP (p-values between 0.3 and 0.6), as well as for the Myo/Med (p-values range from 0.4 to 0.6) ratios (data not illustrated). Moreover, no relationship was found using the ratios calculated with SUV_{max} values for the Myo/ivBP and Myo/Med versus the molar activity or the respective injected mass, or the sum of both compounds (p-value > 0.2, Figure 5).

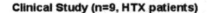
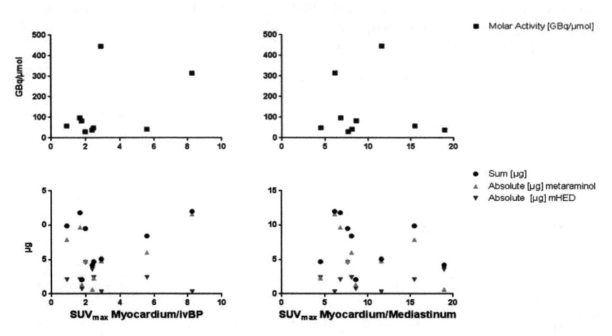

Figure 5. Correlation of the myocardium/intra-ventricular blood pool ratio (**left**) and correlation between the myocardium/mediastinum ratio (**right**) and the molar activity, the mass of residual precursor and non-labelled mHED, as well as the sum of both (heart transplantation (HTX) patients).

3. Discussion

In general, [^{11}C]mHED is a cardiac PET tracer with excellent pharmacokinetic properties, and can be used for diverse clinical issues like imaging of cardiac diseases, white-to-brown fat conversion, and oncology. The radiosynthesis is highly robust, as already reported in literature. Since the retention of mHED is strongly affected by minor variations in pH or salt concentration, a major challenge of the [^{11}C]mHED radiosynthesis is the separation and purification from the precursor, side products, and the used methylation agent ([^{11}C]CH$_3$I or [^{11}C]MeOTf). None of the published separation methods using semi-preparative RP-HPLC were reproducible or (long-term) repeatable in our laboratories (see Figure 6).

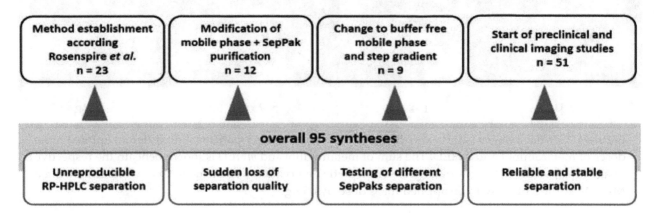

Figure 6. Overview on the radiosynthesis optimization, including the challenges and establishments during the first 44 syntheses and the stable separation process of the last 51 syntheses.

Changes in the separation efficiency occur even by necessary maintenance changes, such as renewing the column of a similar type. Almost 40 syntheses had to be performed to establish long-term stable conditions, and twelve out of these 40 syntheses were used to determine the purification potency via solid phase extraction (SPE). Here, different SPE cartridges were tested (XAD-4, C-18 or SCX), which showed either none or very strong retention of [^{11}C]mHED. The product purification was achieved by removal of the mobile phase via a weakly-cationic ion exchange cartridge, and it was formulated in 3 mL of physiological saline.

The described synthesis procedure is now consistent and has been reproducible for over 50 preparations. None of the fail syntheses was due to poor separation or purification problems. The major achievement of this optimized procedure is the buffer free mobile phase and the utilization of the pH sensitivity of [^{11}C]mHED to elute quickly from the RP-18 column caused by protonation.

Compared to previously published [^{11}C]mHED productions, our method led to a reduced synthesis time, higher molar activities, and the apparent molar activity was discussed for the very first time (see Table 3). However, further comparison of the radiochemical yields or starting activities were not possible, due to insufficient information within the previously published radiosyntheses [5,12,15]. The overall administered doses for patients and animals was calculated in μg/kg bodyweight for metaraminol and mHED and correlated to the myocardium/intraventricular blood pool. To investigate the perfusion effect, a [^{13}N]NH$_3$ scan was performed upfront to the [^{11}C]mHED imaging. However, neither patients nor animals suffered from pharmacological effects, nor any loss in imaging quality could be confirmed. The intra-individual variations and the progress of denervation had a higher impact on [^{11}C]mHED accumulation than the apparent and molar activity. A limit of 50 nmol/kg (8.4 μg/kg) for metaraminol was stated to avoid effect on the imaging quality based solely on blocking studies, and the overall amount of metaraminol and mHED was not taken into account [14]. On the other hand, different doses of mHED were applied with constant concentrations of metaraminol in a recently published study. A washout or decreased time activity curve was observed from an applied concentration of 10 μg/kg bodyweight mHED [16]. The IC$_{50}$ value of mHED towards NET drug inhibition was reported as 0.42 μM (competitive inhibition) by Foley at al. [17]. However, in PET studies, target binding affinities are required in the low nanomolar range to avoid competition to endogenous ligands. Therefore, the imaging mechanism of [^{11}C]mHED is subject to long tissue life caused by several reuptake cycles, metabolic resistance, and rapid pharmacokinetics (Myo/ivBP ratio up to 5 after 10 min) [6,17]. With our new synthesis method, this limiting concentration was never reached, and by the correlation we could prove that higher doses of metaraminol, mHED, or the sum of both are necessary for observing impact on the image quality. Therefore, we could confirm that our administered amounts are too low for any effect on image quality or to trigger pharmacological effects.

Table 3. Comparison of radiosynthetic parameters of previously published and our optimized [11C]mHED method.

	Rosenspire et al. 1990	Nagren et al. 1995	Van Dort et al. 2000	Law et al. 2010	This work
Methylation agent	[11C]CH$_3$I	[11C]CH$_3$OTf	[11C]CH$_3$I	According to Rosenspire et al.	[11C]CH$_3$OTf
	250 μL DMF:DMSO (3:1)	100 μL ACN	anhydrous DMF 150 μL	250 μL DMF:DMSO (3:1)	DMF:DMSO (4:1, v/v%)
[c] Precursor	1 mg metaraminol free base, freshly prepared from metaraminol bitartrate	1 mg free base	0.6 mg free base	1 mg free base	1 mg free base
Formulation	10% EtOH + 0.24 M NaH$_2$PO$_4$, ~7 mL	physiological phosphate buffer 8 mL	0.04 M NaH$_2$PO$_4$ 10 mL	According to Rosenspire et al.	0.9% saline 3 mL
[c] Metaraminol	21 μg mean	Not reported	Not reported	2 μM	8 ± 7 μg/mL
[c] mHED		Not reported	Not reported	9 μM	3 ± 8 μg/mL
Radiochemical purity%	98 2% unidentified RI	Not reported	>98	95 ± 5	98 ± 2
Time of synthesis (EOB)	45 min without evaporation	Approx. 41 min	40 min	According to Rosenspire et al.	30–35 min
Molar activity (EOS) [GBq/μmol]	33 ± 18 (n = 19)	Not reported	47–60 (mean = 51) (n = 8)	10–30	126 ± 97 (n = 32)

4. Material and Methods

4.1. Radiosynthesis

The $[^{11}C]CO_2$ was produced within a GE PETtrace cyclotron (General Electric Medical System, Uppsala, Sweden) by a $^{14}N(p,\alpha)^{11}C$ nuclear reaction under irradiation of a gas target filled with N_2 (+1% O_2) (Air Liquide Austria, GmbH, Schwechat, Austria). The conversion of $[^{11}C]CO_2$ to $[^{11}C]CH_3I$ was performed in the GE Tracerlab FX C Pro synthesizer. Therefore, the cyclotron production of $[^{11}C]CO_2$ was terminated at desired target activities between 67–127 GBq using a current of 45 µA for ~30 min, and the activity was trapped upon delivery on a molecular sieve (4 Å) within the synthesizer. Subsequently, $[^{11}C]CO_2$ was converted into $[^{11}C]CH_4$ by a Ni-catalyzed reduction with H_2 at 400 °C. The $[^{11}C]CH_3I$ was produced using gas phase conversion, as described in a previous study [18]. In short, the resulting $[^{11}C]CH_4$ was reacted with sublimated iodine at 738 °C in a recirculating process for 5 min to give $[^{11}C]CH_3I$. The produced $[^{11}C]CH_3I$ was trapped on-line on a Porapak® N column and finally released by heating the trap to 190 °C. The $[^{11}C]CH_3OTf$ was prepared on-line at the passage of $[^{11}C]CH_3I$ through a silver triflate column (containing 300 mg impregnated graphitized carbon), pre-heated to 200 °C, at a flow rate of 40 mL/min. The $[^{11}C]CH_3OTf$ was trapped in a glass reactor containing 1 mg metaraminol in 500 µL of a DMF:DMSO mixture (4/1 %v/v) and heated to 75 °C for 2 min (Figure 7). After the reaction time, the reactor was cooled to 35 °C and the reaction was quenched by adding 1 mL of RP-HPLC solvent (mobile phase A). The entire volume of the crude mixture was automatically transferred to a semi-preparative RP-HPLC column (see section semi-preparative scale purification). The $[^{11}C]mHED$ peak was collected in a round-bottom flask containing 10 mL of distilled water to increase the volume for subsequent solid-phase extraction, which was performed using a weakly-cationic ion exchange cartridge (Sep-Pak Accell Plus Short Cartridge, Waters [WAT020550]). After rinsing the cartridge with 10 mL water for complete removal of residual acetonitrile from the HPLC solvent, the pure product was eluted with 3 mL of 0.9% saline and filter sterilized (0.22 µm) under aseptic conditions (laminar air flow hot cell, class A).

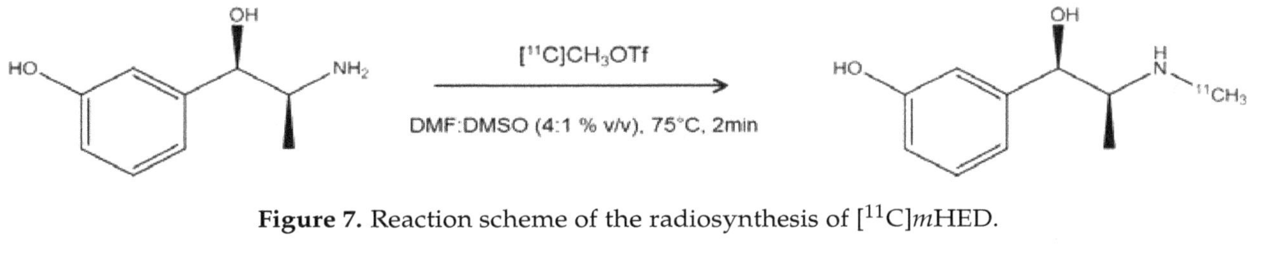

Figure 7. Reaction scheme of the radiosynthesis of $[^{11}C]mHED$.

4.2. Semi-Preparative Purification

Purification of the crude mixture was performed using a semi-preparative RP-HPLC (Supelcosil TMLC-ABZ+Plus, 5 µm, 250 × 10 mm (Supelco®, Bellefonte, PA, USA)) with a step gradient method. For the step gradient, two solvents were used: solvent A consisted of acetonitrile and water (58/42), and solvent B of a mixture of acetonitrile/water (50/50) mixture, which has been acidified (~pH 3, 0.1% H_3PO_4). The column was conditioned with solvent A, at a flow rate of 6 mL/min for injection, and then the flow was raised immediately to 8 mL/min. After the elution of $[^{11}C]CH_3OTf$, non-converted $[^{11}C]CH_3I$, precursor, as well as the DMF/DMSO mixture (approx. 6 min.), the mobile phase was switched to solvent mixture B. Subsequently, the $[^{11}C]mHED$ could be eluted with a retention time of 8–10 min (see Figure 8). After the completion of the RP-HPLC separation (after around 12 min), the mobile phase was set back to 100% solvent A to elongate column separation stability and lifespan, as long-time storage under acidic conditions should be avoided.

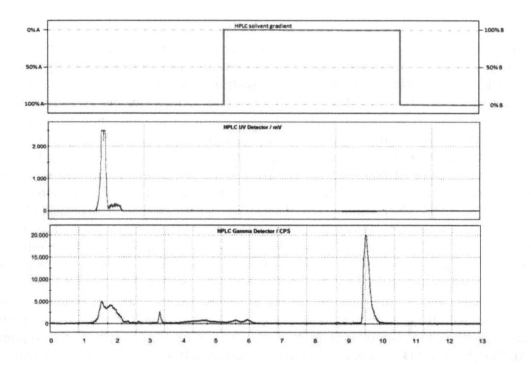

Figure 8. Typical chromatogram of the semi-preparative RP-HPLC purification of the crude mixture: The $[^{11}C]m$HED elutes after 9.5 min from the C-18 RP column after using a step gradient, as illustrated at the top of the graphic. Solvent A consists of an acetonitrile:water mixture (58:42) and solvent B is a mixture of acetonitrile and acidified water (50:50; 0.004% H_3PO_4, conc).

4.3. Quality Control

Radiochemical and chemical purities were assessed using analytical radio- and UV/Vis-RP-HPLC. Identity of $[^{11}C]m$HED was confirmed by co-injection with the respective reference standard. In detail, an Agilent 1260 system (Agilent Technologies GmbH; Santa Clara, CA, USA) equipped with a quaternary pump (G1311B), a multi wavelength UV-detector (G1365D) set to 220 and 275 nm (reference wavelength 450 nm), a NaI (Tl) detector from Berthold Technologies (Bad Wildbad, Germany), and GINA Star controlling software (Elysia-Raytest; Straubenhardt, Germany) were used. As the stationary phase, an analytical RP-HPLC column, X-Bridge BEH Shield RP-18, 4.6 × 50 mm, 2.5 µm, 130 Å (Waters GmbH) was used [19]. Precursor and mHED concentrations were determined, and subsequently, the molar activity was calculated. The concentrations of the calibration curve were in the range of 0.1–5.0 µg/mL with R^2 = 0.996 ± 0.002 (see Figure 9). The limit of detection for mHED was 0.22 µg/mL (220 nm) and 0.27 µg/mL (275 nm), and 0.23 µg/mL (220 nm) and 0.32 µg/mL (275 nm) for metaraminol. Sterility, absence of endotoxins, pH, osmolality, and residual solvents were determined by standard procedures routinely performed at the PET Centre of the Vienna General Hospital/Medical University of Vienna, and following similar monographs to the European Pharmacopoeia.

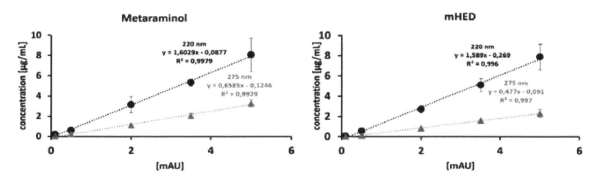

Figure 9. Calibration curve for metaraminol and *m*HED. Concentrations were chosen in the range of 0.1–5 μg/mL.

4.4. Animal Preparation

All procedures and protocols involving animals were conducted in compliance with and approval by the Institutional Animal Care and Use Committee of the Medical University of Vienna, Austria, as well as by the Austrian Ministry of Science, Research, and Economy (ZI. 1413/115-97/98 2014/2015). The manuscript adheres to the Directive European law (2010/63/EU) and to the ARRIVE guidelines for reporting animal experiments.

4.5. Imaging of μPET/μCT

In vivo imaging experiments were conducted with a small animal-cone beam-computed tomography (μCT) and positron emission tomography (μPET) scanner (Siemens Inveon Multimodal μSPECT/μCT, dedicated μPET; Siemens Medical Solutions, Knoxville, TN, USA). Twelve to fourteen weeks old male Sprague Dawley rats (HIM:OFA, Himberg, Austria) underwent the scans 14–15 days after chirurgical intervention (myocardial infarction model), weighing 373 ± 45 g (n = 11), and were kept under controlled laboratory conditions (22 ± 1 °C; 12 h light/dark cycle), with food and water access ad libitum. Rats were anesthetized (1.5–2.0% isoflurane vaporized in oxygen 1.0–1.5 L/min) and positioned in the center of the field of view (FOV). Physiological parameters and the depth of anesthesia were constantly monitored and adapted throughout the experiment. All animals received [^{11}C]*m*HED in 100% physiological saline (78 ± 12 MBq, molar activity: 211 ± 152 GBq/μmol (range: 38–446 GBq/μmol)). Once the radiotracer was administered through the lateral tail vein, μPET data acquisition took 30 min to allow tracer kinetics to attain full equilibrium. Three-dimensional static sinograms were generated from the list files, which were further reconstructed by an OSEM-3D/MAP algorithm (4 OSEM and 18 MAP iterations). All μPET data were corrected for attenuation, scatter, and decay. The image matrix was 256×256 pixels in the transversal plane. The μCT data were acquired within a full rotation and 360 projections with a FOV of 100×100 mm^2. Furthermore, 80 kV, 500 μA, and 200 ms exposure time were used for the protocol settings. CT raw data was reconstructed with a Feldkamp algorithm, including ramp filtration and beam-hardening correction, resulting in a final image matrix of 1024×1024 pixels in the transversal plane. Data pre- and post-processing was performed by means of PMOD 3.8 (PMOD Technologies Ltd., Zurich, Switzerland). A 3D Gaussian filter with kernel size 1 mm $\times$ 1 mm $\times$ 1 mm was applied to the μPET data and a $2 \times 2 \times 2$ reduction to the matrix was performed for the μCT data, in order to prevent excessive computing time. Rigid multimodal registration was performed to align both image datasets. A delineation of the volumes of interest (VOI), namely myocardium and intra-ventricular blood pool, was performed. We defined a good image quality, by the differentiability of myocardium and blood, respectively. Therefore, the ratio between myocardium/intra-ventricular blood pool was calculated. All animal data were excluded from the correlation when there was an incomplete data set available, due to technical problems or vitality of the animals.

4.6. PET/MRI Imaging

Institutional review board approval was gained for this prospective pilot study (IRB No.: 2301/2016 and 1562/2018). All patients gave written an informed consent prior to study inclusion. Patients were allowed to eat until 4 hours prior to the examination, but were asked to abstain from caffeine intake for 36 hours prior to PET/MRI imaging. None of the patients received medication that interferes with the presynaptic sympathetic nervous system (e.g., antidepressants, clonidine, etc.), beta-, or alpha blockade. All PET/MRI examinations (frames: 6×30 s, 2×60, 2×150, 2×300, 2×600) were conducted on a simultaneous PET/MR system (Biograph mMR; Siemens, Erlangen, Germany) according to a study published in 2013 [20]. Patients were positioned head first and supine. An ECG device was used for cardiac triggering. The [^{11}C]mHED was injected through a venous cannula. A 40 min dynamic PET acquisition was performed for all patients.

All Morbus Fabry patients (n = 5) received [^{11}C]mHED as well as [^{13}N]NH$_3$ for perfusion monitoring. Applied [^{11}C]mHED activities were 320 ± 47 MBq, with molar activities of 155 ± 85 GBq/µmol (range: 61–279) formulated in 0.9% saline solution, and further diluted with saline to a standard volume of 17 mL. For the heart transplanted patients (HTX), the tracer formulation and scan procedure were the same, with applied activities of 470 ± 102 MBq (128 ± 148 GBq/µmol). From ten overall HTX patients, one had to be excluded due to a shorter scanning time. The myocardium/intra-ventricular blood pool ratio was calculated according to Bonfiglioli et al. [5].

4.7. Statistical Analysis

All data is shown as mean ± standard deviation, if not stated otherwise. The limit of detection was calculated according to ICH guidelines, and was defined as LOD = $(3 \times \sigma)$/slope.

All ratios were correlated with the absolute applied concentration of mHED and metaraminol, the apparent and molar activity (pearson correlation, two-tailed p-value, and a confidence interval of 95%), and the p-values were determined using GraphPadPrism 6.01 (GraphPad Software 7825 Fay Avenue, Suite 230 La Jolla, CA 92037, USA).

5. Conclusions

Due to the optimized synthesis procedure of [^{11}C]mHED, the overall synthesis time was reduced as well as the amount of the precursor metaraminol and mHED, and consequently a higher molar activity. Indeed, the beneficial feature is the buffer free RP-HPLC assay and the formulation through a weakly-cationic ion exchange cartridge. Therefore, a highly reproducible and repeatable, fully-automated radiosynthetic procedure could be developed. Furthermore, it was shown that the administrated molar and apparent activities are distinctly lower, and therefore no effect on the imaging quality was observed using this separation and purification method. Therefore, this robust production procedure is appropriate for preclinical as well as clinical studies without showing blocking or pharmacological effects in patients or animals.

Author Contributions: C.V.: conceptualization, methodology, writing/original draft preparation, interpretation; V.P. conceptualization, methodology, writing; N.B.-I.: radiosynthesis and methodology; T.W.: patient study and post-processing & quantification of human data, A.P.: post processing and quantification of animal experiments; M.H.: imaging and animal handling; L.F. imaging and animal handling, data post processing; D.B.: supervisor of human studies, clinical ethic, review and editing; X.L.: providing the animal model and the ethic, animal preparation; C.P.: radiosynthesis; K.P.: methodology and review and editing; M.M.: resources and editing; M.H.: resources, project supervisor; W.W.: resources and editing.

Acknowledgments: This scientific project was performed with the support of the Medical Imaging Cluster of the Medical University of Vienna. We gratefully acknowledge Monika Dumanic, MSc for her qualified expertise in cardiac imaging, and the whole Preclinical Imaging Laboratory team, namely Anna Zacher, Elena Krstevska-Vulic, and Stefanie Marie Bugayong, as well as former members Markus Zeilinger and Florian Pichler, who were involved in this project. We further want to thank Ingrid Leitinger for the radiosynthesis of [^{11}C]mHED and her support, as well as the whole PET/MRI team, namely Daniela Senn, Benedikt Schmiedinger, Julia Kesselbacher,

Rainer Bartosch, and Iulia Ponce. Furthermore, we want to thank Thomas Zenz und Andreas Krcal for their technical support.

References

1. WHO. Cardiovascular Disease. Available online: https://www.who.int/cardiovascular_diseases/en/ (accessed on 30 November 2018).
2. WHO. Fact Sheet. Available online: https://www.who.int/mediacentre/factsheets/fs310.pdf (accessed on 30 November 2018).
3. Någren, K.; Müller, L.; Halldin, C.; Swahn, C.G.; Lehikoinen, P. Improved synthesis of some commonly used PET radioligands by the use of [11C]methyl triflate. *Nucl. Med. Biol.* **1995**, *22*, 235–239. [CrossRef]
4. Rosenspire, K.C.; Haka, M.S.; Van Dort, M.E.; Jewett, D.M.; Gildersleeve, D.L.; Schwaiger, M.; Wieland, D.M. Synthesis and preliminary evaluation of carbon-11-meta-hydroxyephedrine: A false transmitter agent for heart neuronal imaging. *J. Nucl. Med.* **1990**, *31*, 1328–1334.
5. Bonfiglioli, R.; Nanni, C.; Martignani, C.; Zanoni, L.; La Donna, R.; Diemberger, I.; Boriani, G.; Pettinato, C.; Sambuceti, G.; Fanti, S.; et al. 11C-mHED for PET/CT: Principles of synthesis, methodology and first clinical applications. *Curr. Radiopharm.* **2014**, *7*, 79–83. [CrossRef] [PubMed]
6. Todeschini, P.; Carpinelli, A.; Savi, A.; Manca, E.; Picchio, M.; Gianolli, L. [11C]Meta-Hydroxyephedrine PET/CT. *Curr. Radiopharm.* **2010**, *3*, 1–9. [CrossRef]
7. Kunze, K.P.; Nekolla, S.G.; Rischpler, C.; Zhang, S.H.; Hayes, C.; Langwieser, N.; Ibrahim, T.; Laugwitz, K.-L.; Schwaiger, M. Myocardial perfusion quantification using simultaneously acquired $^{13}NH_3$-ammonia PET and dynamic contrast-enhanced MRI in patients at rest and stress. *Magn. Reson. Med.* **2018**, *80*, 2641–2654. [CrossRef] [PubMed]
8. Quarta, C.; Lodi, F.; Mazza, R.; Giannone, F.; Boschi, L.; Nanni, C.; Nisoli, E.; Boschi, S.; Pasquali, R.; Fanti, S.; et al. (11)C-meta-hydroxyephedrine PET/CT imaging allows in vivo study of adaptive thermogenesis and white-to-brown fat conversion. *Mol. Metab.* **2013**, *2*, 153–160. [CrossRef] [PubMed]
9. Izzi-Engbeaya, C.; Salem, V.; Atkar, R.S.; Dhillo, W.S. Insights into Brown Adipose Tissue Physiology as Revealed by Imaging Studies. *Adipocyte* **2015**, *4*, 1–12. [CrossRef] [PubMed]
10. Li, J.; Yang, C.-H. Improvement of preoperative management in patients with adrenal pheochromocytoma. *Int. J. Clin. Exp. Med.* **2014**, *7*, 5541–5546. [PubMed]
11. Mann, G.N.; Link, J.M.; Pham, P.; Pickett, C.A.; Byrd, D.R.; Kinahan, P.E.; Krohn, K.A.; Mankoff, D.A. [11C]metahydroxyephedrine and [18F]fluorodeoxyglucose positron emission tomography improve clinical decision making in suspected pheochromocytoma. *Ann. Surg. Oncol.* **2006**, *13*, 187–197. [CrossRef] [PubMed]
12. Lodi, F.; Rizzello, A.; Carpinelli, A.; Di Pierro, D.; Cicoria, G.; Mesisca, V.; Marengo, M.; Boschi, S. Automated synthesis of [11C]meta hydroxyephedrine, a PET radiopharmaceutical for studying sympathetic innervation in the heart. In Proceedings of the Computers in Cardiology, Bologna, Italy, 14–17 September 2008; Volume 35, pp. 341–343.
13. Dort, M.E.V.; Tluczek, L. Synthesis and carbon-11 labeling of the stereoisomers of meta-hydroxyephedrine (HED) and meta-hydroxypseudoephedrine (HPED). *Off. J. Int. Isot. Soc.* **2000**, *43*, 603–612.
14. Law, M.P.; Schäfers, K.; Kopka, K.; Wagner, S.; Schober, O.; Schäfers, M. Molecular imaging of cardiac sympathetic innervation by 11C-mHED and PET: From man to mouse? *J. Nucl. Med.* **2010**, *51*, 1269–1276. [CrossRef] [PubMed]
15. Werner, R.A.; Rischpler, C.; Onthank, D.; Lapa, C.; Robinson, S.; Samnick, S.; Javadi, M.; Schwaiger, M.; Nekolla, S.G.; Higuchi, T. Retention Kinetics of the 18F-Labeled Sympathetic Nerve PET Tracer LMI1195: Comparison with 11C-Hydroxyephedrine and 123I-MIBG. *J. Nucl. Med.* **2015**, *56*, 1429–1433. [CrossRef] [PubMed]
16. Werner, R.A.; Chen, X.; Maya, Y.; Eissler, C.; Hirano, M.; Nose, N.; Wakabayashi, H.; Lapa, C.; Javadi, M.S.; Higuchi, T. The Impact of Ageing on 11C-Hydroxyephedrine Uptake in the Rat Heart. *Sci. Rep.* **2018**, *8*, 11120. [CrossRef] [PubMed]
17. Foley, K.F.; Van Dort, M.E.; Sievert, M.K.; Ruoho, A.E.; Cozzi, N.V. Stereospecific inhibition of monoamine uptake transporters by meta-hydroxyephedrine isomers. *J. Neural Transm.* **2002**, *109*, 1229–1240. [CrossRef] [PubMed]

18. Rami-Mark, C.; Berroterán-Infante, N.; Philippe, C.; Foltin, S.; Vraka, C.; Hoepping, A.; Lanzenberger, R.; Hacker, M.; Mitterhauser, M.; Wadsak, W. Radiosynthesis and first preclinical evaluation of the novel norepinephrine transporter pet-ligand [(11)C]ME@HAPTHI. *EJNMMI Res.* **2015**, *5*, 113. [CrossRef] [PubMed]
19. Nics, L.; Steiner, B.; Klebermass, E.-M.; Philippe, C.; Mitterhauser, M.; Hacker, M.; Wadsak, W. Speed matters to raise molar radioactivity: Fast HPLC shortens the quality control of C-11 PET-tracers. *Nucl. Med. Biol.* **2018**, *57*, 28–33. [CrossRef]
20. Torigian, D.A.; Zaidi, H.; Kwee, T.C.; Saboury, B.; Udupa, J.K.; Cho, Z.-H.; Alavi, A. PET/MR Imaging: Technical Aspects and Potential Clinical Applications. *Radiology* **2013**, *267*, 26–44. [CrossRef]

9

Design, Synthesis, In Vitro and Initial In Vivo Evaluation of Heterobivalent Peptidic Ligands Targeting Both NPY(Y$_1$)- and GRP-Receptors— An Improvement for Breast Cancer Imaging?

Alicia Vall-Sagarra [1], **Shanna Litau** [1,2], **Clemens Decristoforo** [3] (ID), **Björn Wängler** [2], **Ralf Schirrmacher** [4] (ID), **Gert Fricker** [5] and **Carmen Wängler** [1,*]

[1] Biomedical Chemistry, Department of Clinical Radiology and Nuclear Medicine, Medical Faculty Mannheim of Heidelberg University, Theodor-Kutzer-Ufer 1-3, 68167 Mannheim, Germany; Alicia.Vall-Sagarra@medma.uni-heidelberg.de (A.V.-S.); Shanna.Litau@medma.uni-heidelberg.de (S.L.)

[2] Molecular Imaging and Radiochemistry, Department of Clinical Radiology and Nuclear Medicine, Medical Faculty Mannheim of Heidelberg University, Theodor-Kutzer-Ufer 1-3, 68167 Mannheim, Germany; Bjoern.Waengler@medma.uni-heidelberg.de

[3] Department of Nuclear Medicine, University Hospital Innsbruck, Medical University Innsbruck, Anichstrasse 35, 6020 Innsbruck, Austria; Clemens.Decristoforo@tirol-kliniken.at

[4] Department of Oncology, Division Oncological Imaging, University of Alberta, 11560 University Avenue, Edmonton, AB T6G 1Z2, Canada; schirrma@ualberta.ca

[5] Institute of Pharmacy and Molecular Biotechnology, University of Heidelberg, Im Neuenheimer Feld 329, 69120 Heidelberg, Germany; gert.fricker@uni-hd.de

* Correspondence: Carmen.Waengler@medma.uni-heidelberg.de

Abstract: Heterobivalent peptidic ligands (HBPLs), designed to address two different receptors independently, are highly promising tumor imaging agents. For example, breast cancer has been shown to concomitantly and complementarily overexpress the neuropeptide Y receptor subtype 1 (NPY(Y$_1$)R) as well as the gastrin-releasing peptide receptor (GRPR). Thus, radiolabeled HBPLs being able to bind these two receptors should exhibit an improved tumor targeting efficiency compared to monospecific ligands. We developed here such bispecific HBPLs and radiolabeled them with ^{68}Ga, achieving high radiochemical yields, purities, and molar activities. We evaluated the HBPLs and their monospecific reference peptides in vitro regarding stability and uptake into different breast cancer cell lines and found that the ^{68}Ga-HBPLs were efficiently taken up via the GRPR. We also performed in vivo PET/CT imaging and ex vivo biodistribution studies in T-47D tumor-bearing mice for the most promising ^{68}Ga-HBPL and compared the results to those obtained for its scrambled analogs. The tumors could easily be visualized by the newly developed ^{68}Ga-HBPL and considerably higher tumor uptakes and tumor-to-background ratios were obtained compared to the scrambled analogs in and ex vivo. These results demonstrate the general feasibility of the approach to use bispecific radioligands for in vivo imaging of breast cancer.

Keywords: breast cancer; ^{68}Ga; GRPR; NPY(Y$_1$)R; peptide heterodimers; PET/CT imaging

1. Introduction

Radiolabeled peptides, being able to specifically bind certain receptors overexpressed on many malignancies, have become standard radiotracers for tumor-specific imaging by positron emission tomography (PET) in a clinical routine. However, these radiolabeled peptides are able to address only one target receptor type, being thus only able to visualize tumors expressing this particular receptor.

As different tumor lesions can however overexpress different receptor types and receptor expression can change upon metastasis and disease progression, a monovalent peptidic radioligand is often not able to visualize all tumor cells with the same efficiency and some lesions might be completely missed by the applied radiopeptide.

Radiolabeled heterobivalent peptide ligands (HBPLs) on the other hand—by their ability to specifically target more than one receptor type—have been proposed to be better-suited agents for tumor imaging as they enable the visualization of the tumor by different receptor types potentially overexpressed by the target cells [1,2].

HBPLs furthermore can have favorable effects for in vivo tumor imaging compared to monovalent ligands such as improved in vivo biodistribution and enhanced avidity caused by simultaneous binding if both receptors are present on the tumor cell surface. In this case, also a higher probability of rebinding is achieved for a heterobivalent binder in case of dissociation from the receptor compared to a monovalent peptide due to "forced proximity" of the second potential binder to the second target receptor.

Furthermore, by being able to target different receptor types on the tumor cell surface, an overall higher number of receptors can be addressed by a heterobivalent ligand, increasing the probability of binding and thus tumor visualization. Thus, HBPLs are also of special interest not only for the imaging of such tumors that express both receptor types concomitantly, but also for tumors exhibiting a heterogeneous target expression with varying receptor densities between different individuals or lesions and for differential target expression during disease progression. A non-uniform distribution of target receptors between lesions results—if using monomeric peptidic radioligands—in the visualization of only some of the lesions whereas others are not depicted. Applying a HBPL for imaging, such lesions can nevertheless be addressed as long as one of the target receptors is present (Figure 1).

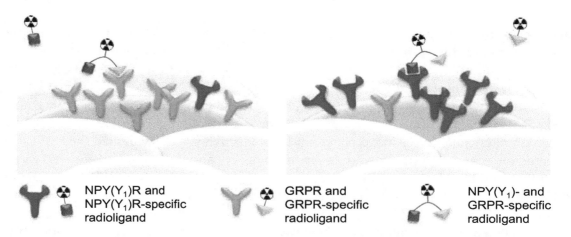

NPY(Y$_1$)R and NPY(Y$_1$)R-specific radioligand

GRPR and GRPR-specific radioligand

NPY(Y$_1$)- and GRPR-specific radioligand

Figure 1. Schematic depiction of the functional principle of radiolabeled NPY(Y$_1$)R- and gastrin-releasing peptide receptor (GRPR)-binding heterobivalent peptidic ligands (HBPLs) for tumor imaging: Monomeric peptide radiotracers can only bind to one receptor type and thus miss tumor tissues or lesions that do not express the respective receptor due to tumor heterogeneity or disease progression whereas the use of radiolabeled HBPLs, which can bind to more than one target receptor type, results in a higher probability of target visualization.

Recently, a radiolabeled HBPL, being able to address the gastrin-releasing peptide receptor as well as integrin $\alpha_v\beta_3$ was successfully translated into the clinics for imaging of prostate cancer with PET/CT, showing a much higher tumor visualization sensitivity compared to the respective GRPR-targeting peptide monomer. This proves the clinical relevance of the heterobivalent peptide targeting concept [3].

To be able to develop a HBPL being able to more efficiently target tumor tissues than the respective peptide monomers, it is necessary to know the receptor expression profile on the target tumor type.

Regarding this point, some excellent systematical work has been carried out, determining the presence of certain receptor types and their densities on different human malignancies [2,4–6].

Human breast cancer, for example, overexpresses in about 75% of all cases the gastrin-releasing peptide receptor (GRPR) [7] and in 66–85% the neuropeptide Y receptor subtype 1 (NPY(Y_1)R) [8]. Both receptors are expressed to an insignificant amount on healthy breast tissue, thus rendering both receptor types well-suited target structures for sensitive and specific breast cancer imaging. Furthermore, Reubi and co-workers could show on 68 human breast cancer samples that 63/68 (93%) overexpressed one or both receptor types. Of these, 32 (51%) expressed both receptors concomitantly, whereas 18 (29%) expressed only the GRPR, and a further 13 (21%) expressed only the NPY(Y_1)R [5]. Thus, the combination of two peptidic ligands being able to specifically bind the NPY(Y_1)R and the GRPR to one radioligand should enable a considerably higher breast cancer visualization efficiency and sensitivity and thus give less false-negative results compared to the respective monovalent radioligands (Figure 1).

To obtain a highly potent bispecific HBPL, it is mandatory that both peptide parts of the construct are still able to bind to their respective target receptor type despite the considerable chemical modifications necessary for peptide heterodimerization. Thus, a suitable molecular design has to be found that enables the binding of both peptides to their respective target receptor.

So far, only one example of a heterobivalent NPY(Y_1)R- and GRPR-targeting ligand has been described [9,10] and for this substance, no descriptions of radiolabeling with a PET isotope, in vitro cell uptake or in vivo imaging data are available. Thus, the general feasibility of the approach has not been demonstrated so far.

Thus, the aims of this study were to: (i) Develop a synthesis strategy yielding different HBPLs varying in molecular design and consisting of a NPY(Y_1)- and a GRPR-affine peptide as well as a chelating agent (for radiolabeling with the positron-emitting radiometal nuclide ^{68}Ga); (ii) Establish the ^{68}Ga-radiolabeling and determine the $\log_D$ and in vitro stability of the resulting ^{68}Ga-HBPLs in human serum; (iii) Evaluate the uptake of the ^{68}Ga-HBPLs into human breast cancer cell lines in vitro to determine if the substances can still interact with both target receptors and are taken up by the tumor cells; (iv) Determine if the particular molecular design used has a measurable influence on tumor cell uptake; and (v) Show the general feasibility of the approach by investigating the tumor uptake of the most potent HBPL in vivo by PET/CT imaging and ex vivo biodistribution in a proof-of-concept study and determine if the tumor uptake profits from the heterodimerization of the receptor-specific peptides.

2. Results and Discussion

2.1. Synthesis of GRPR- and NPY(Y_1)R-Binding HBPLs 22–26, Scrambled HBPL Analogs 24a–c, Blocking Agents 3 and 4 as well as Monomeric Reference Peptides 27 and 28

At first, a suitable synthesis strategy towards the GRPR- and NPY(Y_1)R-binding HBPLs was developed. The target molecular design of the substances is depicted in Figure 2 and was based on the following considerations: (i) The structure was to be based on a symmetrically branched scaffold to obtain homogenous products and the scaffold should comprise the chelator NODA-GA ((1,4,7-triazacyclononane-4,7-diyl)diacetic acid-1-glutaric acid), which is able to stably and efficiently complex ^{68}Ga [11]; (ii) The chelator should be spatially separated from the receptor-affine peptides by a short PEG linker to prevent an interference of the radiometal complex with receptor binding [12]; (iii) As we and others were able to show before for peptide di- and multimers, the distance between the peptides within the same molecule can have a significant influence on the achievable receptor interaction [13–16], thus different distances between both peptidic receptor ligands should be investigated for the target HBPLs by introducing linkers of different length; (iv) Furthermore, as it was proposed that also the rigidity of the molecules might influence cellular uptakes by a conformational stabilization of the spatial orientation of the receptor ligands, the used linker structures did not only differ in length, but also in rigidity.

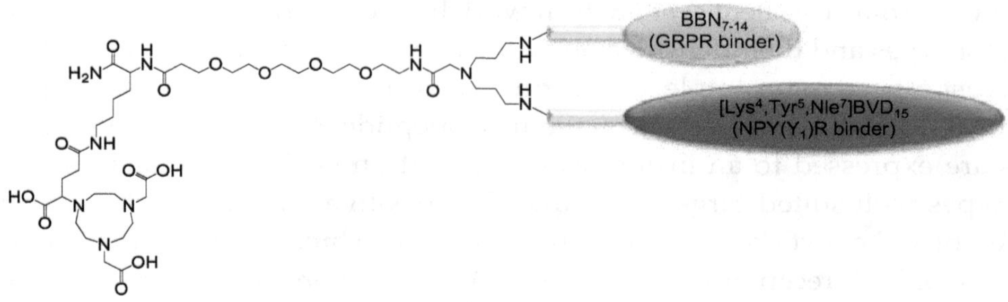

Figure 2. Schematic depiction of the general molecular design of the target HBPLs consisting of a chelating agent (NODA-GA), a short PEG_4-linker between radiometal complex and peptides, the symmetrical branching unit, the linkers of different length and rigidity (green) and the GRPR- and $NPY(Y_1)R$-binding peptides BBN_{7-14} (cyan) and $[Lys^4,Trp^5,Nle^7]BVD_{15}$ (magenta).

2.1.1. Synthesis of the Peptide Monomers 1−6

Aiming at the synthesis of GRPR-and $NPY(Y_1)R$-binding HBPLs and their following in vitro and in vivo evaluation in human breast cancer tumor cells, we first synthesized the respective peptide monomers for subsequent heterodimerization on symmetrically branched scaffolds. As GRPR-affine peptide monomer, we chose the receptor agonist PESIN (PEG_4-BBN_{7-14}), which exhibits a favorably high stability, significant tumor uptake, as well as high tumor to background ratios in vivo [17,18], and can be modified at its N-terminal end without considerably changing its receptor binding affinity [13]. As $NPY(Y_1)R$-affine peptide monomer, we chose $[Lys^4,Trp^5,Nle^7]BVD_{15}$ as this peptide was shown to exhibit good affinities to the $NPY(Y_1)R$ even when further modified in position four [9,19,20].

The peptides were to be conjugated to the symmetrically branched scaffolds by a click chemistry approach to be able to obtain the desired rather complex target HBPLs efficiently. Furthermore, the coupling products have to be stable under physiological conditions. Different click chemistry reactions fulfill these requirements; of these, we chose the oxime formation between aminooxy functionalities and aldehydes.

Both peptides were synthesized by standard solid phase peptide synthesis (SPPS) methods [13,21] by successive conjugation of the respective N_α-Fmoc-amino acids after HBTU activation to the respective rink amide resin and finally modified on resin with *bis*-Boc-aminooxy acetic acid, giving aminooxy-PESIN (1) and $[Lys^4(aminooxy),Trp^5,Nle^7]BVD_{15}$ (2) (Figure 3). In case of PESIN, the aminooxy functionality was introduced at the N-terminal end as the peptide can be modified in this position without considerable alterations in binding affinity. In case of $[Lys^4,Trp^5,Nle^7]BVD_{15}$, the aminooxy functionality was introduced in position 4 (N_ε amine of lysine) as modifications in this position interfere least with receptor binding.

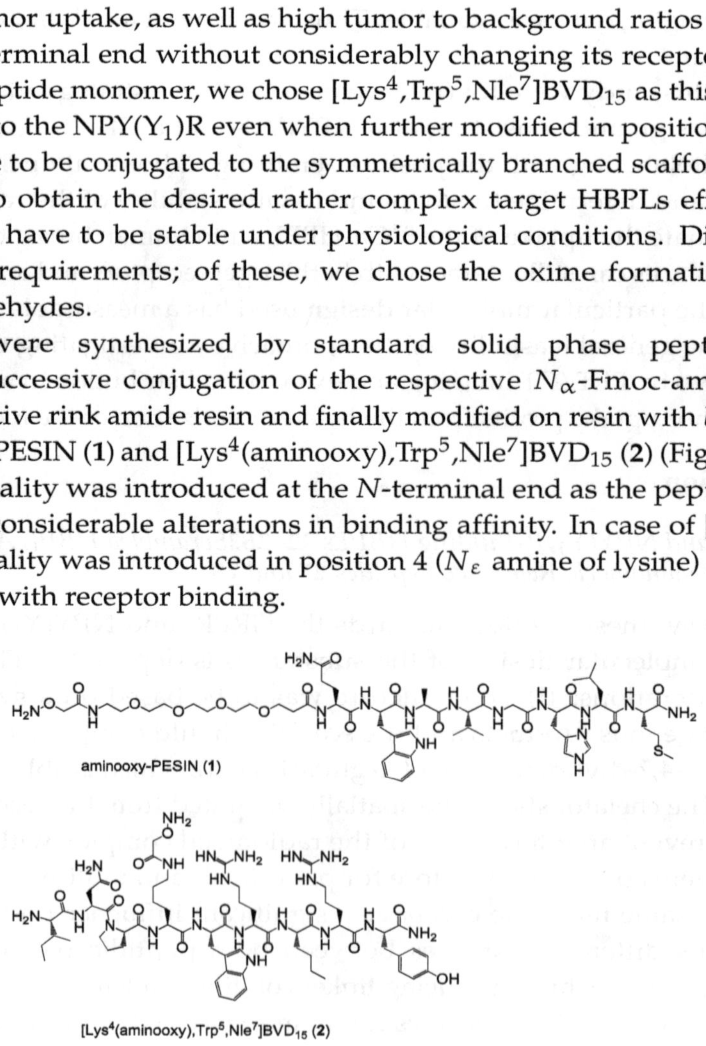

Figure 3. Depiction of the chemical structures of aminooxy-PESIN (1) and $[Lys^4(aminooxy),Trp^5,Nle^7]BVD_{15}$ (2) used for the assembly of the HBPLs.

As the target HBPLs should be evaluated in vitro regarding their ability to be taken up by human breast cancer cell lines and the contribution of both parts of the HBPLs on tumor cell uptake should be assessed, we further synthesized the peptide monomers bombesin (**3**) and [Lys^4,Trp^5,Nle^7]BVD$_{15}$ (**4**) as blocking substances for the GRPR and the NPY(Y$_1$)R during these experiments (Figure 4).

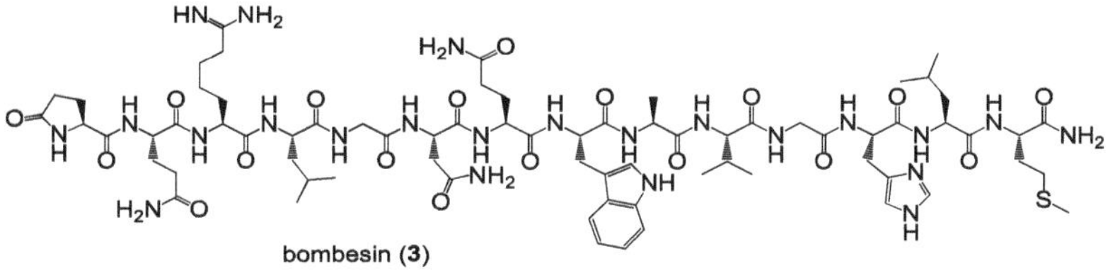

bombesin (**3**)

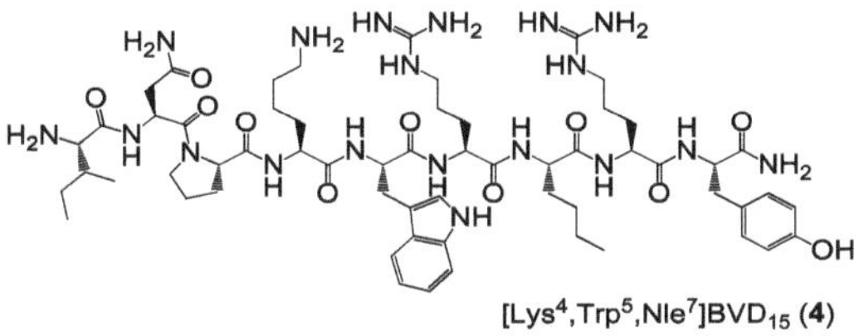

[Lys^4,Trp^5,Nle^7]BVD$_{15}$ (**4**)

Figure 4. Depiction of the chemical structures of bombesin (**3**) and [Lys^4,Trp^5,Nle^7]BVD$_{15}$ (**4**) used as receptor blocking substances during the in vitro tumor cell uptake studies.

Regarding the in vivo evaluation of the HBPLs in tumor-bearing animals and the verification of the receptor specificity of the observed tumor uptakes and the contribution of both peptides of the HBPLs to overall tumor uptakes, two different approaches can be followed. The first one is to block the respective target receptor analogous to the in vitro assays by adding blocking substances **3** or **4** and the other one is to use scrambled HBPL analogs. To compare the in vivo tumor uptake of an HBPL to that of its scrambled analogs instead of performing blocking studies however eliminates possible difficulties that might arise from the low stability of the monomeric receptor ligands.

Thus, three different scrambled HBPL analogs were synthesized: PESIN combined with scrambled [Lys^4(aminooxy),Trp^5,Nle^7]BVD$_{15}$, scrambled PESIN combined with [Lys^4(aminooxy), Trp^5,Nle^7]BVD$_{15}$ and both peptides of the HBPL scrambled. For this purpose, the two scrambled aminooxy-modified peptide monomers aminooxy-PESIN$_{scrambled}$ (**5**) and [Lys^4(aminooxy),Trp^5,Nle^7] BVD$_{15,scrambled}$ (**6**) (Figure 5) were synthesized and analogously to **1** and **2** used during the following HBPL syntheses.

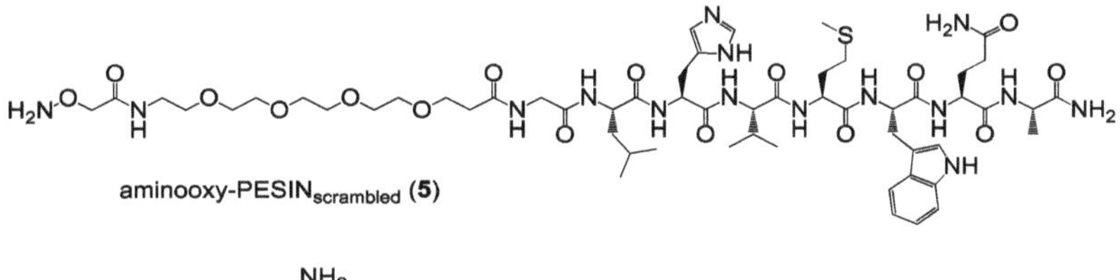

aminooxy-PESIN$_{scrambled}$ (**5**)

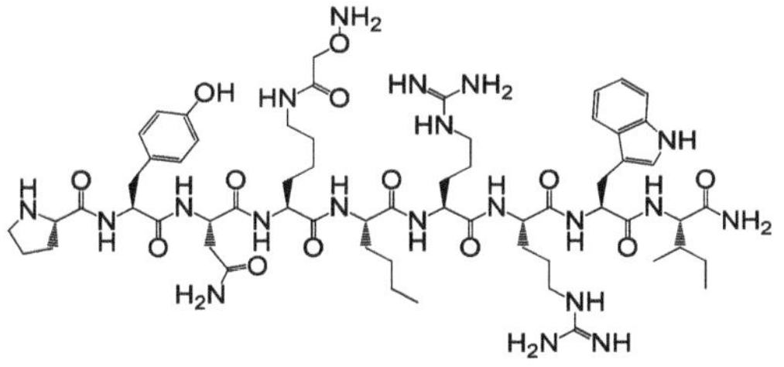

[Lys^4(aminooxy),Trp^5,Nle^7]BVD$_{15,scrambled}$ (**6**)

Figure 5. Depiction of the chemical structures of aminooxy-PESIN$_{scrambled}$ (**5**) and [Lys^4(aminooxy), Trp^5,Nle^7]BVD$_{15,scrambled}$ (**6**) which were used to synthesize partly or fully scrambled HBPL analogs.

2.1.2. Synthesis of the Heterobivalent Ligands 22–26, 24a–c and Monomeric Reference Peptides 27 and 28

The branched *bis*-amines 7−11 and *bis*-aldehydes 12−16 (Scheme 1) were synthesized following a published procedure [22] with minor modifications (see Supplementary Materials for detailed description). In the following, these NODA-GA-modified branched *bis*-aldehyde scaffolds 12−16 were efficiently reacted with aminooxy-PESIN (1) and aminooxy-PESIN$_{scrambled}$ (5) to the monovalent intermediates 17−21 and 19a. These were further reacted with [Lys^4(aminooxy),Trp^5,Nle^7]BVD$_{15}$ (2) and its scrambled analog 6 to the final heterobivalent peptidic target structures 22−26 and their partly or fully scrambled analogs 24a–c (Scheme 1).

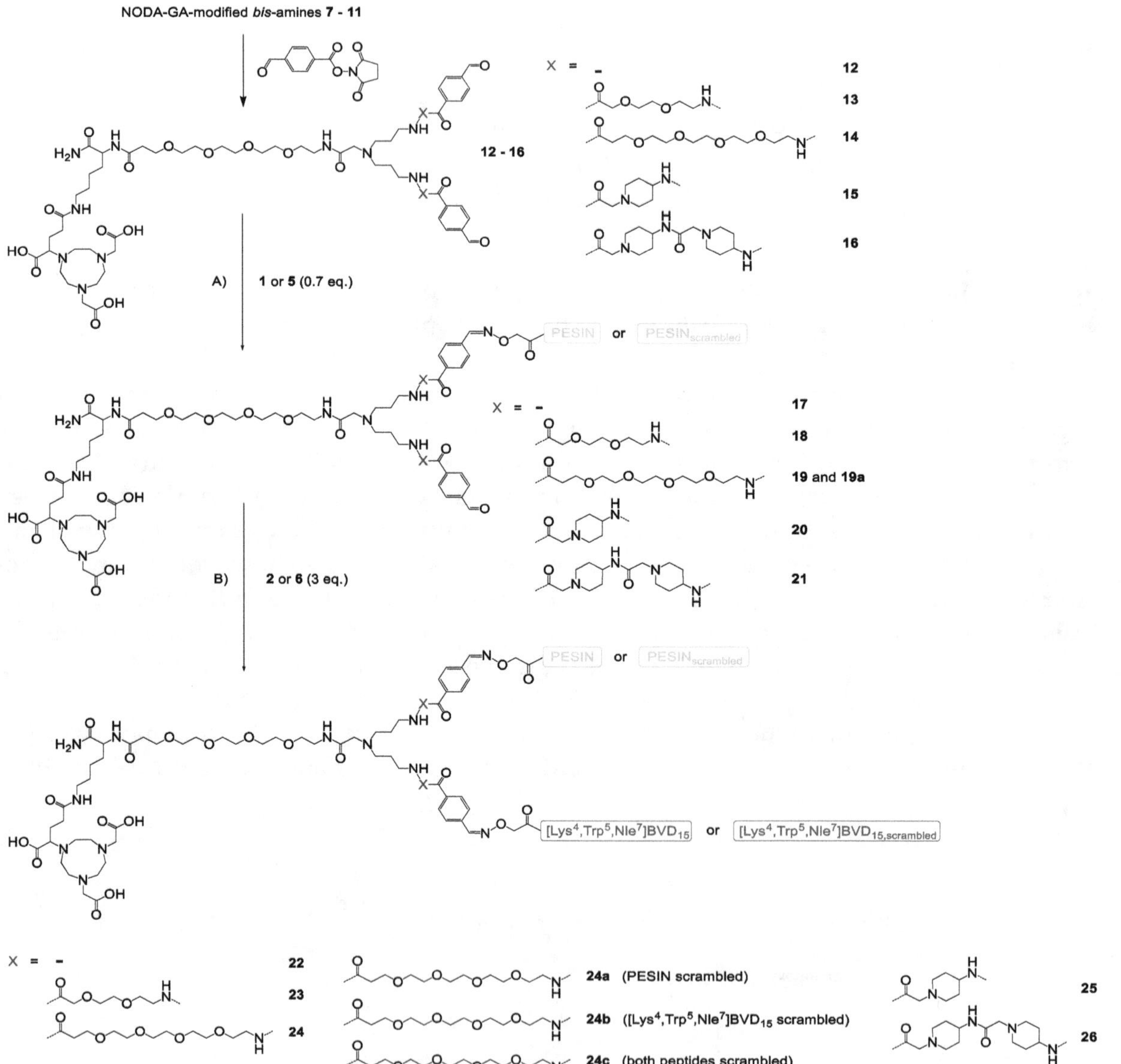

Scheme 1. Schematic depiction of the syntheses of the GRPR- and NPY(Y$_1$)R-affine HBPLs 22−26 and the scrambled analogs 24a–c. Conditions: **(A)** 1, H$_2$O + 0.1% TFA, phosphate buffer, pH 4.0−4.6, RT, 5 min, yields: 47% for 17, 51% for 18, 43% for 19, 44% for 19a, 58% for 20, 55% for 21; **(B)** 2, H$_2$O + 0.1% TFA, phosphate buffer, pH 4.0−4.6, RT, 5 min, yields: 82% for 22, 79% for 23, 66% for 24, 49% for 24a, 63% for 24b, 61% for 24c, 75% for 25, 73% for 26.

1 as well as its scrambled analog **5** reacted efficiently within minutes with the branched *bis*-aldehydes **12−16**, giving the respective monovalent conjugation products **17−21** and **19a** in satisfactory yields of 47% to 58%. Higher yields could not be obtained as **1** and **5** had to be applied in a lower amount than the *bis*-aldehydes **12−16** to minimize the formation of the respective homobivalent PESIN-dimers, being the only observed side products in this reaction. These monovalent intermediates were in the following reacted with **2** or **6**, proceeding equally efficient than the first reaction step within minutes, giving the target HBPLs **22−26** as well as the scrambled analogs **24a–c** in good yields of 49% to 82%.

The HBPLs exhibited—depending on the linker structure used—distances between both peptidic receptor ligands of 46 (no additional linker units used), 64 (PEG_2 linkers), 78 (PEG_4 linkers), 60 (ACMP linkers), and 74 (two successive ACMP linkers) bond lengths.

Besides the target HBPLs and the scrambled analogs, also the monomeric reference compounds DOTA-PESIN (**27**) [18] and [Lys^4(DOTA),Trp^5,Nle^7]BVD_{15} (**28**) [19] (Figure 6) (DOTA = (1,4,7,10-tetraazacyclododecane-1,4,7,10-tetrayl)tetraacetic acid), having been described before to be potent agents efficiently targeting the GRPR and NPY(Y_1)R, were synthesized in yields of 7% and 45%, respectively. These ligands, addressing only one of the target receptors types, served as monomeric reference compounds for the following in vitro evaluations.

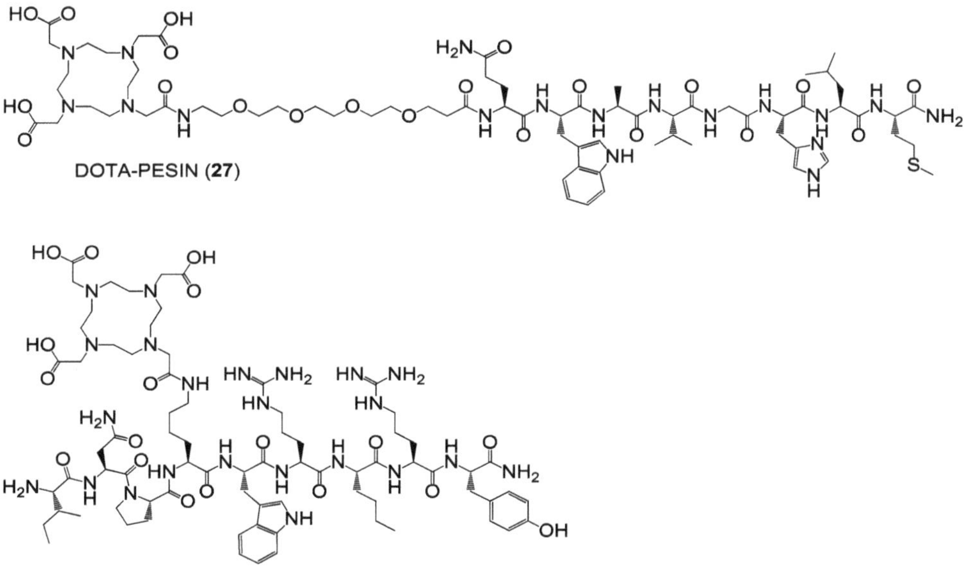

DOTA-PESIN (**27**)

[Lys^4(DOTA),Trp^5,Nle^7]BVD_{15} (**28**)

Figure 6. Depiction of the structures of DOTA-PESIN (**27**) and [Lys^4(DOTA),Trp^5,Nle^7]BVD_{15} (**28**), serving as mono-specific reference substances for the HBPLs in the following in vitro tumor cell uptake studies.

2.2. ^{68}Ga-Radiolabeling, log$_D$ and Stability Determination of Peptide Heterodimers [^{68}Ga]22−[^{68}Ga]26 and Monomeric Reference Peptides [^{68}Ga]27 and [^{68}Ga]28

The heterobivalent ligands **22−26** and the reference substances **27** and **28** were in the following radiolabeled with ^{68}Ga^{3+}. The ^{68}Ga^{3+} was obtained via elution of an itG or Eckert & Ziegler IGG100 ^{68}Ge/^{68}Ga generator system. After adjusting the pH of the solution to 3.5 to 4.0, the NODA-GA-comprising HBPLs **22−26** were incubated at 40–45 °C for 10 min. The DOTA-comprising reference compounds **27** and **28** were reacted at 99 °C under otherwise identical conditions. The ^{68}Ga-labeled products [^{68}Ga]22−[^{68}Ga]26, [^{68}Ga]27 and [^{68}Ga]28 were obtained in radiochemical yields and purities of 95−99% (Figure S1A) as well as non-optimized molar activities of 10−15 GBq/μmol (used for in vitro assays and obtained by using an itG generator system) or

40−46 GBq/µmol (used for in vivo evaluations, obtained by using an Eckert & Ziegler IGG100 generator system), starting from 110−150 or 420–460 MBq of $^{68}Ga^{3+}$, respectively.

Regarding a favorable in vivo biodistribution of the radioligands, the $\log_D$ of the HBPLs should be in a comparable range as that of the lead peptide monomers as we and others were able to show before that a high lipophilicity negatively influences tumor uptake, organ distribution, and unspecific background accumulation, resulting in a limited usefulness of the radiopeptides for tumor visualization [23–25]. Consequently, we determined the $\log_D$ of the developed HBPLs [^{68}Ga]22−[^{68}Ga]26 in comparison to the monomeric reference peptides [^{68}Ga]27 and [^{68}Ga]28 via the distribution coefficient of the respective radiotracer between phosphate buffer and 1-octanol. The results of these evaluations are depicted in Figure S2. The results showed a comparatively high hydrophilicity for all of the tested substances (-1.857 ± 0.054 for [^{68}Ga]27, -1.982 ± 0.162 for [^{68}Ga]28, -1.569 ± 0.111 for [^{68}Ga]22, -1.527 ± 0.109 for [^{68}Ga]23, -1.672 ± 0.086 for [^{68}Ga]24, -1.550 ± 0.114 for [^{68}Ga]25 and -1.518 ± 0.089 for [^{68}Ga]26). This indicates that the in vivo pharmacokinetics of the developed HBPLs [^{68}Ga]22−[^{68}Ga]26 should, in terms of hydrophilicity, be similar to that of the parent monomeric radiopeptides [^{68}Ga]27 and [^{68}Ga]28.

Besides lipophilicity, the stability of peptidic radioligands is an important parameter regarding their applicability for in vivo imaging. Thus, the stability of the ^{68}Ga-labeled HBPLs [^{68}Ga]22−[^{68}Ga]26 and the reference compounds [^{68}Ga]27 and [^{68}Ga]28 was determined in human serum. Typical radio-HPLC chromatograms for each substance (obtained after 90 min incubation with human serum) are depicted in Figure S1B. All of the tested compounds were stable over the testing period of 90 min, showing only a negligible degradation after this time: $3 \pm 0.2\%$ for [^{68}Ga]27, $4 \pm 0.8\%$ for [^{68}Ga]28, $2 \pm 1.6\%$ for [^{68}Ga]22, $1 \pm 0.5\%$ for [^{68}Ga]23, no observable fragmentation for [^{68}Ga]24, $2 \pm 0.3\%$ for [^{68}Ga]25 and $2 \pm 0.5\%$ for [^{68}Ga]26. From the serum stability point of view—which can however only give a rough estimation of stability under in vivo conditions [26]—all of the radioligands are applicable for in vivo tumor imaging with PET/computed tomography (CT).

2.3. In Vitro Cell Uptake Studies: Tumor Cell Uptake of [^{68}Ga]22−[^{68}Ga]26 in Comparison to the Reference Peptides [^{68}Ga]27 and [^{68}Ga]28 in Different Human Breast Cancer Cell Lines

In the following, we intended to determine if we could observe an independent binding of both peptide parts of the HBPLs to both target receptor types, being the prerequisite for improved/more likely tumor uptake (→ Figure 1). This can be achieved by tumor cell uptake studies of the radiotracers as it was shown before for radiolabeled somatostatin analogs that the in vitro cell uptake directly correlates to in vivo tumor uptakes [27], demonstrating the relevance of such in vitro tumor cell uptake studies.

The human breast cancer cell line T-47D was described to express both the GRPR [9,28] as well as the NPY(Y$_1$)R [29,30] (where β-estradiol in the medium increases NPY(Y$_1$)R-expression) and thus should be the ideal cell line to determine if both parts of the developed HBPLs bind to their respective receptor and if a synergistic effect of peptide heterodimerization on tumor cell uptake can be achieved. Of course, it would also have been feasible to use different cells lines expressing either the GRPR or the NPY(Y$_1$)R to demonstrate that both peptides of the HBPLs are still able to address their respective target receptor, but a cell line expressing both receptors concomitantly is far more advantageous to showcase the potential beneficial effects of heterodimerization and to determine the part each of the peptides contributes to tumor cell uptake in case of a concomitant receptor expression.

Thus, we first determined the uptake of the HBPLs [^{68}Ga]22−[^{68}Ga]26 in comparison to the peptide monomers [^{68}Ga]27 and [^{68}Ga]28 in T-47D cells. The results of the cell uptake studies of the radioligands are shown in Figure 7a (overall specific cell uptake of [^{68}Ga]22−[^{68}Ga]26, [^{68}Ga]27 and [^{68}Ga]28) and Figure 7b (uptake of [^{68}Ga]24, differentiated by overall uptake, internalization and surface binding; the results for the other tested radioligands were comparable and can be found in the Supplementary Materials in Figures S3–S7).

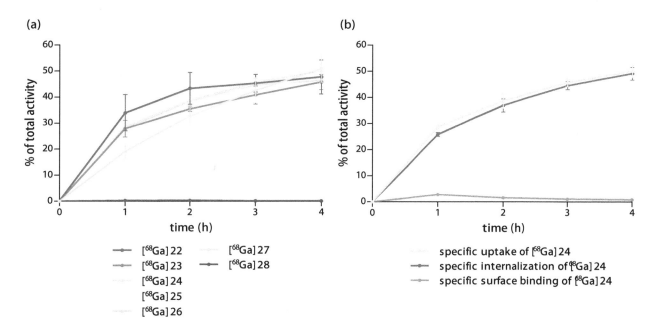

Figure 7. (a) Specific cell uptake of [^{68}Ga]**22**−[^{68}Ga]**26**, [^{68}Ga]**27** and [^{68}Ga]**28** in T-47D cells over 4 h of incubation; **(b)** Uptake of [^{68}Ga]**24** in the same cells, differentiated by overall uptake, internalization, and surface binding.

As expected, a high and constant specific uptake of the monovalent GRPR-specific peptide [^{68}Ga]**27** of 51.0 ± 5.2% was observed into the T-47D cells after 4 h. Also, the HBPLs [^{68}Ga]**22**−[^{68}Ga]**26** demonstrated a comparably high specific uptake into these cells of 47.8 ± 6.5%, 45.8 ± 2.9%, 50.1 ± 2.4%, 48.2 ± 2.8% and 46.4 ± 2.4%, respectively, after the same time. Interestingly, the monovalent, NPY(Y$_1$)-binding peptide [^{68}Ga]**28** showed no specific uptake (0.2 ± 0.03%). This means that the uptake of the HBPLs [^{68}Ga]**22**−[^{68}Ga]**26** into the T-47D cells is exclusively mediated by the GRPR.

These results indicate that the heterodimerization and the resulting significant chemical modification of the peptides as well as the compounds' complexity and size do not affect the GRPR-specific tumor cell uptake of the HBPLs compared to the monomeric reference [^{68}Ga]**27**. Also, the molecular design of the heterobivalent ligands comprising linkers of different length and rigidity does not seem to have a significant effect on the GRPR-mediated cellular uptake of the respective HBPL radiotracer.

In the following, we tested the uptake of the peptide monomers [^{68}Ga]**27** and [^{68}Ga]**28** in three further standard cell lines of breast cancer: BT-474, MCF-7 and MDA-MB-231 cells. Of these, the BT-474 cells were also described to express both the GRPR [31] and the NPY(Y$_1$)R [31], whereas MCF-7 cells were described to be NPY(Y$_1$)R positive [30,32] but expressing the GRPR only to a low extent [9] and MDA-MB-231 cells were described to be GRPR positive [33] but expressing the NPY(Y$_1$)R to a low extent [29,30]. The results of these experiments can be found in the Supplementary Materials (Figures S8–S10) and demonstrated contrary to the expectations only negligible uptakes of both peptide monomers in all cell lines.

As the HBPLs [^{68}Ga]**22**−[^{68}Ga]**26** and the respective monomer [^{68}Ga]**27** were however shown to be efficiently taken up by GRPR-positive T-47D cells, these results indicate that the GRPR is present to an only low amount on BT-474, MCF-7, and MDA-MB-231 cells. Concerning the missing uptake of [^{68}Ga]**28** into all tested cell lines, three explanations are possible: (i) The NPY(Y$_1$)R is present on at least some of the cells but the peptide sequence [Lys^4,Trp^5,Nle^7]BVD$_{15}$, being the NPY(Y$_1$)R-targeting sequence in monomer [^{68}Ga]**28** as well as the HBPLs [^{68}Ga]**22**−[^{68}Ga]**26**, is not able to efficiently address the NPY(Y$_1$)R; (ii) The NPY(Y$_1$)R is expressed in such low amounts that the tested radioligands cannot be efficiently taken up by the cells by this receptor; or (iii) The molar activities of the tested radioligands were too low and a significant self-blocking of the NPY(Y_1)R-mediated uptake took place, preventing the cell uptake.

In order to determine if the NPY(Y_1)R is actually present on T-47D, MCF-7 and BT-474 cells and if the molar activity of monomer [^{68}Ga]28 and the HBPLs [^{68}Ga]22–[^{68}Ga]26 prevented their cellular uptake via the NPY(Y_1)R, the cell uptake studies were repeated using commercially available ^{125}I-PYY, binding the NPY(Y_1)R [29] and exhibiting a high molar activity of 81.4 GBq/μmol. In these experiments, an about 100-fold lower amount of substance was used for the cell uptake studies compared to the ^{68}Ga-labeled ligands ([^{68}Ga]22–[^{68}Ga]26, [^{68}Ga]27 and [^{68}Ga]28: 0.37–0.40 pmol per 1.5×10^6 cells; ^{125}I-PYY: 0.003–0.005 pmol per 1.5×10^6 cells) in order to exclude the eventuality of self-blocking. In all of the three tested cell lines, the specific uptake of ^{125}I-PYY showed to be negligibly low (between 0.2 and 2.5% of the total activity applied), confirming that the target NPY(Y_1) receptor might be present on the cells but if so, then only to a very low amount, being too low to give useful results in the cell uptake studies.

Furthermore, this low receptor density prevents a successful determination of the receptor affinity of the developed radioligands. This is in contrast to other studies, using identically treated MCF-7 cells to determine NPY(Y_1)R affinities of newly developed NPY(Y_1)R-affine radioligands [9,19]. We could however not reproduce these results using MCF-7 cells of different suppliers due to the observed low expression of NPY(Y_1)R on the cells.

As it was described that MCF-7 cells can express the target NPY(Y_1)R to a much higher extent in vivo than under in vitro conditions [34], this might also be the case for the T-47D cell line, expressing besides the NPY(Y_1)R also the for our scientific question important GRPR. Thus, we in the following performed initial in vivo evaluations of HBPL [^{68}Ga]24, showing highly promising results in the preceding evaluations. Of the developed HBPLs, [^{68}Ga]24 showed the highest stability and hydrophilicity as well as a slightly higher tumor cell uptake than the other analogs in vitro and thus represents a potent representative of the developed HBPLs for a following proof-of-concept in vivo evaluation.

2.4. Proof-of-Concept: Evaluation of HBPL [^{68}Ga]24 and Its Scrambled Analogs [^{68}Ga]24a and [^{68}Ga]24b via In Vivo PET/CT Imaging in T-47D-Bearing Nude Mice and Ex Vivo Biodistribution

To investigate the in vivo pharmacokinetic properties of the most potent HBPL [^{68}Ga]24, we performed small animal PET/CT imaging studies in T-47D tumor-bearing immunodeficient mice. Likewise, also the scrambled variants of [^{68}Ga]24, [^{68}Ga]24a (PESIN$_{scrambled}$ combined with [Lys^4(aminooxy),Trp^5,Nle^7]BVD$_{15}$) and [^{68}Ga]24b (PESIN combined with [Lys^4(aminooxy),Trp^5,Nle^7]BVD$_{15,scrambled}$), were evaluated under the same conditions for comparison.

By evaluating these radioligands under the same conditions, the proportion of both peptide binders on the uptake of [^{68}Ga]24 and also the receptor-specificity of the uptake of the radioligand via both receptors should be determined. The evaluation of the partly scrambled monovalent analogs instead of the monomeric peptides, which would also have been possible, exhibits the advantage that all evaluated radioligands show a similar pharmacokinetic distribution and also a similar possible degradation pattern. Using the monovalent peptides bombesin or NPY/BVD for receptor blocking (to show the receptor specificity of both peptide parts of [^{68}Ga]24 and to determine the contribution of both peptide parts of the HBPL to overall tumor uptake) might have resulted in an incomplete blocking of the respective receptor as the GRPR-affine bombesin as well as the NPY(Y_1)R-affine peptides NPY and BVD are known for their limited in vivo stability.

For the PET/CT imaging studies, 5.5–8.0 MBq of the respective ^{68}Ga-radioligand were administered via the lateral tail vein under isoflurane anesthesia to the tumor-bearing animals. Directly after completion of the diagnostic scans, the animals were sacrificed, the organs were collected and measured in a gamma-counter. The results of these in vivo PET/CT imaging studies and the ex vivo biodistribution data are given in Figure 8 and Table S1.

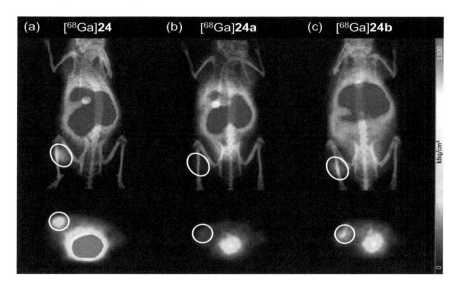

Figure 8. Representative small animal positron emission tomography/computed tomography (PET/CT) imaging results for [^{68}Ga]**24** (**a**); [^{68}Ga]**24a** (**b**) and [^{68}Ga]**24b** (**c**). The images show coronal (**upper row**) and transaxial (**lower row**) slices for all tracers at 37.5 min p.i. The same scaling was used for all images and 4 animals were examined per radioligand. The tumor is encircled in each image.

As can easily be seen from the in vivo PET/CT imaging as well as the ex vivo biodistribution data, all developed ligands showed a rather high kidney and liver uptake. Thus, further improvements in ligand design must be carried out to result in clinically relevant imaging agents for improved breast cancer visualization with PET/CT.

Compared to the bispecific ligand [^{68}Ga]**24** with which the tumor can easily be delineated via PET/CT, the scrambled analogs [^{68}Ga]**24a** and [^{68}Ga]**24b** showed a considerably less efficient tumor visualization ability (Figure 8).

This results from a lower absolute tumor uptake for [^{68}Ga]**24a** and [^{68}Ga]**24b** compared to [^{68}Ga]**24** over the course of PET imaging (Figure 9a, SUVs$_{(85min)}$ of 122.03 $\pm$ 16.27 kBq/cm^3 for [^{68}Ga]**24**, 42.95 $\pm$ 26.38 kBq/cm^3 for [^{68}Ga]**24a** and 70.29 $\pm$ 16.09 kBq/cm^3 for [^{68}Ga]**24b** were observed), which was also confirmed in the ex vivo biodistribution experiments (Figure 9b).

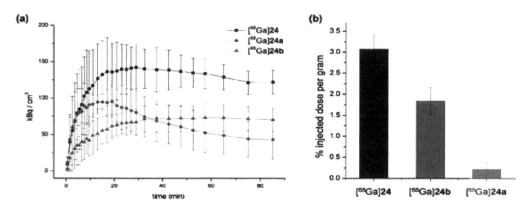

Figure 9. Absolute tumor uptakes as determined by in vivo PET imaging as well as ex vivo biodistribution experiments ($n = 4$). (**a**) Time-activity-curves are depicted, showing tumor uptakes over the course of PET imaging for [^{68}Ga]**24** (black), [^{68}Ga]**24a** (purple) and [^{68}Ga]**24b** (green); (**b**) Tumor uptakes (% injected dose per gram) are shown for [^{68}Ga]**24** (black), [^{68}Ga]**24a** (purple) and [^{68}Ga]**24b** (green) as determined by ex vivo biodistribution directly after the completed diagnostic scans.

This indicates that both parts of HBPL [^{68}Ga]**24** contributed to in vivo tumor uptake and that its uptake into the tumor was GRPR- and also NPY(Y$_1$)R-specific.

As can be observed from the time-activity-curves obtained by PET imaging (Figure 9a), those ligands comprising an intact variant of the GRPR-targeting ligand BBN$_{7-14}$ showed a stable plateau phase in tumor accumulation ([^{68}Ga]**24b**) or only a slight decrease ([^{68}Ga]**24**) whereas [^{68}Ga]**24a**, comprising a scrambled variant of BBN$_{7-14}$, shows a surge in tumor uptake followed by a decline of activity in the tumor. This might be attributable to the limited stability of BVD analogs under in vivo conditions, which has been described before [35] and might result in radioligand metabolization during imaging. If then the GRPR-binding peptide is still able to bind to its target receptor, the tumor uptake nevertheless remains largely stable due to a GRPR-mediated uptake. However, if only a scrambled variant of BBN$_{7-14}$ is present, no receptor-affine peptide binder remains for continuous radiotracer uptake into the tumor, resulting in an overall decrease in tumor accumulation.

Further, high and considerably improved tumor-to-background ratios could be achieved for [^{68}Ga]**24** (tumor-to-muscle: 11.81 ± 1.83, tumor-to-blood: 2.72 ± 0.43) compared to [^{68}Ga]**24a** (tumor-to-muscle: 1.07 ± 1.14, tumor-to-blood: 0.50 ± 0.47) and [^{68}Ga]**24b** (tumor-to-muscle: 3.83 ± 0.80, tumor-to-blood: 0.91 ± 0.24) as determined by ex vivo biodistribution at 130 min p.i. This indicates that both peptide parts of the HBPL contributed to tumor uptake and thus tumor visualization.

In summary, we were able to show here for the first time that the general concept to assemble a GRPR- and a NPY(Y$_1$)R-affine peptide to one combined radioligand is in general feasible regarding a contribution of both peptides of the HBPL to in vivo tumor uptake and thus is beneficial with regard to overall tumor uptake and tumor visualization probability compared to the monospecific agents.

3. Materials and Methods

General. All commercially available chemicals were of analytical grade and were used without further purification. Resins for solid phase-based syntheses, PyBOP (Benzotriazole-1-yl-oxy-*tris*-pyrrolidino-phosphonium hexafluorophosphate), Fmoc-protected standard amino acids as well as *bis*-Boc-aminooxy acetic acid were purchased from NovaBiochem (Darmstadt, Germany). SFB (Succinimidyl-*p*-formyl-benzoate) was synthesized according to a published procedure [36]. Fmoc-ACMP-OH (Fmoc-4-amino-1-carboxymethyl-piperidine) was obtained from Iris Biotech (Marktredwitz, Germany), respectively. Fmoc-L-Lys(Boc$_2$-Aoa)-OH, mono-Fmoc ethylene diamine hydrochloride, HBTU (O-(Benzotriazol-1-yl)-N,N,N',N'-tetramethyluronium hexafluorophosphate), Tracepur water and N,N-bis(N'-Fmoc-3-aminopropyl)-glycine potassium hemisulfate ((Fmoc-NH-Propyl)$_2$-Gly-OH) were purchased from Iris Biotech, SigmaAldrich (Schnelldorf, Germany), Carl Roth (Karlsruhe, Germany), VWR (Bruchsal, Germany) and PolyPeptide (Strasbourg, France), respectively. NODA-GA-(tBu)$_3$ and DOTA-(tBu)$_3$ were obtained from CheMatech (Dijon, France).

Bis-amines **7–11** and *bis*-aldehydes **12–16** were synthesized according to published procedures [22] with minor modifications of the synthesis protocols. Details of these syntheses can be found in the supplementary information.

Unless otherwise stated, the coupling reactions during solid phase-based syntheses were usually carried out in DMF for 30 min using 4 eq. of acid, 3.9 eq. of HBTU as coupling reagent and 4 eq. of DIPEA (N,N-Diisopropylethylamine) as base. Fmoc protecting groups were removed using 50% (*v/v*) piperidine in DMF.

For analytical and semipreparative HPLC chromatography, Dionex UltiMate 3000 systems equipped with a Chromolith Performance (RP-18e, 100-4.6 mm, Merck, Darmstadt, Germany) and a Chromolith SemiPrep (RP-18e, 100-10 mm, Merck) column were used, operated with a flow rate of 4 mL/min and H$_2$O + 0.1% TFA and MeCN + 0.1% TFA as eluents. For radio-analytical HPLC chromatography, a Dionex UltiMate 3000 system equipped with a Chromolith Performance (RP-18e, 100-4.6 mm, Merck) column and a GabiStar radioactivity detector (Raytest, Straubenhardt, Germany) or an Agilent 1200 system equipped with a Chromolith Performance (RP-18e, 100-4.6 mm, Merck) column and a GabiStar radioactivity detector (Raytest) were used and operated with a flow rate of 4 mL/min and H_2O + 0.1% TFA and MeCN + 0.1% TFA as eluents. MALDI (Matrix-Assisted Laser Desorption/Ionization) spectra were obtained with a Bruker Daltonics Microflex spectrometer (Bremen, Germany).

The human breast cancer cell lines T-47D, MDA-MB-231 and MCF-7 were purchased from SigmaAldrich (Schnelldorf, Germany), whereas the cell line BT-474 was obtained from the Leibniz-Institute DSMZ (Braunschweig, Germany). Dulbecco's Modified Eagle Medium (DMEM), RPMI-1640 medium, 200 mM L-glutamine, 0.05% trypsin/EDTA and 0.25% trypsin/EDTA were purchased from Life Technologies. Fetal calf serum (FCS) was obtained from GE Healthcare Life Sciences and phosphate buffered saline (PBS) as well as β-estradiol were purchased from Sigma Aldrich. Bovine serum albumin (BSA) was purchased from CarlRoth (Karlsruhe, Germany).

The human ^{125}I-labeled NPY(Y_1)-binding peptide [^{125}I]-Peptide-YY was obtained from PerkinElmer in a molar activity of 81.4 GBq/μmol. The γ-counter used was a 2480 WIZARD[2] system (PerkinElmer, Rodgau, Germany).

For the in vivo evaluations, five week old female Fox Chase SCID mice were obtained from Janvier and implanted with estradiol pellets (0.36 mg/60 days; obtained from Innovative Research of America) one week prior to tumor cell inoculation. Tumor cells were inoculated using Matrigel basal membrane matrix with reduced growth factor (obtained from VWR). For PET/CT measurements, a small animal Albira II PET/SPECT/CT system (Bruker, Eggenstein-Leopoldshafen, Germany) was used.

Synthesis of aminooxy-PESIN (1) and aminooxy-PESIN$_{scrambled}$ (5). The peptides were synthesized on solid support by standard Fmoc solid-phase peptide synthesis using a commercially available standard Rink amide MBHA resin, HBTU as coupling reagent, standard N_α-Fmoc-amino acids, N_ω-Fmoc-PEG$_4$-OH and *bis*-Boc-aminooxy acetic acid. All amino acids (apart from *bis*-Boc-aminooxy acetic acid which was reacted for 60 min) were coupled within 30 min. The crude aminooxy-modified peptides were cleaved from the solid support using a mixture of TFA:TIS:H_2O of 95:2.5:2.5 (*v/v*) for 60 min, suspended in diethyl ether and purified by semipreparative HPLC.

1 was purified using a gradient of 15–30% MeCN + 0.1% TFA in 8 min (R_t = 6.35 min) and isolated as white solid after lyophilization in yields of 27% (85.0 mg; 67.4 μmol). MALDI-MS (*m/z*) using 2,5-dihydroxybenzoic acid as matrix substance for $[M + H^+]^+$ (calculated): 1260.23 (1260.46); $[M + Na^+]^+$ (calculated): 1282.21 (1282.62); $[M + K^+]^+$ (calculated): 1298.16 (1298.60). MALDI-MS (*m/z*) using α-cyano-4-hydroxycinnamic acid as matrix substance for $[M + H^+]^+$ (calculated): 1260.63 (1260.46); $[M + Na^+]^+$ (calculated): 1282.56 (1282.62); $[M + K^+]^+$ (calculated): 1298.54 (1298.60).

5 was purified using a gradient of 10–60% MeCN + 0.1% TFA in 8 min (R_t = 5.42 min) and isolated as white solid after lyophilization in yields of 22% (28.1 mg, 22.2 μmol). MALDI-MS (*m/z*) using α-cyano-4-hydroxycinnamic acid as matrix substance for $[M + H^+]^+$ (calculated): 1260.81 (1260.46); $[M + Na^+]^+$ (calculated): 1282.84 (1282.62); $[M + K^+]^+$ (calculated): 1298.78 (1298.60).

Synthesis of [Lys⁴(aminooxy),Trp⁵,Nle⁷]BVD15 (2) and [Lys⁴(aminooxy),Trp⁵,Nle⁷]BVD15$_{scrambled}$ (6). The peptides were synthesized on solid support by standard Fmoc solid-phase peptide synthesis using a commercially available Rink amide MBHA resin, HBTU as coupling reagent, standard N_α-Fmoc-amino acids and N_α-Fmoc-L-Lys(Boc$_2$-Aoa)-OH. The crude aminooxy-modified peptides were cleaved from the solid support using a mixture of TFA:TIS:H_2O of 95:2.5:2.5 (*v/v*) for 90 min, suspended in diethyl ether and purified by semipreparative HPLC.

2 was purified using a gradient of 10–60% MeCN + 0.1% TFA in 8 min (R_t = 3.71 min) and isolated as white solid after lyophilization in yields of 35% (114.2 mg; 86.7 μmol). MALDI-MS (*m/z*) using 2,5-dihydroxybenzoic acid as matrix substance for $[M + H^+]^+$ (calculated): 1317.02 (1317.54); $[M + Na^+]^+$ (calculated): 1339.13 (1339.74); $[M + K^+]^+$ (calculated): 1355.03 (1355.71). MALDI-MS (*m/z*) using α-cyano-4-hydroxycinnamic acid as matrix substance for $[M + H^+]^+$ (calculated): 1317.89 (1317.54); $[M + Na^+]^+$ (calculated): 1339.89 (1339.74); $[M + K^+]^+$ (calculated): 1355.86 (1355.71).

6 was purified using a gradient of 10–50% MeCN + 0.1% TFA in 8 min (R_t = 4.31 min) and isolated as white solid after lyophilization in yields of 20% (26.0 mg; 19.7 μmol). MALDI-MS (*m/z*) using

α-cyano-4-hydroxycinnamic acid as matrix substance for [M + H$^+$]$^+$ (calculated): 1317.37 (1317.54); [M + Na$^+$]$^+$ (calculated): 1339.38 (1339.74).

Synthesis of bombesin (3). The peptide was synthesized on solid support by standard Fmoc solid-phase peptide synthesis using a commercially available standard Rink amide resin, HBTU as coupling reagent and standard N_α-Fmoc-amino acids. All amino acids were coupled within 35 min. The crude peptide was cleaved from the solid support using a mixture of TFA:TIS:H$_2$O of 95:2.5:2.5 (v/v) for 90 min, suspended in diethyl ether and purified by semipreparative HPLC using a gradient of 15–60% MeCN + 0.1% TFA in 5.5 min (R$_t$ = 3.40 min) and isolated as white solid after lyophilization in yields of 22% (35.2 mg, 21.6 µmol). MALDI-MS (m/z) using α-cyano-4-hydroxycinnamic acid as matrix substance for [M + H$^+$]$^+$ (calculated): 1618.56 (1618.82); [M + Na$^+$]$^+$ (calculated): 1640.55 (1640.81); [M + K$^+$]$^+$ (calculated): 1656.57 (1656.78).

Synthesis of [Lys^4,Trp^5,Nle^7]BVD15 (4). The peptide was synthesized on solid support by standard Fmoc solid-phase peptide synthesis using a commercially available standard Rink amide resin, HBTU as coupling reagent and standard N_α-Fmoc-amino acids. All amino acids were coupled within 30 min. The crude peptide was cleaved from the solid support using a mixture of TFA:TIS:H$_2$O of 95:2.5:2.5 (v/v) for 120 min, suspended in diethyl ether and purified by semipreparative HPLC using a gradient of 10–60% MeCN + 0.1% TFA in 5.5 min (R$_t$ = 3.05 min) and isolated as white solid after lyophilization in yields of 40% (49.2 mg; 39.5 µmol). MALDI-MS (m/z) using α-cyano-4-hydroxycinnamic acid as matrix substance for [M + H$^+$]$^+$ (calculated): 1244.63 (1244.73); [M + Na$^+$]$^+$ (calculated): 1266.65 (1266.72); [M + K$^+$]$^+$ (calculated): 1282.60 (1282.69).

General synthesis of NODA-GA-PESIN-aldehydes (17—21) and NODA-GA-PESIN$_{scrambled}$-aldehyde (19a). To a solution of the respective branched NODA-GA-*bis*-aldehyde (12—16) in H$_2$O + 0.1% TFA (250—500 µL) was added a solution of aminooxy-PESIN (1) or aminooxy-PESIN$_{scrambled}$ (5) (0.7 eq.) in H$_2$O + 0.1% TFA (250—500 µL). The pH of the solutions was adjusted to 4.0–4.6 by addition of phosphate buffer (0.1 M, pH 7.2, ~150 µL) and the reaction progress was monitored by analytical HPLC. The reactions were found to be finished within 5 min and the products were purified by semipreparative HPLC. The products were isolated as white solids after lyophilization. Gradients used for HPLC purification and synthesis yields for each compound are given below.

17: gradient: 20–45% MeCN + 0.1% TFA in 5 min (R$_t$ = 4.45 min), yield: 47%. MALDI-MS (m/z) using α-cyano-4-hydroxycinnamic acid as matrix substance for [M + H$^+$]$^+$ (calculated): 2427.33 (2427.22); [M + Na$^+$]$^+$ (calculated): 2449.30 (2449.21); [M + K$^+$]$^+$ (calculated): 2465.49 (2465.18). MALDI-MS (m/z) using 2,5-dihydroxybenzoic acid as matrix substance for [M + H$^+$]$^+$ (calculated): 2426.69 (2427.22); [M + Na$^+$]$^+$ (calculated): 2448.99 (2449.21); [M + K$^+$]$^+$ (calculated): 2464.93 (2465.18). MALDI-MS (m/z) using sinapic acid as matrix substance for [M + H$^+$]$^+$ (calculated): 2427.38 (2427.22); [M + Na$^+$]$^+$ (calculated): 2449.25 (2449.21).

18: gradient: 25–45% MeCN + 0.1% TFA in 5 min (R$_t$ = 3.76 min), yield: 51%. MALDI-MS (m/z) using α-cyano-4-hydroxycinnamic acid as matrix substance for [M + H$^+$]$^+$ (calculated): 2717.48 (2717.37); [M + Na$^+$]$^+$ (calculated): 2739.21 (2739.36); [M + K$^+$]$^+$ (calculated): 2755.49 (2755.33). MALDI-MS (m/z) using 2,5-dihydroxybenzoic acid as matrix substance for [M + H$^+$]$^+$ (calculated): 2717.18 (2717.37); [M + Na$^+$]$^+$ (calculated): 2739.60 (2739.36); [M + K$^+$]$^+$ (calculated): 2755.13 (2755.33).

19: gradient: 25–45% MeCN + 0.1% TFA in 5 min (R$_t$ = 4.26 min), yield: 43%. MALDI-MS (m/z) using α-cyano-4-hydroxycinnamic acid as matrix substance for [M + H$^+$]$^+$ (calculated): 2921.63 (2921.50); [M + Na$^+$]$^+$ (calculated): 2943.64 (2943.49); [M + K$^+$]$^+$ (calculated): 2959.46 (2959.47). MALDI-MS (m/z) using 2,5-dihydroxybenzoic acid as matrix substance for [M + H$^+$]$^+$ (calculated): 2921.63 (2921.50); [M + Na$^+$]$^+$ (calculated): 2943.34 (2943.49); [M + K$^+$]$^+$ (calculated): 2959.57 (2959.47).

19a (PESIN scrambled): gradient: 25–45% MeCN + 0.1% TFA in 5.5 min (R$_t$ = 4.18 min), yield: 44%. MALDI-MS (m/z) using α-cyano-4-hydroxycinnamic acid as matrix substance for [M + H$^+$]$^+$ (calculated): 2921.59 (2921.50); [M + Na$^+$]$^+$ (calculated): 2943.56 (2943.49); [M + K$^+$]$^+$ (calculated): 2959.52 (2959.47).

20: gradient: 20–45% MeCN + 0.1% TFA in 5 min (R_t = 3.93 min), yield: 58%. MALDI-MS (m/z) using α-cyano-4-hydroxycinnamic acid as matrix substance for $[M + H^+]^+$ (calculated): 2707.24 (2707.41); $[M + Na^+]^+$ (calculated): 2729.30 (2729.40); $[M + K^+]^+$ (calculated): 2745.58 (2745.37). MALDI-MS (m/z) using 2,5-dihydroxybenzoic acid as matrix substance for $[M + H^+]^+$ (calculated): 2706.98 (2707.41); $[M + Na^+]^+$ (calculated): 2728.88 (2729.40); $[M + K^+]^+$ (calculated): 2744.78 (2745.37).

21: gradient: 25–45% MeCN + 0.1% TFA in 5 min (R_t = 2.85 min), yield: 55%. MALDI-MS (m/z) using α-cyano-4-hydroxycinnamic acid as matrix substance for $[M + H^+]^+$ (calculated): 2987.39 (2987.60); $[M + Na^+]^+$ (calculated): 3009.40 (3009.59); $[M + K^+]^+$ (calculated): 3025.80 (3025.56). MALDI-MS (m/z) using 2,5-dihydroxybenzoic acid as matrix substance for $[M + H^+]^+$ (calculated): 2987.03 (2987.60). MALDI-MS (m/z) using sinapic acid as matrix substance for $[M + H^+]^+$ (calculated): 2987.81 (2987.60).

General synthesis of heterobivalent ligands 22−26 and scrambled analogs 24a–c. To a solution of the respective NODA-GA-PESIN-aldehyde (**17−21** or **19a**) in H_2O + 0.1% TFA (250−500 μL) was added a solution of **2** or **6** (3 eq.) in H_2O + 0.1% TFA (250−500 μL). The pH of the solutions was adjusted to 4.0–4.6 by addition of phosphate buffer (0.1 M, pH 7.2, ~150 μL) and the reaction progress was monitored by analytical HPLC. The reactions were found to be finished within 5 min and the products were purified by semipreparative HPLC. The products were isolated as white solids after lyophilization. Gradients used for HPLC purification and synthesis yields for each compound are given below.

22: gradient: 25–50% MeCN + 0.1% TFA in 5 min (R_t = 3.19 min), yield: 82%. MALDI-MS (m/z) using α-cyano-4-hydroxycinnamic acid as matrix substance for $[M + H^+]^+$ (calculated): 3728.21 (3728.29); $[M + Na^+]^+$ (calculated): 3750.49 (3750.28). MALDI-MS (m/z) using 2,5-dihydroxybenzoic acid as matrix substance for $[M + H^+]^+$ (calculated): 3728.71 (3728.29); $[M + Na^+]^+$ (calculated): 3750.76 (3750.28).

23: gradient: 25–45% MeCN + 0.1% TFA in 5 min (R_t = 3.65 min), yield: 79%. MALDI-MS (m/z) using α-cyano-4-hydroxycinnamic acid as matrix substance for $[M + H^+]^+$ (calculated): 4018.99 (4018.61); $[M + Na^+]^+$ (calculated): 4040.69 (4040.60). MALDI-MS (m/z) using 2,5-dihydroxybenzoic acid as matrix substance for $[M + H^+]^+$ (calculated): 4018.95 (4018.61); $[M + Na^+]^+$ (calculated): 4040.02 (4040.60).

24: gradient: 25–45% MeCN + 0.1% TFA in 6 min (R_t = 3.86 min), yield: 66%. MALDI-MS (m/z) using α-cyano-4-hydroxycinnamic acid as matrix substance for $[M + H^+]^+$ (calculated): 4222.98 (4222.87). MALDI-MS (m/z) using 2,5-dihydroxybenzoic acid as matrix substance for $[M + H^+]^+$ (calculated): 4222.48 (4222.87); $[M + Na^+]^+$ (calculated): 4244.96 (4244.86); $[M + K^+]^+$ (calculated): 4260.51 (4260.97). MALDI-MS (m/z) using sinapic acid as matrix substance for $[M + H^+]^+$ (calculated): 4222.87 (4222.87).

24a (PESIN scrambled): gradient: 25–45% MeCN + 0.1% TFA in 6 min (R_t = 3.55 min), yield: 49%. MALDI-MS (m/z) using α-cyano-4-hydroxycinnamic acid as matrix substance for $[M + H^+]^+$ (calculated): 4222.54 (4222.87). MALDI-MS (m/z) using 2,5-dihydroxybenzoic acid as matrix substance for $[M + H^+]^+$ (calculated): 4222.17 (4222.87); $[M + Na^+]^+$ (calculated): 4244.94 (4244.86).

24b ([Lys^4,Trp^5,Nle^7]BVD$_{15}$ scrambled): gradient: 25–40% MeCN + 0.1% TFA in 5.5 min (R_t = 4.58 min), yield: 63%. MALDI-MS (m/z) using α-cyano-4-hydroxycinnamic acid as matrix substance for $[M + H^+]^+$ (calculated): 4222.35 (4222.87). MALDI-MS (m/z) using 2,5-dihydroxybenzoic acid as matrix substance for $[M + H^+]^+$ (calculated): 4222.29 (4222.87); $[M + Na^+]^+$ (calculated): 4244.99 (4244.86); $[M + K^+]^+$ (calculated): 4260.49 (4260.97).

24c (PESIN and [Lys^4,Trp^5,Nle^7]BVD$_{15}$ scrambled): gradient: 25–45% MeCN + 0.1% TFA in 5.5 min (R_t = 4.36 min), yield: 61%. MALDI-MS (m/z) using α-cyano-4-hydroxycinnamic acid as matrix substance for $[M + H^+]^+$ (calculated): 4222.67 (4222.87); $[M + K^+]^+$ (calculated): 4260.98 (4260.97). MALDI-MS (m/z) using 2,5-dihydroxybenzoic acid as matrix substance for $[M + H^+]^+$ (calculated): 4222.48 (4222.87); $[M + Na^+]^+$ (calculated): 4244.90 (4244.86).

25: gradient: 25–50% MeCN + 0.1% TFA in 6 min (R_t = 2.76 min), yield: 75%. MALDI-MS (m/z) using α-cyano-4-hydroxycinnamic acid as matrix substance for [M + H⁺]⁺ (calculated): 4008.53 (4008.66); [M + Na⁺]⁺ (calculated): 4030.76 (4030.65); [M + K⁺]⁺ (calculated): 4046.33 (4046.76). MALDI-MS (m/z) using 2,5-dihydroxybenzoic acid as matrix substance for [M + H⁺]⁺ (calculated): 4009.12 (4008.66).

26: gradient: 25–45% MeCN + 0.1% TFA in 6 min (R_t = 2.83 min), yield: 73%. MALDI-MS (m/z) using 2,5-dihydroxybenzoic acid as matrix substance for [M + H⁺]⁺ (calculated): 4288.72 (4289.03). MALDI-MS (m/z) using sinapic acid as matrix substance for [M + H⁺]⁺ (calculated): 4289.59 (4289.03).

Synthesis of DOTA-PESIN (27). The peptide was synthesized on solid support by standard Fmoc solid-phase peptide synthesis using a commercially available standard Rink amide MBHA resin, HBTU as coupling reagent, standard N_α-Fmoc-amino acids, and N_ω-Fmoc-PEG₄-OH. After the conjugation of the PEG₄ linker to the peptide sequence, DOTA-(tBu)₃ was coupled within 120 min using an excess of the synthon of 2.7 eq. together with 2.6 eq. HBTU and 4 eq. DIPEA. The crude product was cleaved from the solid support using a mixture of TFA:TIS:H₂O of 95:2.5:2.5 (v/v) for 3 h, suspended in diethyl ether and purified by semipreparative HPLC using a gradient of 20–35% MeCN + 0.1% TFA in 8 min (R_t = 4.34 min) and isolated as white solid after lyophilization in yields of 7% (10.7 mg; 6.8 μmol). MALDI-MS (m/z) using 2,5-dihydroxybenzoic acid as matrix substance for [M + H⁺]⁺ (calculated): 1573.02 (1573.80); [M + Na⁺]⁺ (calculated): 1595.06 (1595.79); [M + K⁺]⁺ (calculated): 1610.94 (1611.76). MALDI-MS (m/z) using α-cyano-4-hydroxycinnamic acid as matrix substance for [M + H⁺]⁺ (calculated): 1573.75 (1573.80); [M + Na⁺]⁺ (calculated): 1595.85 (1595.79).

Synthesis of [Lys⁴(DOTA),Trp⁵,Nle⁷]BVD₁₅ (28). The peptide was synthesized on solid support by standard Fmoc solid-phase peptide synthesis using a commercially available standard Rink amide MBHA resin, HBTU as coupling reagent, standard N_α-Fmoc-amino acids and Fmoc-Lys(Mtt)-OH. After conjugation of the last amino acid, the lysine side chain Mtt-protecting group was removed with diluted TFA (TFA:DCM 1:99 (v/v)) within 2 h and DOTA-(tBu)₃ was coupled in this position within 120 min using an excess of the synthon of 2.7 eq. together with 2.6 eq. HBTU and 4 eq. DIPEA. The crude DOTA-modified peptide was cleaved from the solid support using a mixture of TFA:TIS:H₂O of 95:2.5:2.5 (v/v) for 3 h, suspended in diethyl ether and purified by semipreparative HPLC using a gradient of 20–25% MeCN + 0.1% TFA in 8 min (R_t = 2.58 min) and isolated as white solid after lyophilization in yields of 45% (73.4 mg; 45.0 μmol). MALDI-MS (m/z) using 2,5-dihydroxybenzoic acid as matrix substance for [M + H⁺]⁺ (calculated): 1630.38 (1630.91); [M + Na⁺]⁺ (calculated): 1652.59 (1652.90); [M + K⁺]⁺ (calculated): 1668.39 (1668.87). MALDI-MS (m/z) using α-cyano-4-hydroxycinnamic acid as matrix substance for [M + H⁺]⁺ (calculated): 1630.54 (1630.91). MALDI-MS (m/z) using sinapic acid as matrix substance for [M + H⁺]⁺ (calculated): 1630.53 (1630.91).

⁶⁸Ga-radiolabeling of NODAGA-modified peptide heterodimers (22−26) and peptide monomers 27 and 28 for in vitro evaluations. The respective labeling precursor (10 nmol, dissolved in 10 μL of Tracepur water) was reacted with 110–150 MBq of ⁶⁸Ga³⁺ obtained by an itG ⁶⁸Ge/⁶⁸Ga generator system (Garching, Germany). The generator was eluted with HCl (0.05 M, 3 mL) and the eluate was trapped on a cation exchange cartridge (Macherey-Nagel, Chromafix PS-H⁺). The ⁶⁸Ga³⁺ was eluted from the cartridge using a NaCl solution (5 M, 1.5 mL) and the pH was adjusted to 3.5–4.0 by addition of sodium acetate solution (1.25 M, ~50 μL). After reaction for 10 min at 45 °C (**22−26**) or 99 °C (**27 and 28**), the reaction mixtures were analyzed by analytical radio-HPLC. The radiolabeled products were found to be 95–99% pure and obtained in molar activities of 10–15 GBq/μmol (non-optimized).

⁶⁸Ga-radiolabeling of NODAGA-modified peptide heterodimers (24 and 24a–c) for in vivo evaluations. The respective labeling precursor (10 nmol, dissolved in 10 μL of Tracepur water) was reacted with 420–460 MBq of ⁶⁸Ga³⁺ obtained by fractioned elution of an Eckert & Ziegler ⁶⁸Ge/⁶⁸Ga generator system (IGG100, Eckert & Ziegler, Berlin, Germany). The generator was eluted with HCl (0.1 M, 1.4 mL) and the pH was adjusted to 3.5–4.0 by addition of sodium acetate solution (1.25 M, 90–95 μL). After reaction for 10 min at 45 °C, the reaction mixtures were analyzed by analytical radio-HPLC. The radiolabeled products were found to be 95–99% pure and obtained in molar activities of 40–46 GBq/μmol (non-optimized). The pH of the radiotracer solution was adjusted to 6.0–7.0 using HEPES buffer (2.0 M, pH 8.0, 200 μL) and used for the in vivo studies.

Determination of radiotracer lipophilicity. The heterobivalent ligands (**22**–**26**) as well as the monomeric reference compounds (**27** and **28**) were radiolabeled with ^{68}Ga as described before and 2 μL of the product solution (~65 pmol of the respective radioligand) were added to a mixture of phosphate buffer (0.05 M, pH 7.4, 800 μL) and 1-octanol (800 μL) and incubated for 5 min at ambient temperature under vigorous shaking. Both phases were separated by centrifugation and 100 μL of each phase were measured for radioactivity in a gamma-counter. From these data, the distribution coefficient $\log_D$ was calculated from the following equation: $\log D_{o/w} = \log(\text{cpm}_o/\text{cpm}_w)$, where: cpm_o = activity in the 1-octanol phase [cpm] (cpm = counts per minute), cpm_w = activity in the aqueous phase [cpm]. These experiments were performed six times independently.

Determination of the stability of the ligands in human serum. The heterobivalent ligands (**22**–**26**) as well as the monomeric reference compounds (**27** and **28**) were radiolabeled with ^{68}Ga as described before and 125 μL of the product solution were added to 500 μL of human serum and incubated at 37 °C. At defined time-points of 5, 15, 30, 60 and 90 min, aliquots of 75 μL of the mixture were added to 75 μL of ethanol and the precipitation of serum proteins was enhanced by ice-cooling for 2 min. After centrifugation, supernatant and precipitate were measured for radioactivity and the supernatant was analyzed by analytical radio-HPLC. These experiments were performed thrice.

Cell culture. All cell lines were grown in suitable culture medium at 37 °C in a humidified CO_2 (5%) atmosphere. The human breast cancer cell lines T-47D, MDA-MB-231 and MCF-7 were grown in Dulbecco's Modified Eagle Medium (DMEM), supplemented with 10% (v/v) fetal calf serum (FCS) and 1% (v/v) L-Glutamine. For a high expression of the NPY(Y_1) receptor on T-47D cells, the medium for this cell line was further supplemented with 0.15% (w/v) β-estradiol. The BT-474 and PC-3 cell lines were grown in RPMI-1640 medium, also supplemented with 10% (v/v) fetal calf serum (FCS) and 1% (v/v) L-Glutamine.

Internalization studies. Cells (T-47D, MDA-MB-231, MCF-7, BT-474 and PC-3, 1.5×10^6 cells per well) were seeded into 6-well plates and incubated overnight at 37 °C in a humidified CO_2 (5%) atmosphere. The next day, the medium was removed and the cells were washed twice with the respective medium without supplements (ice-cold, 1 mL) and incubated with 3.7–4.0 kBq (0.37–4.0 pmol) of the respective ^{68}Ga-radiolabeled ligand [^{68}Ga]**22**–[^{68}Ga]**26**, [^{68}Ga]**27** or [^{68}Ga]**28** (in 1.5 mL medium, containing 0.5% (w/v) BSA) for defined time-points of 1, 2, 3 or 4 h at 37 °C in a humidified CO_2 (5%) atmosphere. A 1000-fold excess of the respective peptide (**3** or **4**) was used for blocking to determine the non-specific cell uptake. At each time point, the medium was removed and the cells were washed twice with the respective medium without supplements (ice-cold, 1 mL). Cells were treated twice with 1 mL glycine buffer (ice-cold, 50 mM glycine, 100 mM NaCl, pH 2.8) for 5 min at room temperature, followed by 2 mL NaOH solution (1 M) for 10 min at 37 °C. The supernatants were collected and the radioactivity measured in a gamma counter. The internalized and surface bound activity was expressed as percentage of measured to total added activity. Each data point was generated thrice in triplicates.

These internalization studies were performed accordingly on T-47D, MCF-7, BT-474 and PC-3 (negative control) cells with ^{125}I-PYY (PerkinElmer, molar activity 81.4 GBq/μmol, 0.3 kBq, 0.0032 pmol). The cells were incubated for 1 h with the radioligand and additional blocking experiments were performed using a 1000-fold excess of **4**, **28** and **24**.

In vivo experiments. All animal experiments were performed in compliance with the German animal protection laws and protocols of the local committee (Regierungspräsidium Karlsruhe, approval number: 35-9185.81/G-206/15). 20, six week old female immunodeficient Fox Chase SCID (CB17/Icr-Prkdc^{scid}/IcrIcoCrl) mice with an average weight of 20 g were subcutaneously implanted with 17β-estradiol pellets (0.36 mg/60 days). 4 days later, the tumors were induced by subcutaneous inoculation of 5×10^6 T-47D cells into the left flank of the approval number s. After induction, the tumors were allowed to grow for 8–10 weeks and reached a diameter of about 0.5 cm.

For imaging, the animals were anaesthetized with isoflurane and injected with 5.5–8.0 MBq of the respective radioligand ([^{68}Ga]24, [^{68}Ga]24a or [^{68}Ga]24b) into the lateral tail vein. Dynamic PET images were acquired over 90 min and CT images were obtained within further 30 min. After the end of the diagnostic scan, the animals were sacrificed, the organs were collected and measured in a gamma-counter.

The dynamic PET images were reconstructed using the Albira Suite Reconstructor (Bruker) with an iterative dynamic reconstruction with 12 iterations using an 2D-Maximum-Likelihood Expectation-Maximization (MLEM) algorithm and a cubic image voxel size of 0.5 mm after scatter and decay correction. Data were divided into time frames from 1 to 10 min (10×1 min, 10×2 min, 6×5 min and 3×10 min) for the assessment of temporal changes in regional tracer accumulation. The CT images were obtained at 45 kVp, with currents of 0.4 mA (high dose, good resolution). Acquisitions of 400 projections were taken and a 250 μm isotropic voxel size image was reconstructed via filtered back projection. The reconstructed PET data were manually fused with the CT images using PMOD 3.6.1.1. and analyzed. Volumes of interest (VOIs) were defined for the quantification of tracer accumulation in heart, liver, kidneys, tumor, and muscle. The results for each VOI were calculated as SUV (kBq/cm^3) averaged for each time frame.

4. Conclusions

We were able to show that is chemically and radiochemically feasible to synthesize radiolabeled heterobivalent peptides consisting of a GRPR- and a NPY(Y$_1$)R-affine peptide on symmetrically branched scaffolds, resulting in bispecific heterobivalent peptidic PET radiotracers. The compounds demonstrated high stabilities in human serum, hydrophilicities comparable to the monomeric lead peptides and high GRPR-mediated tumor cell uptakes in vitro.

The performed in vivo imaging and ex vivo biodistribution studies indicated a contribution of both peptides of the evaluated HBPL to overall in vivo tumor uptake, showing the feasibility of the general concept to develop GRPR- and NPY(Y$_1$)R-bispecific PET radiotracers with regard to an improved and more sensitive tumor visualization of human breast cancer.

Nevertheless, the results also show that further work is required to obtain GRPR- and NPY(Y$_1$)R-bispecific imaging agents being useful for clinical application due to the high kidney and liver accumulation of the agents developed so far.

Author Contributions: Conceptualization, C.D., B.W., R.S., G.F. and C.W.; Methodology, C.W.; Investigation, A.V.-S., S.L., C.D.; Writing, A.V.-S., R.S., C.W.; Supervision, C.W.

Acknowledgments: O. Prante (Erlangen, Germany) is acknowledged for the valuable discussions about NPY(Y$_1$)R-expression on breast cancer cell lines.

References

1.   Fischer, G.; Schirrmacher, R.; Wangler, B.; Wangler, C. Radiolabeled heterobivalent peptidic ligands: An approach with high future potential for in vivo imaging and therapy of malignant diseases. *ChemMedChem* **2013**, *8*, 883–890. [CrossRef] [PubMed]
2.   Reubi, J.C.; Maecke, H.R. Approaches to multireceptor targeting: Hybrid radioligands, radioligand cocktails, and sequential radioligand applications. *J. Nucl. Med.* **2017**, *58*, 10s–16s. [CrossRef] [PubMed]

3. Zhang, J.J.; Niu, G.; Lang, L.X.; Li, F.; Fan, X.R.; Yang, X.F.; Yao, S.B.; Yan, W.G.; Huo, L.; Chen, L.B.; et al. Clinical translation of a dual integrin alpha(v)beta(3)- and gastrin-releasing peptide receptor-targeting pet radiotracer, ga-68-bbn-rgd. *J. Nucl. Med.* **2017**, *58*, 228–234. [CrossRef] [PubMed]

4. Reubi, J.C.; Fleischmann, A.; Waser, B.; Rehmann, R. Concomitant vascular grp-receptor and vegf-receptor expression in human tumors: Molecular basis for dual targeting of tumoral vasculature. *Peptides* **2011**, *32*, 1457–1462. [CrossRef] [PubMed]

5. Reubi, J.C.; Gugger, M.; Waser, B. Co-expressed peptide receptors in breast cancer as a molecular basis for in vivo multireceptor tumour targeting. *Eur. J. Nucl. Med. Mol. Imaging* **2002**, *29*, 855–862. [CrossRef] [PubMed]

6. Reubi, J.C.; Waser, B. Concomitant expression of several peptide receptors in neuroendocrine tumours: Molecular basis for in vivo multireceptor tumour targeting. *Eur. J. Nucl. Med. Mol. Imaging* **2003**, *30*, 781–793. [CrossRef] [PubMed]

7. Gugger, M.; Reubi, J.C. Gastrin-releasing peptide receptors in non-neoplastic and neoplastic human breast. *Am. J. Pathol.* **1999**, *155*, 2067–2076. [CrossRef]

8. Reubi, J.C.; Gugger, M.; Waser, B.; Schaer, J.C. Y-1-mediated effect of neuropeptide y in cancer: Breast carcinomas as targets. *Cancer Res.* **2001**, *61*, 4636–4641. [PubMed]

9. Shrivastava, A.; Wang, S.H.; Raju, N.; Gierach, I.; Ding, H.M.; Tweedle, M.F. Heterobivalent dual-target probe for targeting grp and y1 receptors on tumor cells. *Bioorg. Med. Chem. Lett.* **2013**, *23*, 687–692. [CrossRef] [PubMed]

10. Ghosh, A.; Raju, N.; Tweedle, M.; Kumar, K. In vitro mouse and human serum stability of a heterobivalent dual-target probe that has strong affinity to gastrin-releasing peptide and neuropeptide y1 receptors on tumor cells. *Cancer Biother. Radio* **2017**, *32*, 24–32. [CrossRef] [PubMed]

11. Wängler, C.; Wängler, B.; Lehner, S.; Elsner, A.; Todica, A.; Bartenstein, P.; Hacker, M.; Schirrmacher, R. A universally applicable (68)ga-labeling technique for proteins. *J. Nucl. Med.* **2011**, *52*, 586–591. [CrossRef] [PubMed]

12. Liu, Z.F.; Yan, Y.J.; Chin, F.T.; Wang, F.; Chen, X.Y. Dual integrin and gastrin-releasing peptide receptor targeted tumor imaging using f-18-labeled pegylated rgd-bombesin heterodimer f-18-fb-peg(3)-glu-rgd-bbn. *J. Med. Chem.* **2009**, *52*, 425–432. [CrossRef] [PubMed]

13. Lindner, S.; Michler, C.; Wängler, B.; Bartenstein, P.; Fischer, G.; Schirrmacher, R.; Wängler, C. Pesin multimerization improves receptor avidities and in vivo tumor targeting properties to grpr-overexpressing tumors. *Bioconjug. Chem.* **2014**, *25*, 489–500. [CrossRef] [PubMed]

14. Fischer, G.; Lindner, S.; Litau, S.; Schirrmacher, R.; Wangler, B.; Wangler, C. Next step toward optimization of grp receptor avidities: Determination of the minimal distance between bbn(7–14) units in peptide homodimers. *Bioconjug. Chem.* **2015**, *26*, 1479–1483. [CrossRef] [PubMed]

15. Josan, J.S.; Handl, H.L.; Sankaranarayanan, R.; Xu, L.P.; Lynch, R.M.; Vagner, J.; Mash, E.A.; Hruby, V.J.; Gillies, R.J. Cell-specific targeting by heterobivalent ligands. *Bioconjug. Chem.* **2011**, *22*, 1270–1278. [CrossRef] [PubMed]

16. Vagner, J.; Xu, L.P.; Handl, H.L.; Josan, J.S.; Morse, D.L.; Mash, E.A.; Gillies, R.J.; Hruby, V.J. Heterobivalent ligands crosslink multiple cell-surface receptors: The human melanocortin-4 and delta-opioid receptors. *Angew. Chem. Int. Ed.* **2008**, *47*, 1685–1688. [CrossRef] [PubMed]

17. Ananias, H.J.; de Jong, I.J.; Dierckx, R.A.; van de Wiele, C.; Helfrich, W.; Elsinga, P.H. Nuclear imaging of prostate cancer with gastrin-releasing-peptide-receptor targeted radiopharmaceuticals. *Curr. Pharm. Des.* **2008**, *14*, 3033–3047. [CrossRef] [PubMed]

18. Schroeder, R.P.J.; Muller, C.; Reneman, S.; Melis, M.L.; Breeman, W.A.P.; de Blois, E.; Bangma, C.H.; Krenning, E.P.; van Weerden, W.M.; de Jong, M. A standardised study to compare prostate cancer targeting efficacy of five radiolabelled bombesin analogues. *Eur. J. Nucl. Med. Mol. Imaging* **2010**, *37*, 1386–1396. [CrossRef] [PubMed]

19. Guerin, B.; Dumulon-Perreault, V.; Tremblay, M.C.; Ait-Mohand, S.; Fournier, P.; Dubuc, C.; Authier, S.; Benard, F. [lys(dota)(4)]bvd15, a novel and potent neuropeptide y analog designed for y-1 receptor-targeted breast tumor imaging. *Bioorg. Med. Chem. Lett.* **2010**, *20*, 950–953. [CrossRef] [PubMed]

20. Chatenet, D.; Cescato, R.; Waser, B.; Erchegyi, J.; Rivier, J.E.; Reubi, J.C. Novel dimeric dota-coupled peptidic y1-receptor antagonists for targeting of neuropeptide y receptor-expressing cancers. *EJNMMI Res.* **2011**, *1*, 21. [CrossRef] [PubMed]

21. Litau, S.; Niedermoser, S.; Vogler, N.; Roscher, M.; Schirrmacher, R.; Fricker, G.; Wangler, B.; Wangler, C. Next generation of sifalin-based tate derivatives for pet imaging of sstr-positive tumors: Influence of molecular design on in vitro sstr binding and in vivo pharmacokinetics. *Bioconjug. Chem.* **2015**, *26*, 2350–2359. [CrossRef] [PubMed]

22. Lindner, S.; Fiedler, L.; Wängler, B.; Bartenstein, P.; Schirrmacher, R.; Wängler, C. Design, synthesis and in vitro evaluation of heterobivalent peptidic radioligands targeting both grp- and vpac1-receptors concomitantly overexpressed on various malignancies—Is the concept feasible? *Eur. J. Med. Chem.* **2018**, *155*, 84–95. [CrossRef] [PubMed]

23. Glaser, M.; Morrison, M.; Solbakken, M.; Arukwe, J.; Karlsen, H.; Wiggen, U.; Champion, S.; Kindberg, G.M.; Cuthbertson, A. Radiosynthesis and biodistribution of cyclic rgd peptides conjugated with novel [18f]fluorinated aldehyde-containing prosthetic groups. *Bioconjug. Chem.* **2008**, *19*, 951–957. [CrossRef] [PubMed]

24. Garayoa, E.G.; Schweinsberg, C.; Maes, V.; Brans, L.; Blauenstein, P.; Tourwe, D.A.; Schibli, R.; Schubiger, P.A. Influence of the molecular charge on the biodistribution of bombesin analogues labeled with the [tc-99m(co)(3)]-core. *Bioconjug. Chem.* **2008**, *19*, 2409–2416. [CrossRef] [PubMed]

25. Niedermoser, S.; Chin, J.; Wängler, C.; Kostikov, A.; Bernard-Gauthier, V.; Vogler, N.; Soucy, J.P.; McEwan, A.J.; Schirrmacher, R.; Wängler, B. In vivo evaluation of f-18-sifalin-modified tate: A potential challenge for ga-68-dotatate, the clinical gold standard for somatostatin receptor imaging with pet. *J. Nucl. Med.* **2015**, *56*, 1100–1105. [CrossRef] [PubMed]

26. Sparr, C.; Purkayastha, N.; Yoshinari, T.; Seebach, D.; Maschauer, S.; Prante, O.; Hubner, H.; Gmeiner, P.; Kolesinska, B.; Cescato, R.; et al. Syntheses, receptor bindings, in vitro and in vivo stabilities and biodistributions of dota-neurotensin(8-13) derivatives containing beta-amino acid residues—A lesson about the importance of animal experiments. *Chem. Biodivers.* **2013**, *10*, 2101–2121. [CrossRef] [PubMed]

27. Storch, D.; Behe, M.; Walter, M.A.; Chen, J.H.; Powell, P.; Mikolajczak, R.; Macke, H.R. Evaluation of [tc-99m/edda/hynic0]octreotide derivatives compared with [in-111-dota(0),tyr(3), thr(8)]octreotide and [in-111-dtpa(0)]octreotide: Does tumor or pancreas uptake correlate with the rate of internalization? *J. Nucl. Med.* **2005**, *46*, 1561–1569. [PubMed]

28. Fournier, P.; Dumulon-Perreault, V.; Ait-Mohand, S.; Tremblay, S.; Benard, F.; Lecomte, R.; Guerin, B. Novel radiolabeled peptides for breast and prostate tumor pet imaging: Cu-64/and ga-68/nota-peg-[d-tyr(6),beta ala(11),thi(13),nle(14)]bbn(6-14). *Bioconjug. Chem.* **2012**, *23*, 1687–1693. [CrossRef] [PubMed]

29. Amlal, H.; Faroqui, S.; Balasubramaniam, A.; Sheriff, S. Estrogen up-regulates neuropeptide yy1 receptor expression in a human breast cancer cell line. *Cancer Res.* **2006**, *66*, 3706–3714. [CrossRef] [PubMed]

30. Rennert, R.; Weber, L.; Richter, W. Receptor Ligand Linked Cytotoxic Molecules. WO2014040752A1, 20 March 2014.

31. Liu, Z.; Yan, Y.; Liu, S.; Wang, F.; Chen, X. (18)f, (64)cu, and (68)ga labeled rgd-bombesin heterodimeric peptides for pet imaging of breast cancer. *Bioconjug. Chem.* **2009**, *20*, 1016–1025. [CrossRef] [PubMed]

32. Memminger, M.; Keller, M.; Lopuch, M.; Pop, N.; Bernhardt, G.; von Angerer, E.; Buschauer, A. The neuropeptide y y-1 receptor: A diagnostic marker? Expression in mcf-7 breast cancer cells is down-regulated by antiestrogens in vitro and in xenografts. *PLoS ONE* **2012**, *7*, e51032. [CrossRef] [PubMed]

33. Chao, C.; Ives, K.; Hellmich, H.L.; Townsend, C.M.; Hellmich, M.R. Gastrin-releasing peptide receptor in breast cancer mediates cellular migration and interleukin-8 expression. *J. Surg. Res.* **2009**, *156*, 26–31. [CrossRef] [PubMed]

34. Keller, M.; Maschauer, S.; Brennauer, A.; Tripal, P.; Koglin, N.; Dittrich, R.; Bernhardt, G.; Kuwert, T.; Wester, H.J.; Buschauer, A.; et al. Prototypic f-18-labeled argininamide-type neuropeptide y y1r antagonists as tracers for pet imaging of mammary carcinoma. *ACS Med. Chem. Lett.* **2017**, *8*, 304–309. [CrossRef] [PubMed]

35. Ait-Mohand, S.; Dumulon-Perreault, V.; Benard, F.; Guerin, B. Design optimization of a new 64cu/nota truncated npy analog with improved stability and y1 affinity, the first step toward successful breast cancer pet imaging. *J. Nucl. Med.* **2016**, *57*, S1076.

36. Ebner, A.; Wildling, L.; Kamruzzahan, A.S.M.; Rankl, C.; Wruss, J.; Hahn, C.D.; Holzl, M.; Zhu, R.; Kienberger, F.; Blaas, D.; et al. A new, simple method for linking of antibodies to atomic force microscopy tips. *Bioconjug. Chem.* **2007**, *18*, 1176–1184. [CrossRef] [PubMed]

10

Radioligands for Tropomyosin Receptor Kinase (Trk) Positron Emission Tomography Imaging

Ralf Schirrmacher [1],* ⓘ, Justin J. Bailey [1], Andrew V. Mossine [2], Peter J. H. Scott [2,3] ⓘ, Lena Kaiser [4] ⓘ, Peter Bartenstein [4], Simon Lindner [4], David R. Kaplan [5], Alexey Kostikov [6], Gert Fricker [7], Anne Mahringer [7], Pedro Rosa-Neto [8], Esther Schirrmacher [1], Carmen Wängler [9], Björn Wängler [10], Alexander Thiel [6,11], Jean-Paul Soucy [6] and Vadim Bernard-Gauthier [12,13],*

[1]   Department of Oncology, Division of Oncological Imaging, University of Alberta, Edmonton, Alberta T6G 2R3, Canada; jjbailey@ualberta.ca (J.J.B.); eschirrm@ualberta.ca (E.S.)

[2]   Division of Nuclear Medicine, Department of Radiology, The University of Michigan Medical School, Ann Arbor, MI, 48109, USA; amossine@med.umich.edu (A.V.M.); pjhscott@med.umich.edu (P.J.H.S.)

[3]   The Interdepartmental Program in Medicinal Chemistry, University of Michigan, Ann Arbor, MI 48109, USA

[4]   Department of Nuclear Medicine, Ludwig-Maximilians-University of Munich, Marchioninistrasse 15, Munich 81377, Germany; Lena.Kaiser@med.uni-muenchen.de (L.K.); Peter.Bartenstein@med.uni-muenchen.de (P.B.); Simon.Lindner@med.uni-muenchen.de (S.L.)

[5]   Program in Neurosciences and Mental Health, Hospital for Sick Children and Department of Molecular Genetics, University of Toronto, Toronto, ON, Canada M5G 0A4; dkaplan@sickkids.ca

[6]   McConnell Brain Imaging Centre, Montreal Neurological Institute, McGill University, 3801 University Street, Montreal, QC H3A 2B4, Canada; alexey.kostikov@mcgill.ca (A.K.); alexander.thiel@mcgill.ca (A.T.); jean-paul.soucy@mcgill.ca (J.-P.S.)

[7]   Institute of Pharmacy and Molecular Biotechnology, University of Heidelberg, Heidelberg 69120, Germany; gert.fricker@uni-hd.de (G.F.); mahringer@uni-hd.de (A.M.)

[8]   Translational Neuroimaging Laboratory, McGill Centre for Studies in Aging, Douglas Mental Health University Institute, Montreal, QC H4H 1R3, Canada; pedro.rosa.neto@gmail.com

[9]   Biomedical Chemistry, Department of Clinical Radiology and Nuclear Medicine, Medical Faculty Mannheim of Heidelberg University, 68167 Mannheim, Germany; Carmen.Waengler@medma.uni-heidelberg.de

[10] Molecular Imaging and Radiochemistry, Department of Clinical Radiology and Nuclear Medicine, Medical Faculty Mannheim of Heidelberg University, Theodor-Kutzer-Ufer 1-3, Mannheim 68167, Germany; Bjoern.Waengler@medma.uni-heidelberg.de

[11] Jewish General Hospital, Lady Davis Institute, Montreal, QC HT3 1E2, Canada

[12] Azrieli Centre for Neuro-Radiochemistry, Research Imaging Centre, Centre for Addiction and Mental Health, Toronto, ON M5T 1L8, Canada

[13] Department of Psychiatry, University of Toronto, Toronto, ON M5T 1R8, Canada

*   Correspondence: schirrma@ualberta.ca (R.S.); Vadim.bernard-gauthier@camhpet.ca (V.B.-G.);

Abstract: The tropomyosin receptor kinases family (TrkA, TrkB, and TrkC) supports neuronal growth, survival, and differentiation during development, adult life, and aging. TrkA/B/C downregulation is a prominent hallmark of various neurological disorders including Alzheimer's disease (AD). Abnormally expressed or overexpressed full-length or oncogenic fusion TrkA/B/C proteins were shown to drive tumorigenesis in a variety of neurogenic and non-neurogenic human cancers and are currently the focus of intensive clinical research. Neurologic and oncologic studies of the spatiotemporal alterations in TrkA/B/C expression and density and the determination of target engagement of emerging antineoplastic clinical inhibitors in normal and diseased tissue are crucially needed but have remained largely unexplored due to the lack of suitable non-invasive probes. Here, we review the recent development of carbon-11- and fluorine-18-labeled positron emission tomography (PET) radioligands based on specifically designed small molecule kinase catalytic domain-binding inhibitors of TrkA/B/C. Basic developments in medicinal chemistry, radiolabeling and translational PET imaging in multiple species including humans are highlighted.

Keywords: tropomyosin receptor kinase; positron emission tomography; neurodegeneration; oncogenic fusions

1. Introduction

Tropomyosin receptor kinases (TrkA, TrkB, and TrkC) are transmembrane glycoproteins encoded by genes *NTRK1–3*, respectively. These kinases encompass extracellular domains (ECD) interacting specifically with endogenous neurotrophins as well as highly homologous intracellular tyrosine kinase domains (Figure 1A). Nerve growth factor (NGF) binds to TrkA, brain-derived neurotrophic factor (BDNF), neurothrophin-3 (NT-3), and neurotrophin-4 (NT-4) to TrkB, and NT-3 to TrkC [1–3]. Full length TrkB is a 140-kD transmembrane spanning protein, with an extracellular ligand-binding domain containing two cysteine clusters, leucine-rich repeats, and two immunogloblulin-like domains [4]. The intracellular domain encodes a tyrosine kinase domain that when activated transphosphorylates monomers of the TrkB dimer. When transphosphorylated, the Trks engage and phosphorylate their major substrates Shc, Phospholipase C γ1 (PLC-γ 1), and Fibroblast Growth Factor Receptor Substrate 2 (FRS2/SNT1) [5]. The TrkB locus also encodes four variants generated by alternative splicing, of which the most abundant is the 90-kD truncated TrkB.t1 isoform that lacks the kinase domain [6]. Trk signaling occurs primarily through Ras/Mitogen-Activated Protein Kinase 1 (MAPK1), Phosphoinositide-3-Kinase (PI3-K)/Akt and PLC-γ1 [4,7–9] and plays central roles in mediating neuronal survival and differentiation in the embryonic, postnatal, and mature peripheral (PNS) and central nervous system (CNS) [2,3]. Within the CNS, reduced expression, as well as abnormal and impaired signaling of Trk receptors, are associated with a plethora of neuropathologies, including ischemic brain injury, schizophrenia, Rett syndrome, depression, Parkinson's disease (PD), and Alzheimer's disease (AD) [10–16]. In AD, evidence from ex vivo experiments accumulated over the last two decades demonstrates reductions in full length catalytic TrkB/C receptor densities as well as a decline in TrkB/C neurotrophin signaling [17]. Direct evidence for the involvement of alterations in BDNF/TrkB signalling in AD is supported by studies indicating that TrkB levels are profoundly decreased in the hippocampus, frontal and temporal cortex of patients with Alzheimer's [18], although apparently not in the parietal cortex [19]. Furthermore, progressive loss of TrkA, B, and C in basal forebrain cholinergic nuclei is well correlated with the clinical progression of AD [20]. Treatment with agonists of the BDNF/TrkB system of transgenic mouse models of AD increases dendritic spines in the hippocampus and cortex, inhibits neuronal apoptosis and neurodegeneration, and improves spatial memory performance [21–25]. These findings support the use of agents that activate BDNF/TrkB for treating AD [26]. Yet, the in vivo relevance or the spatiotemporal evolution of such changes, as well as the relationships which may exist with known neuropathological hallmarks of neurodegeneration such as plaque deposition and neurofibrillary tangle (NFTs) aggregation in AD—both of which can be visualized using diagnostic positron emission tomography (PET)—are unresolved questions. The potential importance of perturbations of Trk expression, activity and signalling in neurodegeneration hence raises the question of whether these molecular targets can in turn be imaged in vivo and non-invasively using PET. Another potential application for Trk-targeted radioligands stems from the renewed and rapidly growing interest in anti-Trk therapy for cancer. Indeed, important advances in recent years have been made in the treatment of patients with *NTRK* fusion-positive cancers in basket trials using pan-Trk inhibitors [27]. In parallel, remarkable progress has also been achieved in the development of selective pan-Trk and TrkA subtype-selective tyrosine kinase inhibitors (TKIs). *NTRK* fusions are found at low frequency in a number of common cancers and at a relatively high frequency in rare neoplasms—amounting to about 1500–5000 patients with *NTRK* fusions-positive diseases per year in the United States. Current clinical trials assessing *NTRK* fusion-positive patients inherently rely on tumour biopsy (which may not be always achievable) followed by next generation sequencing or fluorescence in situ hybridization for fusion detection. The use of Trk-targeted PET imaging in early clinical stages to assess receptor occupancy, dosing regimen, and *NTRK* fusion-positive status, or to monitor treatment response in place of sequential tumour biopsy may be both achievable and desirable—as previously done with other molecular targeted TKI therapies [28].

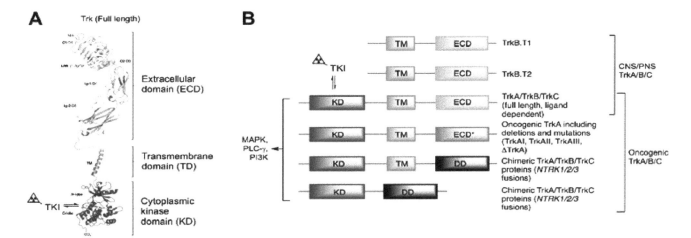

Figure 1. Detailed and representative domains of normally expressed and aberrantly expressed oncogenic tropomyosin receptor kinase (Trk) proteins from *NTRK* fusions (TKI: tyrosine kinase inhibitor). (**A**) Structure overview of the representative full TrkA receptor (D1–D5: domain 1–5; C1/3: cysteine cluster 1/3; LRR: leucine-rich repeat; Ig-1/2: immunoglobulin domain 1/2, TM: transmembrane domain). (**B**) Schematic representation of diverse Trk proteins and domains, including Trk splice variants and Trk fusion proteins. Dimerization and trans-autophosphorylation of Trk kinase domains leads to the activation of the downstream signaling pathways, including MAPK1, PI3-K/Akt and PLC-γ1 (DD: dimerization domain).

Until very recently, suitable imaging lead compounds or quantifiable non-invasive techniques to measure spatiotemporal fluctuations of TrkA/B/C levels have been unavailable. To address this, we undertook in 2014 the task of identifying structural determinants which would enable TrkA/B/C PET imaging. To this end, we developed structurally diverse Trk radiotracers and inhibitor libraries with various levels of potency and kinome selectivity, both from type I and type II inhibitor classes, and exploited diverse radiochemical approaches using carbon-11 and fluorine-18. While our primary objective has been non-oncological neuroimaging in the context of neurodegeneration and most results gathered thus far aimed at meeting this objective, we recognize that with the recent clinical oncological breakthrough in Trk inhibitor therapy comes a clear need for reliable and non-invasive assessment of Trk status in cancer therapy trials. In this short review, we describe the rational design and development of first-in-class Trk-targeted TKI PET radiotracers and delineate imaging validation obtained with these molecular probes to date.

2. The Development of Trk Radioligands for PET Imaging

2.1. Binding Site Considerations

PET radionuclides decay by emission of a positron, which in turn annihilates with a nearby electron, generating two gamma rays of 511 keV (conversion of the positron's and electron's mass into energy). These two gamma rays, emitted in the opposite directions, can then be detected by an outside PET camera, revealing the position of the annihilation events with sufficient spatial resolution (from submillimeter to millimeter in preclinical and clinical settings respectively). Under the assumption of a sufficient tissue target receptor concentration (Bmax), an ideal radiotracer, in this context, needs to meet certain criteria which include: (1) high radioligand concentration in the tissue of interest, (2) radiotracer equilibrium conditions are reached, (3) lack of interfering radiometabolites and (4) high on-target selectivity. Beyond requiring careful studies of possible radiometabolites, this also highlights the importance of targeting suitable domains of a molecular target. This is especially relevant in the case of Trk where various isoforms, splice variants or fusions proteins may be co-expressed within a single tissue in different clinical contexts. For example, in addition to the full length TrkA/B/C, a number of truncated isoforms lacking the intracellular kinase domain have been characterized for TrkB (Figure 1B). Within the brain, the protein expression levels of the truncated isoforms of TrkB present (TrkB.T1 and TrkB.T2) far exceed that of full length TrkB [29]. A radiotracer binding the TrkB extracellular domain (ECD) would consequently map the sum of all TrkB receptors in the brain including the truncated isoforms which as yet have no known reported association with neurodegeneration or as oncogenic drivers. A PET signal originating from such a radiotracer would fail to differentiate catalytically-incompetent truncated from full-length kinase domain-containing receptors and would be unable to engage targets which lack cognate ectodomains such as the many NTRK fusion proteins which are of prime clinical interest (Figure 1B). More pragmatically, another reason to avoid targeting ECDs of Trk for imaging stems from the lack of suitable compounds. Indeed, while the study of nonprotein Trk ECD-binding compounds largely predates the advent of Trk-targeted TKIs, very limited progress has been achieved due to the inherently challenging druggability of the ectodomains compared to the kinase domains of TrkA/B/C and the poor drug-like properties of such compounds. These limitations have been exemplified by our imaging study of radiolabeled 7,8-dihydroxyflavone (7,8-DHF) [30]. This work was based on the initial report by Jang et al. suggesting that 7,8-DHF binds with high affinity to the ECD of TrkB and exhibits agonistic activity in neurons [31]. From this initial work, other more active flavones were described including fluorinated analogs which caught our attention as potential starting points for ^{18}F-PET tracer development [32,33]. Yet, using synthesized or commercially available described flavones we were unable to reproduce any basic biochemical effects in cells (unpublished data). In line with our findings, Boltaev et al. more recently unambiguously demonstrated the lack of direct interaction or TrkB-driven effect of such compounds [34]. In addition, we observed poor in vivo profiles in rats when investigating the radiolabeled isotopologs of these compounds for imaging (including 2-(4-[^{18}F]fluorophenyl)-7,8-dihydroxy-4H-chromen-4-one). Preclinical imaging revealed low-radioactivity overall brain uptake with a maximum standard uptake value (SUV) of 0.64 (whole brain) followed by fast elimination from the brain. These radioligands also were rapidly eliminated from the plasma compartment by hepatic metabolism with an estimated plasma half-life under 4 min suggesting a fast and extensive phase II metabolism and suggesting overall poor druglike properties, as it is known for hydroxyflavones more generally [35,36]. Interestingly, in vitro autoradiography with rat brains revealed apparent specific and BDNF-competitive binding reminiscent of ^{125}I-BDNF binding topology. Yet, we surmise that this binding/blocking effect may have been a consequence of covalent reactivity to nucleophilic cysteines or other non-selective thiol-based reactivity as previously described for pan assay interference flavonoids [37]. Compared to putative ECD binding compounds, inhibitors targeting the ATP binding site of the cytoplasmic Trk kinase domains have been well characterized both functionally and structurally and have been reported alongside detailed crystallographic data enabling derivatization [38]. Targeting the kinase domains however comes with the challenge of selectivity, firstly within the kinome and secondly from within the Trk kinase family itself (TrkA, TrkB and TrkC)—TrkA/B/C display 72–78% and 95–100% sequence identity in their kinase domain and ATP binding sites, respectively. We have strived to detail kinome selectivity using comprehensive kinase screening whenever possible. With the exception of a few compounds, all radiolabeled inhibitors display pan-Trk activities. Yet, owing to the high expression levels of TrkB/C in the CNS compared to TrkA [39–43], and given that the PET signal is driven by target density and ligand affinity, it is to be expected that CNS PET using pan-Trk radioligands will nevertheless detect nearly exclusively TrkB/C-based signal. Another important note pertains to the fact that Trk kinases can adopt both DFG-in (active, targeted by type-I inhibitors) and DFG-out (inactive, targeted by type-II inhibitors) conformations (Figure 2). Conformational changes upon DFG triad rearrangement allow for the access of a deep pocket which can be occupied favorably by lipophilic moieties (Figure 2B,C). Type II Trk inhibitors targeting DFG-out conformation thus also present longer residence times compared to type-I inhibitors. To study potential benefits from each binding modes, we have developed both type-I and II radioligands.

The following paragraphs give an account on our Trk radiotracer development program in chronological order progressing towards first in human PET imaging from preclinical research.

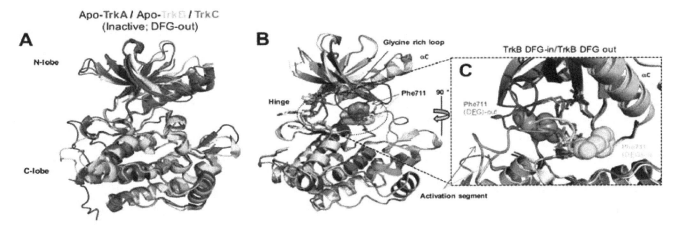

Figure 2. Trk kinase domain. (**A**) Overlap of TrkA, TrkB, and TrkC kinase domain (inactive conformations, PDB ID: 4F0I, 4ASZ, 3V5Q). (**B,C**) Views of the conformational differences between "Asp-Phe-Gly" DFG-in and DFG-out TrkB. The Phe residues of the DFG triad are shown in spheres (PDB ID: 4AT3, 4AT5).

2.1.1. The 4-Aza-2-oxindole Radioligands

PET tracers for neuroimaging have significantly higher chances of achieving high specific binding in brain when displaying certain physicochemical properties. Parameters such as rapid Blood Brain Barrier (BBB) permeation and neuron cell penetration as well as low non-specific binding are mostly determined by the compound's lipophilicity (represented as clogD $_{7.4}$ value, assuming passive diffusion through the cell membrane), reduced susceptibility to active efflux, molecular weight (<350 Da), favorable neuroreceptor binding potential (BP = B_{max}/K_d >10), topological surface area (TSPA) of 30–80 Å^2, and hydrogen bond donor ability (HBD) of >1. These general factors as well as specific properties tend to characterize successful neuroimaging PET tracers [44–47]. With these parameters in mind, we first opted for an inhibitor belonging to the family of 3-arylideneindolin-2-one Trk inhibitors. The 4-aza-2-oxindole inhibitor GW441756 [48] was screened as a compound favorably fulfilling the above mentioned requirements of a potentially successful candidate for brain imaging and was consequently labeled with carbon-11 to provide the radioactive isotopolog for autoradiography and PET imaging (half maximal inhibitory concentration (IC$_{50}$); TrkA = 29.6 nM, TrkB = 6.7 nM, and TrkC = 4.6 nM, Figure 3) [49]. Even though the radiolabeling was straightforward and high yielding, the targeted *Z* isomer, which based on molecular modeling was found to be the active isomer, could not be obtained in pure form after purification of the crude radiolabeling solution. An *E/Z* 1:1 mixture was isolated under all conducted labeling conditions as a result of rapid in situ isomerisation either during the radiosynthesis or during the HPLC purification procedure, reducing the amount of high affinity Trk tracer *Z*-[^{11}C]GW441756 by 50%. The inevitable contamination of the *E*-isomer with *Z*-[^{11}C]GW441756 significantly compromised the merit of this tracer as a potential Trk PET imaging agent, not only from an imaging quality perspective (50% of the PET signal will be the result of the non-specific binding of the Z-isomer) but also from a clinical translational point of view. Autoradiography of the mixed isomers on coronal rat brain sections revealed a displaceable binding in accordance with the ubiquitous distribution of all TrkB/C subtypes. The in vivo evaluation of [^{11}C]GW441756 was performed in Sprague–Dawley rats to evaluate BBB penetration and in vivo biodistribution. In baseline scans the tracer rapidly entered the brain peaking at a SUV of 2 after 30 s, after which the compound was rapidly eliminated from the brain over 30 min. Tracer distribution was uniform in accordance with ubiquitous TrkB/C expression in the rodent brain. A blocking study using unlabeled GW441756 pre-treatment was inconclusive as to whether the tracer specifically engages the

CNS TrkB/C in vivo, however specific binding was indicated from blocking significant lung uptake of the tracer which may be linked to TrkB specific binding in pulmonary tissue [50]. An ^{18}F derivative bearing an ^{18}F-fluoroethyl group at the 5-hydroxy moiety of a new GW441756 derivative, although being highly selective over other kinases and displaying generally favorable in vitro properties (low IC$_{50}$ values in the nanomolar range for all Trk subtypes), showed unexpected susceptibility towards CYP450 metabolism in vitro in contrast to the original GW441756. These findings were corroborated by rapid formation of brain penetrating metabolites and no observable blocking upon pre-treatment with non-radioactive GW441756 in an animal PET experiment in rats. It can be concluded from our data that radioligands for pan-Trk imaging with PET, derived from the 3-indolydene 4-aza-2-oxindole scaffold despite being selective and highly potent inhibitors of Trk, do most probably not lend themselves towards PET tracer development and clinical translation. The main reason is the inevitable presence of the low affinity E-isomer of [^{11}C]GW441756 due to the rapid reaching of a photostationary state, a physicochemical reality that most definitely is not limited to GW441756 but rather extends to all structurally similar derivatives. However, both tracers displayed high specific binding in TrkB expressing neuroblastoma tumour sections in vitro providing a proof of principle of the utility of such radioligands for oncological imaging.

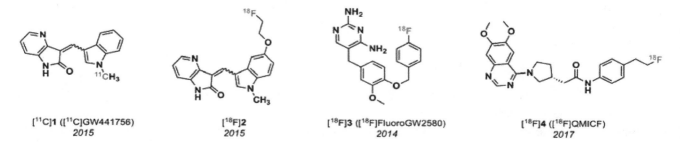

Figure 3. Chemical structures of early Trk-targeted positron emission tomography (PET) radioligands.

2.1.2. 2,4-Diaminopyridmidine and Quinazoline-Based Radioligands

In order to explore the effect of targeting the DFG-out Trk kinase conformation, especially with regard to kinetics [51], we also developed type II radiolabeled inhibitors. In general, type II Trk inhibitors tend to possess mostly elongated structural features, higher molecular weight and HBD count than type-I inhibitors, which may be detrimental for BBB permeation but inconsequential in the context of peripheral imaging. So far we have developed two distinct type-II radiolabeled inhibitors belonging to the class of 2,4-diaminopyridines [52] and quinazoline [53] (Figure 3). Analyses of large kinase inhibitor sets identified GW2580, an orally active dual Trk/colony-stimulating factor-1 receptor (CSF-1R) inhibitor (K_d; CSF-1R = 2 nM, TrkA = 630 nM, TrkB = 36 nM, and TrkC = 120 nM), as one of the most kinome selective inhibitors known [54]. Based on this attribute, and the overall promising preclinical ADME (absorption, distribution, metabolism, and excretion) of this inhibitor, we undertook to identify a radioligand based on this scaffold. We rationalized that since CSF-1R is highly expressed in tumour-infiltrating macrophages, such compounds may be useful in cancer imaging beyond Trk. We synthesized fluorinated derivatives and performed labelling of the most promising lead, 5-(4-((4-[^{18}F]fluorobenzyl)oxy)-3-methoxybenzyl)pyrimidine-2,4-diamine ([^{18}F]3, Figure 3). While inhibitor [^{18}F]3 maintained the excellent kinome selectivity of GW2580, its radiosynthesis was challenging and relied on the synthesis of the prosthetic group 4-[^{18}F]fluorobenzyl bromide [55] followed by subsequent reaction with a phenolic labeling precursor. The multistep procedure only produced low radiochemical yields (RCYs) of [^{18}F]3. This technical shortcoming precluded this tracer from its translation into a clinical setting and only most recent efforts applying Cu-mediated late stage fluorination techniques provided this tracer in high RCYs and high molar activities suitable for human PET scanning (unpublished). More recently, the quinazoline-based type II pan-Trk inhibitor [^{18}F]QMICF ([^{18}F]4) was developed (Figure 3) [53]. Starting from the corresponding racemic quinazoline-based dual FLT3/TrkB inhibitor, a structure–activity relationship study demonstrated that the (R)-enantiomer was primarily responsible for Trk inhibition [56]. To conserve optimal target interaction with the Trk receptor, the position of fluorine introduction was carefully consolidated through molecular modeling. Only one particular position, namely the allosteric pocket fragment, proved adaptable towards structural modifications with the least detrimental effect on binding interaction. We replaced the isopropyl moiety connected in 4-position to a structurally flexible benzene moiety in the original inhibitor with a 2-fluoro ethyl group to facilitate an easy introduction of $^{18}F^-$ via common nucleophilic substitution of a corresponding mesyl derivative. This modification led to an about 10-fold potency reduction but also favorably abrogated FLT3 activity. Kinases profiling of inhibitor **4** revealed excellent selectivity and a Calcein-AM assay in P-gp overexpressing MDCKII cells confirmed only low interaction with P-gp. Radiotracer [^{18}F]QMICF could be straightforwardly synthesized from the corresponding mesyl precursor in RCYs of 18% in one step. The compound is currently being evaluated for Trk brain imaging and tumor imaging in TrkA-TPM3 (IC$_{50}$ = 162 nM) overexpressing colon carcinoma KM12 mice tumor xenografts and other neoplasms bearing diverse *NTKR* fusions.

2.1.3. Imidazo[1,2-*b*]pyridazine-Based Radioligands

In 2014, when we started the syntheses of imidazo[1,2-*b*]pyridazine-based radioligands, it was demonstrated that *NTRK* fusion were actionable drivers in human cancers, however only a few non selective Trk inhibitors had been used in a therapeutic approach. The Trk inhibitor landscape was however rapidly moving from exploratory tool inhibitor (such as GW441756) to more relevant drug leads and there was a clear trend in preclinical work and patent literature towards what has now become one of the most explored chemotypes, specifically imidazo[1,2-*b*]pyridazine and pyrazolo[1,5-a]pyrimidine-based inhibitors (Figure 4). Cognizant of this trend, and expecting that scaffolds selected for clinical oncological studies should display overall excellent druglike properties which could in turn be advantageous for achieving brain and peripheral imaging using PET, we reoriented our effort towards inhibitors of these classes. We found that in comparison to all potential radiotracers described above, the type I pan-Trk inhibitors sharing the (2-pyrrolidin-1-yl)imidazo[1,2-*b*]pyridazine structural motif (Figure 5), share exceptionally high affinities to all three Trk subtype receptors orders of magnitude higher than any other inhibitor described so far.[57] Based on extensive molecular docking studies, a comprehensive PET-oriented library of imidazo[1,2-*b*]pyridazine-based compounds (bearing positions amenable for labeling using carbon-11 and/or fluorine-18) was reported in 2015 [57]. All new pan-Trk inhibitors were subjected to a [γ-^{33}P]ATP-based enzymatic assay to assess activities towards the different Trk subtypes. Remarkably, eight inhibitors from this library displayed <200 pM potency against TrkB/C and were initially regarded as potential candidates for radiotracer development. Two structures, ($\pm$)-IPMICF6 and ($\pm$)-IPMICF10 (Figure 5) lent themselves towards an easy introduction of ^{18}F via simple nucleophilic substitution and were translated into the corresponding ^{18}F-radiotracers. Both compounds displayed favorable in vitro activity and kinome selectivity. Their ^{18}F labeling was straightforward and yielded the corresponding radiotracers in 3% and 8% RCY, respectively. In autoradiography experiments, both compounds were conclusively apt to topologically map the known brain distribution (cortex, striatum, thalamus and cerebellum) of TrkB/C receptors in coronal rat brain sections in accordance with mRNA and protein levels. In an important follow up study, one inhibitor from the reported imidazo[1,2-*b*]pyridazine-based library, IPMICF16, was chosen for radiotracer translation based on the alignment of favorable physicochemical properties (as described above) and optimal pharmacological parameters [58]. Pan-Trk inhibitor IPMICF16's structure is geared towards simple ^{11}C-methylation radiolabeling. In order to confirm that (*R*)-IPMICF16 was the more active and hence more suitable enantiomer for radiotracer development, as expected based on crystal structure and docking analyses, both the *R* and *S* isomers were synthesized and evaluated. Non-radioactive (*R*)-IPMICF16 displayed IC$_{50}$s of 4.0, 0.2 and 0.1 nM for human TrkA, TrkB, and TrkC, respectively and inhibitory constants (K_i) of 2.80, 0.05 and 0.021 nM for TrkA, TrkB, and TrkC, respectively (200,000–500,000-fold over K_m ATP for all Trks). The *S*-enantiomer was significantly less potent which is in line with our docking studies. Interestingly, this study showed that (*R*)-IPMICF16 constitutes a rare example where an ATP-competitive Trk inhibitor displays intra-Trk sub-type selectivity. With regard to TrkA, (*R*)-IPMICF16 showed 56-fold and 133-fold higher selectivity for TrkB and TrkC, respectively. It was further asserted that the compound shows high selectivity towards TrkB/C over >99% of the testable human kinome (369 targets). The radiosynthesis of [^{11}C]-(R)-IPMICF16 was routinely achieved using the corresponding desmethyl-precursor and radioactive [^{11}C]methyl iodide (or alternatively [^{11}C]methyl triflate) in >10% RCYs. Soon thereafter, the robust synthesis was set up according to good manufacturing practices and regulations at four different production sites where [^{11}C]-(R)-IPMICF16 was evaluated in mice, rats, non-human primates, and finally in one healthy human subject (Figure 6).

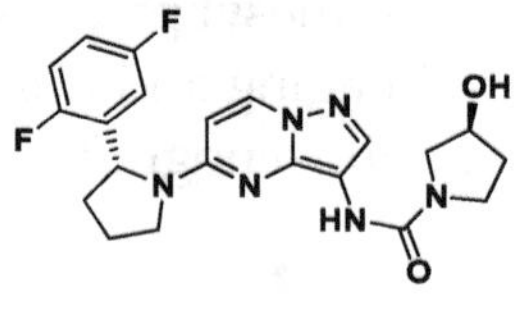

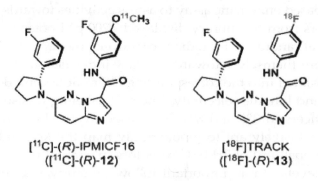

5 (Larotrectinib)
Pyrazolo[1,5a]pyrimidines
Multiple Phase I/II, 2015-

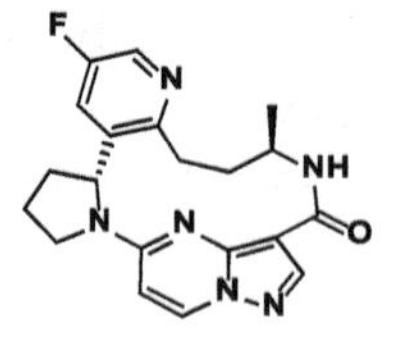

6 (LOXO-195)
Pyrazolo[1,5a]pyrimidines(macrocyclic)
Phase I/II, 2017-

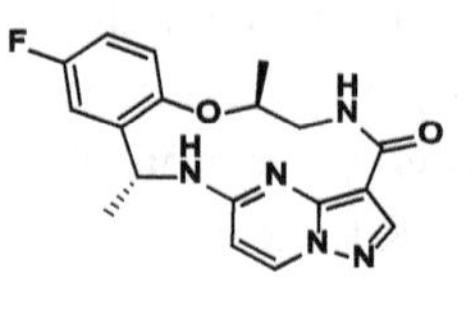

7 (Repotrectinib - TPX-0005)
Pyrazolo[1,5a]pyrimidines
(macrocyclic)
Phase I/II, 2017-

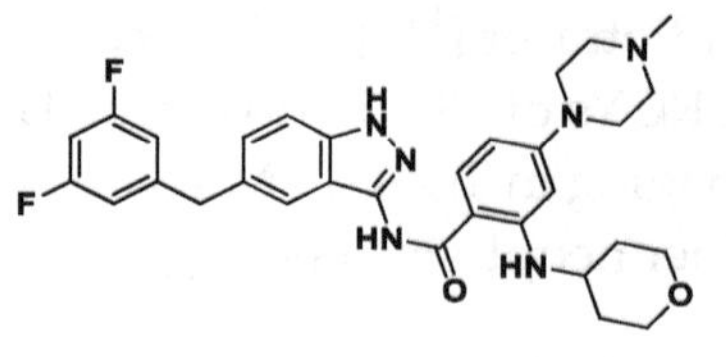

8 (Entrectinib)
Multiple Phase I/II, 2015-

Figure 4. Chemical structures of selected clinical Trk inhibitors.

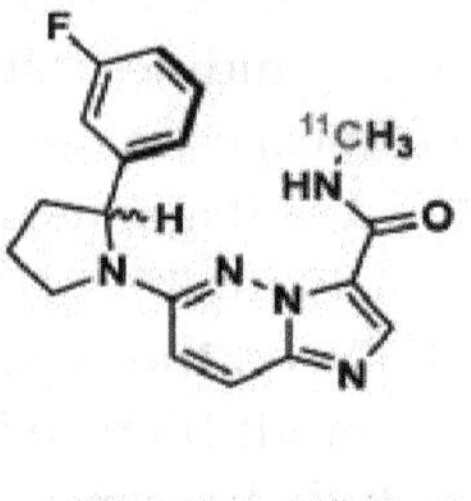

[^{11}C]-(±)-IPMICF22
([^{11}C]9)

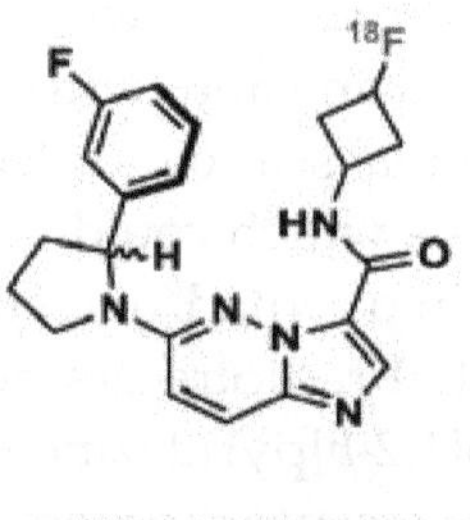

[^{18}F]-(±)-IPMICF6
([^{11}C]10)

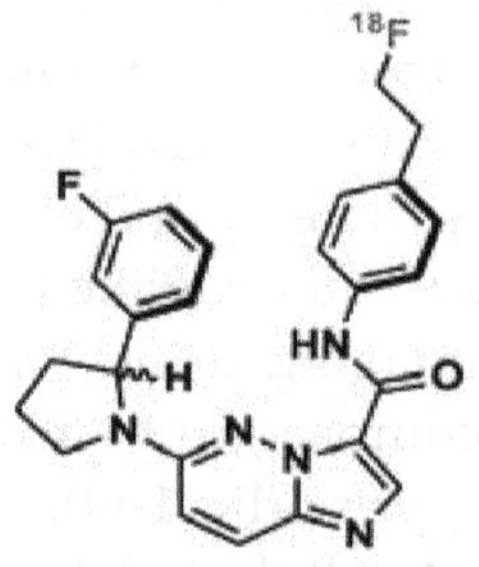

[^{18}F]-(±)-IPMICF10
([^{11}C]11)

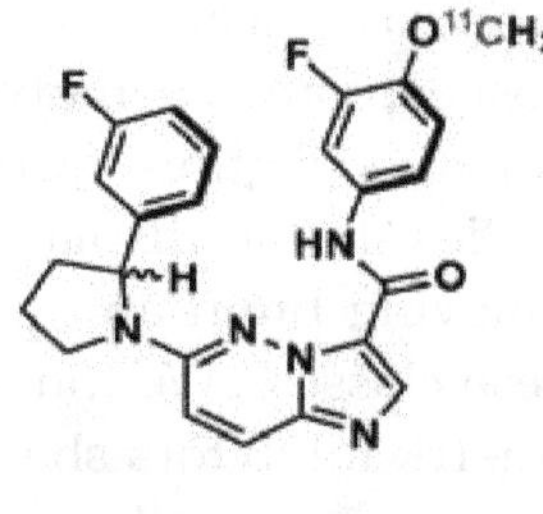

[^{11}C]-(±)-IPMICF16
([^{11}C]12)

Figure 5. Chemical structures of preclinical imidazo[1,2b]pyridazine-based Trk-targeted PET radioligands.

[^{11}C]-(R)-IPMICF16
([^{11}C]-(R)-12)

[^{18}F]TRACK
([^{18}F]-(R)-13)

Figure 6. Chemical structures of clinical imidazo[1,2b]pyridazine-based Trk-targeted PET radioligands.

Despite partial elimination of [^{11}C]-(R)-IPMICF16 from the rat brain due to active efflux transporters in rodents (P-gp and breast cancer resistance protein) as demonstrated in double knockout *Mdr1a/b-Bcrp* mice, SUV after 60-min scan time was still 0.4. The brain TrkB/C specific binding of [^{11}C]-(R)-IPMICF16 in vivo was unambiguously demonstrated by pharmacological challenge with the clinical pan-Trk inhibitor entrectinib. Up to 88% of the radioactivity signal could be blocked after intraperitoneal injection of entrectinib, albeit high blocking doses (350 mg/kg) were required due to the documented low brain uptake of this inhibitor. Encouraged by these promising data, an evaluation of [^{11}C]-(R)-IPMICF16 was performed in non-human primates (NHP). In comparison to rodents, the brain kinetics in NHP was significantly slower with a continuously increasing radioactivity signal in the brain devoid of an observable washout throughout the entire 60 min PET scan. Regional analysis confirmed a heterogenous radioactivity distribution following Trk rich grey matter with highest uptake in thalamus (SUV 0.8). Radioactivity uptake in white matter was comparatively low, as expected and in accordance with low level Trk expression. Although the efflux kinetic profiles of [^{11}C]-(R)-IPMICF16 was notable in rodents, data from NHP PET imaging indicated interspecies differences and suggested that efflux may not be a liability in higher species. Hence, it was decided to move the tracer forward towards human in vivo translation. This decision was further motivated by the demonstration that in vitro [^{11}C]-(R)-IPMICF16 autoradiography was sufficiently sensitive to reproduce the known and significant region-specific hippocampal TrkB/C density reduction found in AD brains (compared to age-matched controls). All radioactivity signals in brain tissues (controls and AD) were blockable using a structurally unrelated pan-Trk inhibitor proving specificity of the observed uptake as a result of TrkB/C receptor engagement. Taken together, these preclinical data justified moving towards a first-in-human tracer evaluation with PET.

Injection of [^{11}C]-(R)-IPMICF16 into a 41-year-old healthy male subject led to brain uptake of the radiotracer which was rapid, with a peak SUV in the thalamus of 1.5 after 25 s post injection, very similar to what was observed in NHP. After reaching equilibrium, the SUV in one of the highest Trk tissues, the thalamus, remained 0.7 after 60 min with low observable washout. In accordance with non-human primate PET data, the radioactivity distribution in human matched the topography of the Trk disposition in grey matter with lowest SUVs in TrkB/C low white matter regions (Figure 7). The overall distribution aligned affirmatively with the known Trk distribution from ex vivo studies with highest uptake in the thalamus, followed by cerebellum and cortex. No adverse effects were observed after the injection of [^{11}C]-(R)-IPMICF16.

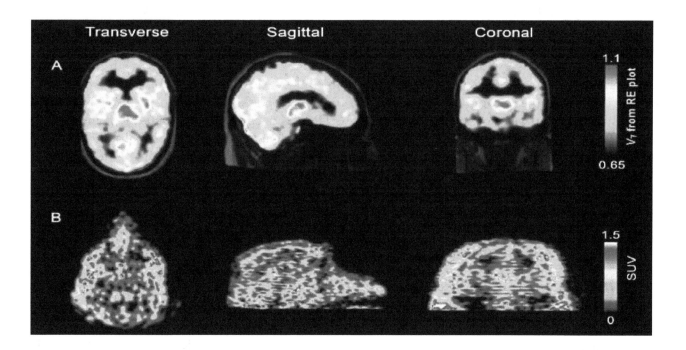

Figure 7. Upper row: PET/T1MP-RAGE MRT in vivo overlay images of [^{11}C]-(R)-12 in a human subject with high SUVs in TrkB/C rich compartments such as thalamus, followed by cerebellum and cortical grey matter and low uptake in Trk devoid white matter areas; Bottom row: In vivo PET images of [^{18}F]-(R)-13 (high A_m of 245 GBq/μmol) in rhesus monkey brain matching the expected TrkB/C distribution.

Owing to the detailed structure-activity study conducted in the first phase of this project, we intended to modify the structure of [^{11}C]-(R)-IPMICF16 to enable labeling with fluorine-18 based on the recently introduced Cu catalysed late stage fluorination of non-activated aromatic boronic esters [59–61]. Despite several shortcomings such as the inevitable side formation of protodeboronation side products, consequently contaminating the ^{18}F-labeled target molecule and therefore significantly reducing the effective molar activity (A_m) (the ^{18}F and H substitution product have very similar physicochemical as well as pharmacodynamics properties), the Cu-catalyzed ^{18}F fluorination of boronic esters and the introduction of mesityl aryl iodonium salts as labeling precursors can be easily regarded as being among the most important developments of modern ^{18}F-radiochemistry [62,63]. [^{11}C]-(R)-IPMICF16 originally bore a methoxy group directly adjacent to the fluorine atom at the aromatic amide fragment (Figure 6) which was identified as one contributor for the overall P-gp liability observed. That methoxy group was removed resulting in a pan-Trk inhibitor with further improved subtype selectivity but slightly reduced affinity for TrkB/C to reach binding equilibrium faster than [^{11}C]-(R)-IPMICF16. The efflux of the corresponding fluorinated inhibitor was also noticeably reduced in cells. This radiotracer, called [^{18}F]TRACK (the R isomer), was conveniently obtained in one step via Cu mediated radio-fluorination of a corresponding boronic ester precursor (the Bpin derivative) in satisfactory RCYs for further translation [64]. During the ^{18}F-fluorination, the protodeboronation product was formed which reduced the effective A_m to a low value of 15 GBq/μmol, an order of magnitude below what was expected. After extensive screening, this problem could be solved by employing a pentafluorophenyl (PFP) HPLC column for tracer purification—which constitutes currently the standard method used to achieve separation [65]. The column material showed improved stationary phase affinity interaction with the fluorinated TRACK tracer over standard octadecylsilane reversed phase, leading to a base-line separation of [^{18}F]TRACK from all impurities—including the protodeboronation side product. This improved the A_m to >100 GBq/μmol. In vivo evaluation in rhesus monkey confirmed uptake of [^{18}F]TRACK in TrkB/C-rich regions with SUVs in the grey matter ranging from 0.9 for the cerebellum, 0.8 for the thalamus, and 0.6 for the cortex (Figure 7). White matter uptake was comparably low (0.2 SUV). The brain kinetics of [^{18}F]TRACK were significantly different than what has been observed for [^{11}C]-(R)-IPMICF16, displaying characteristics of a more reversibly binding radiotracer. Injections of [^{18}F]TRACK of varying A_m (low, medium and high) into the same monkey illustrated the paramount importance of high A_m for Trk PET imaging. The PET signal was obviously reduced in cases of sub-optimal A_m. [^{18}F]TRACK is currently evaluated in human healthy controls and first in human PET data will be reported in due course. First obtained results with [^{18}F]TRACK in a healthy human volunteer are in line with the data obtained with [^{11}C]-(R)-IPMICF16 in terms of PET image quality and ease of production (unpublished).

3. Conclusions

The analysis, investigation and quantification of Trk receptors in neurodegenerative diseases and cancer is currently limited to ex vivo post-mortem analysis or invasive methods. While these kinases constitute important molecular targets which can be visualized using non-invasive PET imaging, Trk PET imaging is still in its infancy. Whether prototypical radioligands such as [^{11}C]-(R)-IPMICF16 and [^{18}F]TRACK, which display moderate brain uptake in humans, will be suitable for clinical neuroimaging and can provide reliable CNS TrkB/C measurements or adequately detect reductions in receptor density remain to be established. While tracers with higher brain penetration, volume of distribution (V_T) values or binding potentials are desirable for temporally and spatially assessing Trk expression in conditions such as AD, the current tracers could certainly be beneficial in cases where Trk is overexpressed such as in numerous human cancers, both in the periphery and CNS. Further research is currently aimed at identifying structural determinants improving overall brain uptake of current type I and II tracers, including cyclic derivatives such as LOXO 195 and derivatives thereof.

References

1. Lessmann, V.; Gottmann, K.; Malcangio, M. Neurotrophin secretion: Current facts and future prospects. *Progr. Neurobiol.* **2003**, *69*, 341–374. [CrossRef]
2. Chao, M.V. Neurotrophin receptors: A window into neuronal differentiation. *Neuron* **1992**, *9*, 583–593. [CrossRef]
3. Chao, M.V. Neurotrophins and their receptors: A convergence point for many signalling pathways. *Nat. Rev. Neurosci.* **2003**, *4*, 299–309. [CrossRef] [PubMed]
4. Huang, E.J.; Reichardt, L.F. Trk Receptors: Roles in Neuronal Signal Transduction. *Annu. Rev. Biochem.* **2003**, *72*, 609–642. [CrossRef] [PubMed]
5. Kaplan, D.R.; Miller, F.D. Neurotrophin signal transduction in the nervous system. *Curr. Opin. Neurobiol.* **2000**, *10*, 381–391. [CrossRef]
6. Fenner, B.M. Truncated TrkB: Beyond a dominant negative receptor. *Cytokine Growth Factor Rev.* **2012**, *23*, 15–24. [CrossRef] [PubMed]
7. Yan, W.; Lakkaniga, N.R.; Carlomagno, F.; Santoro, M.; McDonald, N.Q.; Lv, F.; Gunaganti, N.; Frett, B.; Li, H.-Y. Insights into Current Tropomyosin Receptor Kinase (TRK) Inhibitors: Development and Clinical Application. *J. Med. Chem.* **2018**. [CrossRef]
8. Huang, E.J.; Reichardt, L.F. Neurotrophins: Roles in neuronal development and function. *Annu. Rev. Neurosci.* **2001**, *24*, 677–736. [CrossRef]
9. Poo, M.-M. Neurotrophins as synaptic modulators. *Nat. Rev. Neurosci.* **2001**, *2*, 24–32. [CrossRef]
10. Zhang, F.; Kang, Z.; Li, W.; Xiao, Z.; Zhou, X. Roles of brain-derived neurotrophic factor/tropomyosin-related kinase B (BDNF/TrkB) signalling in Alzheimer's disease. *J. Clin. Neurosci.* **2012**, *19*, 946–949. [CrossRef]
11. Song, J.-H.; Yu, J.-T.; Tan, L. Brain-Derived Neurotrophic Factor in Alzheimer's Disease: Risk, Mechanisms, and Therapy. *Mol. Neurobiol.* **2015**, *52*, 1477–1493. [CrossRef] [PubMed]
12. Murer, M.G.; Yan, Q.; Raisman-Vozari, R. Brain-derived neurotrophic factor in the control human brain, and in Alzheimer's disease and Parkinson's disease. *Progr. Neurobiol.* **2001**, *63*, 71–124. [CrossRef]
13. Reinhart, V.; Bove, S.E.; Volfson, D.; Lewis, D.A.; Kleiman, R.J.; Lanz, T.A. Evaluation of TrkB and BDNF transcripts in prefrontal cortex, hippocampus, and striatum from subjects with schizophrenia, bipolar disorder, and major depressive disorder. *Neurobiol. Dis.* **2015**, *77*, 220–227. [CrossRef] [PubMed]
14. Oyesiku, N.M.; Evans, C.-O.; Houston, S.; Darrell, R.S.; Smith, J.S.; Fulop, Z.L.; Dixon, C.E.; Stein, D.G. Regional changes in the expression of neurotrophic factors and their receptors following acute traumatic brain injury in the adult rat brain. *Brain Res.* **1999**, *833*, 161–172. [CrossRef]
15. Deng, V.; Matagne, V.; Banine, F.; Frerking, M.; Ohliger, P.; Budden, S.; Pevsner, J.; Dissen, G.A.; Sherman, L.S.; Ojeda, S.R. FXYD1 is an MeCP2 target gene overexpressed in the brains of Rett syndrome patients and Mecp2-null mice. *Hum. Mol. Genet.* **2007**, *16*, 640–650. [CrossRef] [PubMed]
16. Gupta, V.K.; You, Y.; Gupta, V.B.; Klistorner, A.; Graham, S.L. TrkB Receptor Signalling: Implications in Neurodegenerative, Psychiatric and Proliferative Disorders. *Int. J. Mol. Sci.* **2013**, *14*, 10122–10142. [CrossRef]
17. Ferrer, I.; Marín, C.; Rey, M.J.; Ribalta, T.; Goutan, E.; Blanco, R.; Tolosa, E.; Martí, E. BDNF and Full-length and Truncated TrkB Expression in Alzheimer Disease. Implications in Therapeutic Strategies. *J. Neuropathol. Exp. Neurol.* **1999**, *58*, 729–739. [CrossRef]
18. Allen, S.J.; Wilcock, G.K.; Dawbarn, D. Profound and Selective Loss of Catalytic TrkB Immunoreactivity in Alzheimer's Disease. *Biochem. Biophys. Res. Commun.* **1999**, *264*, 648–651. [CrossRef]
19. Savaskan, E.; Müller-Spahn, F.; Olivieri, G.; Bruttel, S.; Otten, U.; Rosenberg, C.; Hulette, C.; Hock, C. Alterations in Trk A, Trk B and Trk C Receptor Immunoreactivities in Parietal Cortex and Cerebellum in Alzheimer's Disease. *Eur. Neurol.* **2000**, *44*, 172–180. [CrossRef]
20. Ginsberg, S.D.; Che, S.; Wuu, J.; Counts, S.E.; Mufson, E.J. Down regulation of trk but not p75NTR gene expression in single cholinergic basal forebrain neurons mark the progression of Alzheimer's disease. *J. Neurochem.* **2006**, *97*, 475–487. [CrossRef]
21. Castello, N.A.; Nguyen, M.H.; Tran, J.D.; Cheng, D.; Green, K.N.; LaFerla, F.M. 7,8-Dihydroxyflavone, a Small Molecule TrkB Agonist, Improves Spatial Memory and Increases Thin Spine Density in a Mouse Model of Alzheimer Disease-Like Neuronal Loss. *PLoS ONE* **2014**, *9*, e91453. [CrossRef] [PubMed]
22. Li, N.; Liu, G.-T. The novel squamosamide derivative FLZ enhances BDNF/TrkB/CREB signaling and inhibits neuronal apoptosis in APP/PS1 mice. *Acta Pharmacol. Sin.* **2010**, *31*, 265–272. [CrossRef] [PubMed]

23. Massa, S.M.; Yang, T.; Xie, Y.; Shi, J.; Bilgen, M.; Joyce, J.N.; Nehama, D.; Rajadas, J.; Longo, F.M. Small molecule BDNF mimetics activate TrkB signaling and prevent neuronal degeneration in rodents. *J. Clin. Investig.* **2010**, *120*, 1774–1785. [CrossRef] [PubMed]

24. Nagahara, A.H.; Tuszynski, M.H. Potential therapeutic uses of BDNF in neurological and psychiatric disorders. *Nat. Rev. Drug Discov.* **2011**, *10*, 209–219. [CrossRef] [PubMed]

25. Devi, L.; Ohno, M. TrkB reduction exacerbates Alzheimer's disease-like signaling aberrations and memory deficits without affecting β-amyloidosis in 5XFAD mice. *Transl. Psychiatry* **2015**, *5*, e562. [CrossRef] [PubMed]

26. Géral, C.; Angelova, A.; Lesieur, S. From Molecular to Nanotechnology Strategies for Delivery of Neurotrophins: Emphasis on Brain-Derived Neurotrophic Factor (BDNF). *Pharmaceutics* **2013**, *5*, 127–167. [CrossRef] [PubMed]

27. Cocco, E.; Scaltriti, M.; Drilon, A. NTRK fusion-positive cancers and TRK inhibitor therapy. *Nat. Rev. Clin. Oncol.* **2018**, *15*, 731–747. [CrossRef] [PubMed]

28. Sun, X.; Xiao, Z.; Chen, G.; Han, Z.; Liu, Y.; Zhang, C.; Sun, Y.; Song, Y.; Wang, K.; Fang, F.; et al. A PET imaging approach for determining EGFR mutation status for improved lung cancer patient management. *Sci. Transl. Med.* **2018**, *10*. [CrossRef]

29. Tejeda, G.S.; Díaz-Guerra, M. Integral Characterization of Defective BDNF/TrkB Signalling in Neurological and Psychiatric Disorders Leads the Way to New Therapies. *Int. J. Mol. Sci.* **2017**, *18*, 268. [CrossRef]

30. Bernard-Gauthier, V.; Boudjemeline, M.; Rosa-Neto, P.; Thiel, A.; Schirrmacher, R. Towards tropomyosin-related kinase B (TrkB) receptor ligands for brain imaging with PET: Radiosynthesis and evaluation of 2-(4-[^{18}F]fluorophenyl)-7,8-dihydroxy-4H-chromen-4-one and 2-(4-([N-methyl-11C]-dimethylamino)phenyl)-7,8-dihydroxy-4H-chromen-4-one. *Bioorganic Med. Chem.* **2013**, *21*, 7816–7829. [CrossRef]

31. Jang, S.-W.; Liu, X.; Yepes, M.; Shepherd, K.R.; Miller, G.W.; Liu, Y.; Wilson, W.D.; Xiao, G.; Blanchi, B.; Sun, Y.E.; et al. A selective TrkB agonist with potent neurotrophic activities by 7,8-dihydroxyflavone. *Proc. Natl. Acad. Sci. USA* **2010**, *107*, 2687–2692. [CrossRef]

32. Liu, X.; Chan, C.-B.; Jang, S.-W.; Pradoldej, S.; Huang, J.; He, K.; Phun, L.H.; France, S.; Xiao, G.; Jia, Y.; et al. A Synthetic 7,8-Dihydroxyflavone Derivative Promotes Neurogenesis and Exhibits Potent Antidepressant Effect. *J. Med. Chem.* **2010**, *53*, 8274–8286. [CrossRef]

33. Liu, X.; Chan, C.-B.; Qi, Q.; Xiao, G.; Luo, H.R.; He, X.; Ye, K. Optimization of a Small Tropomyosin-Related Kinase B (TrkB) Agonist 7,8-Dihydroxyflavone Active in Mouse Models of Depression. *J. Med. Chem.* **2012**, *55*, 8524–8537. [CrossRef] [PubMed]

34. Boltaev, U.; Meyer, Y.; Tolibzoda, F.; Jacques, T.; Gassaway, M.; Xu, Q.; Wagner, F.; Zhang, Y.-L.; Palmer, M.; Holson, E.; et al. Multiplex quantitative assays indicate a need for reevaluating reported small-molecule TrkB agonists. *Sci. Signal.* **2017**, *10*. [CrossRef] [PubMed]

35. Shia, C.-S.; Tsai, S.-Y.; Kuo, S.-C.; Hou, Y.-C.; Chao, P.-D.L. Metabolism and Pharmacokinetics of 3,3′,4′,7-Tetrahydroxyflavone (Fisetin), 5-Hydroxyflavone, and 7-Hydroxyflavone and Antihemolysis Effects of Fisetin and Its Serum Metabolites. *J. Agric. Food Chem.* **2009**, *57*, 83–89. [CrossRef] [PubMed]

36. Jäger, A.; Saaby, L. Flavonoids and the CNS. *Molecules* **2011**, *16*, 1471–1485. [CrossRef]

37. Aldrich, C.; Bertozzi, C.; Georg, G.I.; Kiessling, L.; Lindsley, C.; Liotta, D.; Merz, K.M., Jr.; Schepartz, A.; Wang, S. The Ecstasy and Agony of Assay Interference Compounds. *ACS Cent. Sci.* **2017**, *3*, 143–147. [CrossRef]

38. Bothwell, M. Recent advances in understanding neurotrophin signaling. *F1000Research* **2016**, *5*. [CrossRef]

39. Altar, C.A.; Burton, L.E.; Bennett, G.L.; Dugich-Djordjevic, M. Recombinant human nerve growth factor is biologically active and labels novel high-affinity binding sites in rat brain. *Proc. Nat. Acad. Sci. USA* **1991**, *88*, 281–285. [CrossRef]

40. Altar, C.; Dugich-Djordjevic, M.; Armanini, M.; Bakhit, C. Medial-to-lateral gradient of neostriatal NGF receptors: Relationship to cholinergic neurons and NGF-like immunoreactivity. *J. Neurosci.* **1991**, *11*, 828–836. [CrossRef]

41. Merlio, J.P.; Ernfors, P.; Jaber, M.; Persson, H. Molecular cloning of rat trkC and distribution of cells expressing messenger RNAs for members of the trk family in the rat central nervous system. *Neuroscience* **1992**, *51*, 513–532. [CrossRef]

42. Anderson, K.D.; Alderson, R.F.; Altar, C.A.; DiStefano, P.S.; Corcoran, T.L.; Lindsay, R.M.; Wiegand, S.J. Differential distribution of exogenous BDNF, NGF, and NT-3 in the brain corresponds to the relative abundance and distribution of high-affinity and low-affinity neurotrophin receptors. *J. Comp. Neurol.* **1995**, *357*, 296–317. [CrossRef] [PubMed]

43. Altar, C.A.; Siuciak, J.A.; Wright, P.; Ip, N.Y.; Lindsay, R.M.; Wiegand, S.J. In Situ Hybridization of trkB and trkC Receptor mRNA in Rat Forebrain and Association with High-affinity Binding of [^{125}I]BDNF, [^{125}I]NT-4/5 and [^{125}I]NT-3. *Eur. J. Neurosci.* **1994**, *6*, 1389–1405. [CrossRef]

44. Zhang, L.; Villalobos, A.; Beck, E.M.; Bocan, T.; Chappie, T.A.; Chen, L.; Grimwood, S.; Heck, S.D.; Helal, C.J.; Hou, X.; et al. Design and Selection Parameters to Accelerate the Discovery of Novel Central Nervous System Positron Emission Tomography (PET) Ligands and Their Application in the Development of a Novel Phosphodiesterase 2A PET Ligand. *J. Med. Chem.* **2013**, *56*, 4568–4579. [CrossRef] [PubMed]

45. Pike, V.W. PET radiotracers: Crossing the blood-brain barrier and surviving metabolism. *Trends Pharmacol. Sci.* **2009**, *30*, 431–440. [CrossRef] [PubMed]

46. Rankovic, Z. CNS Drug Design: Balancing Physicochemical Properties for Optimal Brain Exposure. *J. Med. Chem.* **2015**, *58*, 2584–2608. [CrossRef] [PubMed]

47. Wager, T.T.; Hou, X.; Verhoest, P.R.; Villalobos, A. Moving beyond Rules: The Development of a Central Nervous System Multiparameter Optimization (CNS MPO) Approach to Enable Alignment of Druglike Properties. *ACS Chem. Neurosci.* **2010**, *1*, 435–449. [CrossRef] [PubMed]

48. Wood, E.R.; Kuyper, L.; Petrov, K.G.; Hunter, R.N.; Harris, P.A.; Lackey, K. Discovery and in vitro evaluation of potent TrkA kinase inhibitors: Oxindole and aza-oxindoles. *Bioorg. Med. Chem. Lett.* **2004**, *14*, 953–957. [CrossRef]

49. Bernard-Gauthier, V.; Aliaga, A.; Aliaga, A.; Boudjemeline, M.; Hopewell, R.; Kostikov, A.; Rosa-Neto, P.; Thiel, A.; Schirrmacher, R. Syntheses and Evaluation of Carbon-11- and Fluorine-18-Radiolabeled pan-Tropomyosin Receptor Kinase (Trk) Inhibitors: Exploration of the 4-Aza-2-oxindole Scaffold as Trk PET Imaging Agents. *ACS Chem. Neurosci.* **2015**, *6*, 260–276. [CrossRef]

50. Prakash, Y.; Thompson, M.A.; Meuchel, L.; Pabelick, C.M.; Mantilla, C.B.; Zaidi, S.; Martin, R.J. Neurotrophins in lung health and disease. *Expert Rev. Respir. Med.* **2010**, *4*, 395–411. [CrossRef]

51. Stachel, S.J.; Sanders, J.M.; Henze, D.A.; Rudd, M.T.; Su, H.-P.; Li, Y.; Nanda, K.K.; Egbertson, M.S.; Manley, P.J.; Jones, K.L.G.; et al. Maximizing Diversity from a Kinase Screen: Identification of Novel and Selective pan-Trk Inhibitors for Chronic Pain. *J. Med. Chem.* **2014**, *57*, 5800–5816. [CrossRef] [PubMed]

52. Bernard-Gauthier, V.; Schirrmacher, R. 5-(4-((4-[^{18}F]fluorobenzyl)oxy)-3-methoxybenzyl)pyrimidine-2,4-diamine: A selective dual inhibitor for potential PET imaging of Trk/CSF-1R. *Bioorg. Med. Chem. Lett.* **2014**, *24*, 4784–4790. [CrossRef] [PubMed]

53. Bernard-Gauthier, V.; Mahringer, A.; Vesnaver, M.; Fricker, G.; Schirrmacher, R. Design and synthesis of a fluorinated quinazoline-based type-II Trk inhibitor as a scaffold for PET radiotracer development. *Bioorg. Med. Chem. Lett.* **2017**, *27*, 2771–2775. [CrossRef] [PubMed]

54. Davis, M.I.; Hunt, J.P.; Herrgard, S.; Ciceri, P.; Wodicka, L.M.; Pallares, G.; Hocker, M.; Treiber, D.K.; Zarrinkar, P.P. Comprehensive analysis of kinase inhibitor selectivity. *Nat. Biotechnol.* **2011**, *29*, 1046–1051. [CrossRef] [PubMed]

55. Lemaire, C.; Libert, L.; Plenevaux, A.; Aerts, J.; Franci, X.; Luxen, A. Fast and reliable method for the preparation of ortho- and para-[^{18}F]fluorobenzyl halide derivatives: Key intermediates for the preparation of no-carrier-added PET aromatic radiopharmaceuticals. *J. Fluor. Chem.* **2012**, *138*, 48–55. [CrossRef]

56. Baindur, N.; Gaul, M.D.; Kreutter, K.D.; Baumann, C.A.; Kim, A.J.; Xu, G.; Tuman, R.W.; Johnson, D.L. Alkylquinoline and Alkylquinazoline Kinase Modulators. U.S. Patent US2006281772, 14 December 2006.

57. Bernard-Gauthier, V.; Bailey, J.J.; Aliaga, A.; Kostikov, A.; Rosa-Neto, P.; Wuest, M.; Brodeur, G.M.; Bedell, B.J.; Wuest, F.; Schirrmacher, R. Development of subnanomolar radiofluorinated (2-pyrrolidin-1-yl)imidazo [1,2-*b*]pyridazine pan-Trk inhibitors as candidate PET imaging probes. *MedChemComm* **2015**, *6*, 2184–2193. [CrossRef]

58. Bernard-Gauthier, V.; Bailey, J.J.; Mossine, A.V.; Lindner, S.; Vomacka, L.; Aliaga, A.; Shao, X.; Quesada, C.A.; Sherman, P.; Mahringer, A.; et al. A Kinome-Wide Selective Radiolabeled TrkB/C Inhibitor for in Vitro and in Vivo Neuroimaging: Synthesis, Preclinical Evaluation, and First-in-Human. *J. Med. Chem.* **2017**, *60*, 6897–6910. [CrossRef]

59. Preshlock, S.; Tredwell, M.; Gouverneur, V. ^{18}F-Labeling of Arenes and Heteroarenes for Applications in Positron Emission Tomography. *Chem. Rev.* **2016**, *116*, 719–766. [CrossRef]

60. Brooks, A.F.; Topczewski, J.J.; Ichiishi, N.; Sanford, M.S.; Scott, P.J.H. Late-stage [(18)F]Fluorination: New Solutions to Old Problems. *Chem. Sci.* **2014**, *5*, 4545–4553.

61. Zlatopolskiy, B.D.; Zischler, J.; Krapf, P.; Zarrad, F.; Urusova, E.A.; Kordys, E.; Endepols, H.; Neumaier, B. Copper-Mediated Aromatic Radiofluorination Revisited: Efficient Production of PET Tracers on a Preparative Scale. *Chem. A Eur. J.* **2015**, *21*, 5972–5979. [CrossRef] [PubMed]

62. Tredwell, M.; Preshlock, S.M.; Taylor, N.J.; Gruber, S.; Huiban, M.; Passchier, J.; Mercier, J.; Génicot, C.; Gouverneur, V. A General Copper-Mediated Nucleophilic ^{18}F Fluorination of Arenes. *Angew. Chem. Int. Ed.* **2014**, *53*, 7751–7755. [CrossRef] [PubMed]

63. Ichiishi, N.; Brooks, A.F.; Topczewski, J.J.; Rodnick, M.E.; Sanford, M.S.; Scott, P.J.H. Copper-catalyzed [^{18}F]fluorination of (mesityl)(aryl)iodonium salts. *Org. Lett.* **2014**, *16*, 3224–3227. [CrossRef] [PubMed]

64. Bernard-Gauthier, V.; Mossine, A.V.; Mahringer, A.; Aliaga, A.; Bailey, J.J.; Shao, X.; Stauff, J.; Arteaga, J.; Sherman, P.; Grand'Maison, M.; et al. Identification of [^{18}F]TRACK, a Fluorine-18-Labeled Tropomyosin Receptor Kinase (Trk) Inhibitor for PET Imaging. *J. Med. Chem.* **2018**, *61*, 1737–1743. [CrossRef] [PubMed]

65. Mossine, A.V.; Brooks, A.F.; Bernard-Gauthier, V.; Bailey, J.J.; Ichiishi, N.; Schirrmacher, R.; Sanford, M.S.; Scott, P.J.H. Automated Synthesis of PET Radiotracers by Copper-mediated ^{18}F-Fluorination of Organoborons: Importance of the Order of Addition and Competing Protodeborylation. *J. Label. Compd. Radiopharm.* **2018**, *63*, 228–236. [CrossRef] [PubMed]

11

Pretargeted Imaging with Gallium-68—Improving the Binding Capability by Increasing the Number of Tetrazine Motifs

Dominik Summer [1][ID], Sonja Mayr [1], Milos Petrik [2], Christine Rangger [1][ID], Katia Schoeler [3], Lisa Vieider [4], Barbara Matuszczak [4][ID] and Clemens Decristoforo [1,*][ID]

[1] Department of Nuclear Medicine, Medical University Innsbruck, Anichstrasse 35, A-6020 Innsbruck, Austria; dominik.summer@i-med.ac.at (D.S.); sonja.mayr@student.uibk.ac.at (S.M.); christine.rangger@i-med.ac.at (C.R.)

[2] Institute of Molecular and Translational Medicine, Faculty of Medicine and Dentistry, Palacky University, CZE-77900 Olomouc, Czech Republic; milos.petrik@seznam.cz

[3] Biocenter—Division of Developmental Immunology, Medical University of Innsbruck, Innrain 80/82, A-6020 Innsbruck, Austria; katia.schoeler@i-med.ac.at

[4] Institute of Pharmacy, Pharmaceutical Chemistry, University of Innsbruck, Center for Chemistry and Biomedicine (CCB), Innrain 80/82, A-6020 Innsbruck, Austria; lisa.vieider@student.uibk.ac.at (L.V.); barbara.matuszczak@uibk.ac.at (B.M.)

* Correspondence: clemens.decristoforo@i-med.ac.at

Abstract: The inverse electron-demand Diels-Alder reaction between 1,2,4,5-tetrazine (Tz) and *trans*-cyclooct-2-ene (TCO) has gained increasing attraction among extensive studies on click chemistry due to its exceptionally fast reaction kinetics and high selectivity for in vivo pretargeting applications including PET imaging. The facile two-step approach utilizing TCO-modified antibodies as targeting structures has not made it into clinics yet. An increase in the blood volume of humans in comparison to mice seems to be the major limitation. This study aims to show if the design of multimeric Tz-ligands by chelator scaffolding can improve the binding capacity and may lead to enhanced PET imaging with gallium-68. We utilized for this purpose the macrocyclic siderophore Fusarinine C (FSC) which allows conjugation of up to three Tz-residues due to three primary amines available for site specific modification. The resulting mono- di- and trimeric conjugates were radiolabelled with gallium-68 and characterized in vitro (logD, protein binding, stability, binding towards TCO modified rituximab (RTX)) and in vivo (biodistribution- and imaging studies in normal BALB/c mice using a simplified RTX-TCO tumour surrogate). The ^{68}Ga-labelled FSC-based Tz-ligands showed suitable hydrophilicity, high stability and high targeting specificity. The binding capacity to RTX-TCO was increased according to the grade of multimerization. Corresponding in vivo studies showed a multimerization typical profile but generally suitable pharmacokinetics with low accumulation in non-targeted tissue. Imaging studies in RTX-TCO tumour surrogate bearing BALB/c mice confirmed this trend and revealed improved targeting by multimerization as increased accumulation in RTX-TCO positive tissue was observed.

Keywords: pretargeting; Fusarinine C; rituximab; click chemistry; multimerization; PET; gallium-68

1. Introduction

Immunoglobulins, in particular monoclonal antibodies (mAbs) are highly attractive targeting structures due to their extraordinary specificity and selectivity and are well established for therapeutic applications, particularly in the field of oncology [1,2]. Because of their favorable targeting abilities and therefore an ever increasing clinical importance, mAbs have regained interest also as imaging agents, in particular for positron emission tomography (PET) applications [3–5]. In principle mAbs can be directly radiolabelled either by direct incorporation of radiohalogens or by attaching a chelator to the protein in case of radiometals. Prolonged circulation time and slow distribution within the organism, however, restricts its use to long-lived radionuclides e.g., zirconium-89 (3.26 d) and iodine-124 (4.18 d). This multiday circulation paired with slow radioactive decay provides unfavorable radiation to healthy tissue and adds significantly to the overall radiation burden of patients.

In order to overcome this problem, various pretargeting methodologies have been reported and reviewed recently [6–8], enabling a straight forward two-step approach. Thereby the modified antibody is administered, allowed to accumulate at the target site and be eliminated from the bloodstream followed by injection of the radioactive payload to form the radioimmunoconjugate in vivo. This provides certain advantages as it facilitates the use of short-lived radioisotopes for PET applications e.g., gallium-68 (1.13 h), fluorine-18 (1.83 h) and copper-64 (12.7 h) and significantly reduces the radiation dose to healthy tissue, since the radioligand either finds its binding partner to form stable conjugates or is rapidly eliminated due to its small size. Furthermore, it allows to apply radiolabelling at high temperatures using high concentrations of organic solvents if necessary—harsh conditions, where the structural integrity of antibodies would be severely in danger when direct labelling was performed.

Among these pretargeting strategies the inverse electron-demand Diels-Alder reaction (IEDDA) between 1,2,4,5-tetrazines (Tz) and *trans*-cyclooct-2-enes (TCO) has gained enormous attention mainly due to the exceptionally fast reaction kinetics and high selectivity between the reaction partners even in complex biological systems as encountered in vivo [9,10]. Various preclinical studies demonstrated the feasibility of this approach for molecular imaging using PET-radioisotopes with promising results [11–14]. The application on humans, however, remains unsuccessful due to the increased blood volume in humans and may therefore lead to insufficient accumulation due to accelerated elimination of the small-sized radioligand.

Related to this, recent study investigated whether an increase of Tz motifs by chelator scaffolding, i.e., multimerization, can improve the binding efficiency and thereby improve imaging contrast. This could contribute in particular to the application of gallium-68 for pretargeted immuno-PET imaging. For this purpose we utilized the macrocyclic chelator Fusarinine C for the design of mono- and multimeric Tz-conjugates as presented in Scheme 1 for a proof-of-concept study, on potentially improved pretargeting for imaging with gallium-68 by applying multimerization. We chose non-internalizing anti-CD20 antibody rituximab (RTX) modified with TCO as targeting vector. Radiolabelling was conducted at room temperature within minutes and the ^{68}Ga-labelled conjugates showed reasonable hydrophilicity and excellent stability in human serum. Protein binding, however, remained comparable within the conjugates but was generally high. The ^{68}Ga-labelled multimeric conjugates showed a higher binding capacity towards TCO-motif bearing RTX. Furthermore, cell-binding studies revealed highly specific targeting properties and the binding of [^{68}Ga]Ga-FSC-Tz multimers to CD20-expressing Raji cells increased with the number of Tz-motifs attached to the chelator. Imaging studies in a simplified pretargeting mouse model proved the trend for improved targeting. We therefore conclude, that multimerization bears a great potential to improve IEDDA related pretargeting when short-lived PET-radioisotopes, particularly gallium-68, are used. Further investigations in established tumor models are warranted to confirm these promising findings.

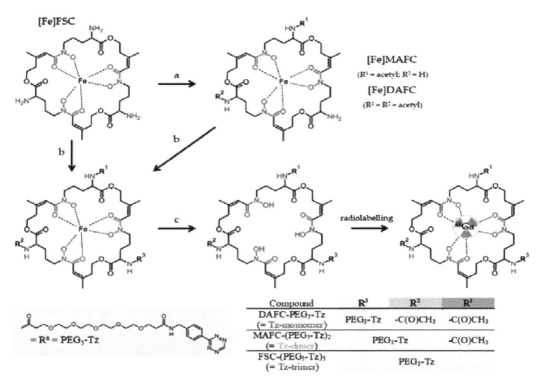

Scheme 1. Synthetic strategy for FSC-based tetrazine (Tz) conjugates [a: methanol and acetic anhydride (MetOH/Ac$_2$O); b: Tz-PEG$_5$-NHS/DMF/DIPEA; c: EDTA] radiolabelled with gallium-68.

2. Results

2.1. (Radio) Chemistry

FSC-based mono- and multimeric Tz-conjugates were accessible in a three-step synthesis to give the corresponding conjugates in good yields and high chemical purity (>95%; analytical RP-HPLC, UV absorption at $\lambda = 220$ nm). The results from mass analysis were in good agreement with the calculated values. The structure of the Tz-conjugates was further confirmed by ^{1}H-NMR spectroscopy. The singlets at 6.30 and 1.86 ppm which can be assigned to the -C=O-CH=C(CH$_3$)C-substructure were used as the marker signals of the FSC subunit. The singlet at 1.83 ppm corresponds to the methyl protons of the acetyl group(s). The singlet at 10.56 ppm is highly characteristic for the tetrazine moiety. The doublets at 8.44 and 7.53 ppm with coupling constants of 8.4 Hz are characteristic for the para-substituted phenyl ring, and the triplet at 8.50 ppm as well as the doublet at 4.40 ppm with a coupling constant of 6.0 Hz can be assigned to the -NH-CH$_2$ group of the PEG$_5$-Tz subunit(s). The ratio of the integrals of these marker signals is summarized in Table 1 and corresponding ^{1}H-NMR spectra are presented in Figures S1–S3. Radiolabelling with gallium-68 was quantitative within minutes at RT, thus exhibiting fast labelling kinetics. Corresponding (radio-)RP-HPLC chromatograms are presented in Figure S4.

Table 1. ^{1}H-NMR data (chemical shifts and integrals) of characteristic signals of FSC-based Tz-conjugates and N,N',N''-triacetylfusarinine (TAFC) as a reference.

	FSC Subunit		Acetyl		PEG$_5$-Tz Subunit			
	$3\times$ CH	$3\times$ CH$_3$	CH$_3$	Tetrazine	p-Phenylen		NH-CH$_2$	NH-CH$_2$
	6.3 ppm	1.86 ppm	1.83 ppm	10.56 ppm	8.44 ppm	7.53 ppm	8.50 ppm	4.40 ppm
Tz-monomer	3 H	9 H	6 H	1 H	2 H	2 H	1 H	2 H
Tz-dimer	3 H	9 H	3 H	2 H	4 H	4 H	2 H	4 H
Tz-trimer	3 H	9 H	none	3 H	6 H	6 H	3 H	6 H
TAFC	3 H	9 H	9 H	none	none	none	none	none

2.2. In Vitro Evaluation

Stability studies of ^{68}Ga-labelled conjugates in fresh human serum and PBS as control revealed high stability as no major degradation was observed over a period of 4 h. Corresponding radio-RP-HPLC chromatograms are presented in Figure S5. The results of logD studies and the ability to bind to serum proteins of ^{68}Ga-labelled conjugates are summarized in Table 2. They revealed suitable hydrophilicity with minor decrease when increasing the number of Tz residues. All conjugates showed very high protein binding with minor differences between mono- and multimeric [^{68}Ga]Ga-Tz-ligands.

Table 2. Distribution coefficient (logD) and protein binding of ^{68}Ga-labelled FSC-based Tz-conjugates.

[68]Ga-Labelled Compound	LogD (pH 7.4)	Protein Binding (%)		
		1 h	2 h	4 h
Tz-monomer	-1.64 ± 0.02	61.8 ± 0.2	63.8 ± 2.1	64.0 ± 1.4
Tz-dimer	-1.35 ± 0.01	67.0 ± 2.4	65.9 ± 1.3	68.4 ± 0.3
Tz-trimer	-1.00 ± 0.06	70.5 ± 0.7	69.5 ± 0.4	67.8 ± 0.4

Data are presented as mean $\pm$ SD ($n = 3$)

The non-internalizing anti-CD20 monoclonal antibody rituximab was modified with the TCO motif similar to a previously published procedure [15] and corresponding FACS analysis of CD20-expressing Raji cells incubated with both, TCO-modified and non-modified RTX showed high target specificity (Figure S6), thus demonstrating that the binding ability was not altered by the TCO modification.

The binding capacity of ^{68}Ga-labelled mono- and multimeric Tz-ligands was assessed via competitive binding on immobilized RTX-TCO using the non-labelled conjugates as competitor and is presented in Figure 1. The binding of the [^{68}Ga]Ga-Tz-monomer was reduced by 50% at a competitor concentration of 486 ± 52 nM when challenged with the non-labelled monomer, whereas the non-labelled dimer (112 ± 6 nM) and trimer (100 ± 10 nM) reduced the binding at significantly lower concentrations. The binding of the [^{68}Ga]Ga-Tz-dimer was reduced by half at 95 ± 25 nM in competition with its non-labelled counterpart and at a comparable concentration with the non-labelled trimer (92 ± 15 nM), whereas a decrease to 50% was only achieved at a much higher concentration in competition with non-labelled monomer (865 ± 263 nM). Binding studies of the [^{68}Ga]Ga-Tz-trimer showed a comparable trend as the non-labelled trimer reduced the binding by 50% at 147 ± 49 nM and the dimer at 258 ± 60 nM; whereby a significantly higher amount of the monomer (2987 ± 1664 nM) was needed for a 50% binding reduction. Overall in all assays improved binding of di- and trimer over monomer was observed.

The results of cell-binding studies on CD20-expressing Raji cells pre-treated with RTX or RTX-TCO prior to incubation with ^{68}Ga-labelled Tz-ligands are presented in Figure 2. All ^{68}Ga-labelled conjugates showed highly specific targeting properties as the amount of unspecific bound radioligand to RTX pre-treated Raji cells was negligible low (<1%). The binding of ^{68}Ga-labelled Tz-ligands on RTX-TCO bound Raji cells increased with the grade of multimerization and was $4.01 \pm 0.24\%$ for [^{68}Ga]Ga-Tz-monomer, $7.35 \pm 0.77\%$ for [^{68}Ga]Ga-Tz-dimer and 15.93 ± 0.88 for [^{68}Ga]Ga-Tz-trimer, respectively.

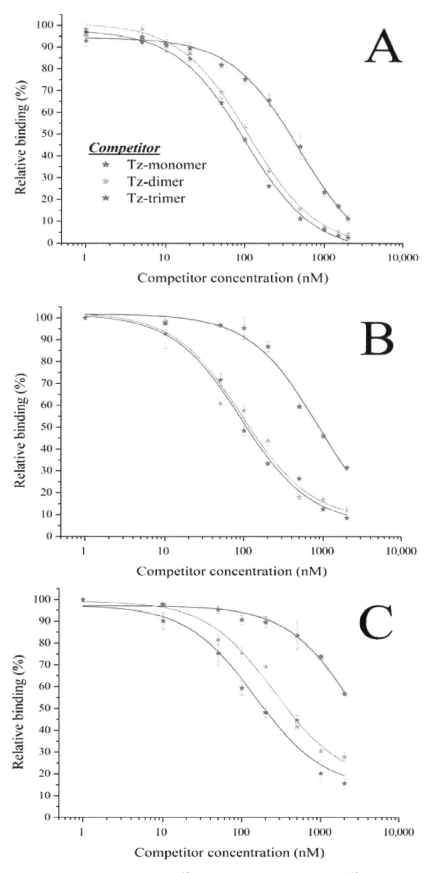

Figure 1. Competitive binding studies of [^{68}Ga]Ga-Tz-monomer (**A**), [^{68}Ga]Ga-Tz-dimer (**B**) and [^{68}Ga]Ga-Tz-trimer (**C**) on immobilized RTX-TCO using the non-labelled counterparts as competitor.

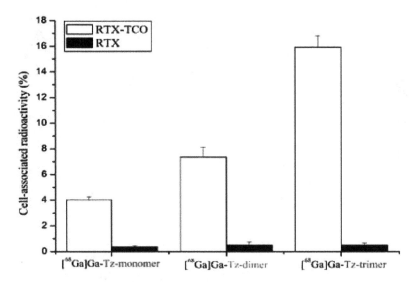

Figure 2. Cell-binding studies of ^{68}Ga-labelled FSC-based Tz-ligands on CD20-expressing Raji cells pre-treated with anti-CD20 antibody RTX (negative control, black bars) and its TCO modified counterpart (white bars).

2.3. In Vivo Evaluation

Biodistribution studies in non-tumour xenografted BALB/c mice 1 h after administration of the ^{68}Ga-labelled Tz-ligands are shown in Figure 3. In general, accumulation in non-targeted tissue was significantly lower for the [^{68}Ga]Ga-Tz-monomer compared to the [^{68}Ga]Ga-Tz-trimer, whereby the difference between the multimers was less pronounced. In particular, the multimeric Tz-ligands showed slower blood clearance and higher accumulation in renal tissue compared to the monomeric conjugate. The conjugates generally showed low accumulation in non-targeted tissue and low retention in critical organs (e.g., muscle, bone).

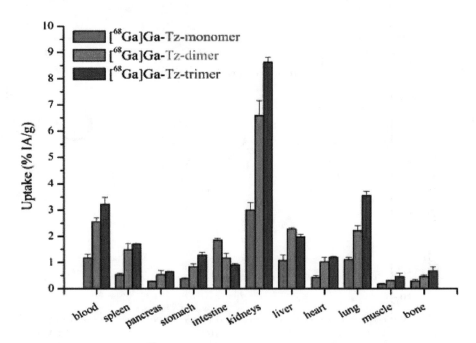

Figure 3. Biodistribution studies of ^{68}Ga-labelled mono- and multimeric FSC-based pretargeting agents in normal BALB/c mice 1 h p.i. presented as percentage of total injected activity per gram tissue ($n = 3$).

Imaging studies using BALB/c mice i.m. injected with RTX and RTX-TCO as tumour surrogate 5 h prior to r.o. administration of the radioligand and imaging performed 90 min p.i. are presented in Figure 4. The results mainly confirmed the suitable in vivo distribution profile of FSC-based Tz-ligands radiolabelled with gallium-68 with main activity in kidneys and bladder and some blood pool activity for the ^{68}Ga-labelled multimers. Moreover, the accumulation in RTX-TCO positive muscle tissue increased with ascending numbers of Tz motifs and was ~1% for the [^{68}Ga]Ga-Tz-monomer, ~2% for the [^{68}Ga]Ga-Tz-dimer and ~3% for the [^{68}Ga]Ga-Tz-trimer. Surprisingly, the accumulation in TCO negative tissue was also approximately 1% showing negligible differences between the different radioligands.

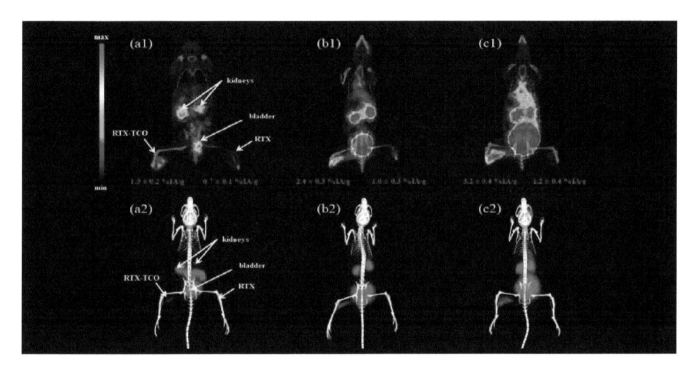

Figure 4. Static μPET/CT image of i.m. RTX(-TCO) pre-treated normal BALB/c mice 5 h after treatment and 90 min p.i. of the ^{68}Ga-labelled Tz-monomer (**a**), Tz-dimer (**b**) and Tz-trimer (**c**). (1 = coronal slice; 2 = 3D volume rendered projections; both prone position).

3. Discussion

IEDDA-based pretargeting has become increasingly popular for molecular imaging as well as radioimmunotherapy over the past few years [16–21]. Despite recent advancements towards structural improvement of cyclen- and TACN-based Tz-probes [22,23] or the synthesis of TCO-bearing dendrimers [24], the design of targeting probes bearing multiple Tz-motifs for potentially improved pretargeting has scarcely been investigated. Devaraj and co-workers reported on polymer modified tetrazines (PMT) radiolabelled with fluorine-18 [25] and gallium-68 [26] for PET applications while Zlatni et al. recently demonstrated the targeting applicability for microbubbles bearing multiple Tz-motifs towards prostate specific membrane antigen for ultrasound related diagnostic purposes [15]. However, investigations on the use of small-sized multimeric Tz-ligands have not been reported yet.

FSC is a suitable chelating scaffold for PET radiometals, particularly gallium-68 and zirconium-89 [27,28]. Its unique structural properties enable straight forward mono- and multimeric tracer design [29–32]. This novel chelator, therefore, represented a very suitable scaffold for the synthesis of mono- and multimeric small-sized Tz-bearing probes for radiolabelling with gallium-68 to evaluate potential benefits for IEDDA-based pretargeting by increasing the number of Tz-residues. The resulting conjugates showed reasonable hydrophilicity and increasing the number of Tz-residues from one to three did not alter the water solubility too much, although being somewhat lower in comparison to linker modified monomeric conjugates [23]. Unexpectedly, all FSC-based Tz-conjugates showed high protein binding with negligible differences between the compounds. This can be related to the introduction of the pegylated Tz residue, since non-modified ^{68}Ga-labelled FSC-based precursors showed a protein binding of <3% (Kaepookum et al. unpublished results). This phenomenon has not been reported in the case of monomeric DOTA- and TACN-based derivatives [22,23] and might be disadvantageous by slowing down the distribution of the tracer to the TCO-interaction site. In vivo results, however, did not really reveal a major problem with too slow pharmacokinetics, since the washout from non-targeted tissue was still sufficiently rapid. Competitive binding assessments showed significantly reduced binding of ^{68}Ga]Ga-Tz-monomer by a factor of five when challenged with the multimeric conjugates in comparison with the non-labelled monomer. This corresponded with the significantly higher amounts of Tz-monomer needed, 8 to 20 fold respectively, to reduce the binding of the ^{68}Ga-labelled multimers by 50%, thus indicating that the binding capacity increased with the number of Tz residues. This was substantiated by the results of the cell binding studies, since the binding to CD20-expressing Raji cells increased by a factor of 1.8 for the ^{68}Ga]Ga-Tz-dimer and 3.9 for the ^{68}Ga]Ga-Tz-trimer in comparison to the ^{68}Ga]Ga-Tz-monomer. Biodistribution studies in non-tumour xenografted healthy BALB/c mice indicated suitable pharmacokinetics and showed a multimerization typical profile exhibiting slower blood clearance and increased kidney retention, similar to prior findings with the FSC-scaffold [31,32]. Imaging studies using a tumour surrogate model confirmed this trend and demonstrated increased binding of the ^{68}Ga-labelled multimeric Tz-conjugates. The accumulation in RTX-TCO pretreated muscle tissue doubled for the ^{68}Ga]Ga-Tz-dimer and was 3-fold higher for the ^{68}Ga]Ga-Tz-trimer compared to the ^{68}Ga]Ga-Tz-monomer.

In regard to imaging in living mice there was a clear improvement of target specific accumulation when switching from mono- to multimers. The use of our simplified tumour surrogate animal model, however, requires further investigations in established animal models to address the limitations of this study:

(1) The accumulation in non-targeted tissue, i.e., i.m. injection of RTX resulted to be ~1%. This effect was even more pronounced when choosing a shorter time interval of 2 h between i.m. administration of the mAb and radioligand injection (data not shown) and was only seen at the injection site but generally not in other tissue. We speculate that this is related to the injection of the antibody leading to tissue damage with increased tissue permeability and unspecific accumulation of the radioligand.

(2) Intravenously injected mAb stimulates accumulation at the target interaction site, but a non-negligible amount remains in circulation, thereby increasing the background signal when administering the radioligand. In order to reduce this amount, high molecular weight TCO-scavenger molecules exhibiting low vascular permeability (clearing agents) have been established with great success, significantly improving target-to-background (TTB) ratios [33,34]. The need for clearing agents was completely neglected in this study and we are fully aware that our animal model does not reflect the real situation regarding TTB ratios.

In summary, we have been able to show that FSC is a suitable scaffold for the design of multimeric Tz-conjugates for radiolabelling with gallium-68. Although multimeric Tz-ligands exhibited significant improvements towards IEDDA-based pretargeting additional studies in tumour models are warranted to explore the full potential of this promising concept. Furthermore, a highly interesting therapeutic approach is the release of drugs directly at the interaction site from antibody-drug conjugates (ADCs) mediated via IEDDA reaction between Tz and TCO [35–37]. It might be of interest for future perspectives if multimeric Tz-conjugates can boost the release of drugs improving this highly promising "click-to-release" strategy.

4. Materials and Methods

4.1. Instrumentation

4.1.1. Analytical [radio]-RP-HPLC

Reversed-phase high-performance liquid chromatography analysis was performed with the following instrumentation: UltiMate 3000 RS UHPLC pump, UltiMate 3000 autosampler, UltiMate 3000 column compartment (25 °C oven temperature), UltiMate 3000 Variable Wavelength Detector (Dionex, Germering, Germany; UV detection at λ = 220 nm) a radio detector (GabiStar, Raytest; Straubenhardt, Germany), Jupiter 5 μm C_{18} 300 Å 150 × 4.6 mm (Phenomenex Ltd. Aschaffenburg, Germany) column with acetonitrile (ACN)/H_2O/0.1% trifluoroacetic acid (TFA) as mobile phase; flow rate of 1 mL/min; gradient: 0.0–1.0 min 10% ACN, 1.0–12.0 min 10–60% ACN, 13.0–15.0 min 60–80% ACN, 15.0–16.0 min 80–10% ACN, 16.0–20.0 min 10% ACN.

4.1.2. Preparative RP-HPLC

Sample purification via RP-HPLC was carried out as follows: Gilson 322 Pump with a Gilson UV/VIS-155 detector (UV detection at λ = 220 nm) using a PrepFC™ automatic fraction collector (Gilson, Middleton, WI, USA), Eurosil Bioselect Vertex Plus 30 × 8 mm 5 μm C_{18A} 300 Å pre-column and Eurosil Bioselect Vertex Plus 300 × 8 mm 5 μm C_{18A} 300 Å column (Knauer, Berlin, Germany) and following ACN/H_2O/0.1% TFA gradients with a flow rate of 2 mL/min: gradient A: 0.0–5.0 min 0% ACN, 5.0–35.0 min 0–50% ACN, 35.0–38.0 min 50% ACN, 38.0–40.0 min 50–0% ACN. Gradient B: 0.0–5.0 min 10% ACN, 5.0–40.0 min 10–60% ACN, 41.0–45.0 min 60% ACN, 46.0–50.0 min. 60–80% ACN, 51.0–55.0 min 80–10% ACN.

4.1.3. MALDI-TOF MS

Mass spectrometry was conducted on a Bruker microflex™ bench-top MALDI-TOF MS (Bruker Daltonics, Bremen, Germany) with a 20 Hz laser source. Sample preparation was performed according to dried-droplet method on a micro scout target (MSP96 target ground steel BC, Bruker Daltonics) using α-cyano-4-hydroxycinnamic acid (HCCA, Sigma-Aldrich, Handels GmbH, Vienna, Austria) as matrix. Flex Analysis 2.4 software was used for processing of the recorded data.

4.1.4. ^{1}H-NMR Spectroscopy

^{1}H-NMR spectra of the FSC-based Tz-conjugates were recorded on a "Saturn" 600 MHz Avance II+ spectrometer and the NMR of the reference compound (TAFC) was recorded on a "Mars" 400 MHz Avance 4 Neo spectrometer, both from Bruker Corporation (Billerica, MA, USA). The centre of the solvent multiplet (DMSO-d_6) was used as internal standard (chemical shifts in δ ppm), which was related to TMS with δ 2.49 ppm. TopSpin 3.5 pl7 software (Bruker) was used for data processing.

4.2. Synthesis

4.2.1. General Information

All chemicals and solvents were purchased as reagent grade from commercial sources unless otherwise stated. *trans*-Cyclooctene-NHS ester and tetrazine-PEG$_5$-NHS ester were bought from Click Chemistry Tools (Scottsdale, AZ, USA). Rituximab (MabThera®, Roche Pharma AG, Grenzach-Wyhlen, Germany) was of pharmaceutical grade and was a kind gift from the University Hospital of Innsbruck.

4.2.2. [Fe]Fusarinine C ([Fe]FSC)

The cyclic siderophore Fusarinine C (FSC) was obtained from iron deficient fungal culture and the extraction of FSC was conducted with a slightly modified method as described before [38]. Briefly, 1 L of iron saturated culture media was flushed through a C_{18}-Reveleris flash cartridge (40 μm, 12 g;

Grace, MD, USA) by using a REGLO tubing pump (Type ISM795, Ismatec SA, Glattbrugg-Zurich, Switzerland) with a flow rate of 10 mL/min. [Fe]FSC fixed on the cartridge was washed with 50 mL of water and eluted afterwards with 50 mL H_2O/ACN (20/80% v/v). After evaporation to dryness ~300 mg [Fe]FSC were obtained as red–brown coloured solid in high purity (>90%). Analytical data: RP-HPLC t_R = 6.95 min; MALDI TOF-MS: m/z [M + H]$^+$ = 779.93 [$C_{33}H_{51}FeN_6O_{12}$; exact mass: 779.63 (calculated)].

4.2.3. Acetylation of [Fe]FSC

[Fe]FSC was dissolved in methanol to a final concentration of 30 mg/mL (38.5 mM). An aliquot of 300 μL was reacted with 10 μL of acetic anhydride for 5 min at room temperature (RT) under vigorous shaking followed by subsequent purification of the resulting mixture of mono-, di- and triacetylfusarinine C via preparative RP-HPLC using gradient A to obtain N-monoacetylfusarinine C ([Fe]MAFC, t_R = 20.1 min) and N,N'-diacetylfusarinine C ([Fe]DAFC, t_R = 24.5 min). Analytical data: [Fe]MAFC: RP-HPLC t_R = 7.67 min; MALDI TOF-MS: m/z [M + H]$^+$ = 822.04 [$C_{35}H_{53}FeN_6O_{13}$; exact mass: 821.67 (calculated)]. [Fe]DAFC: RP-HPLC t_R = 8.49 min; MALDI TOF-MS: m/z [M + H]$^+$ = 864.02 [$C_{37}H_{55}FeN_6O_{14}$; exact mass: 863.71 (calculated)].

4.2.4. Conjugation of Tetrazine-PEG$_5$ Motif

Iron protected FSC (1.0 mg, 1.28 μmol), MAFC (2.0 mg, 2.43 μmol) or DAFC (2.0 mg, 2.32 μmol) were dissolved in 500 μL anhydrous DMF and after addition of Tetrazine-PEG$_5$-NHS ester, 1.5 equivalents (2.10 mg, 3.48 μmol) in case of DAFC, 2.5 equivalents (3.67 mg, 6.08 μmol) in case of MAFC and 3.5 equivalents (2.71 mg, 4.48 μmol) in case of FSC, pH was adjusted to 9.0 using DIPEA and the reaction mixtures were maintained for 4 h at RT. Finally the organic solvent was evaporated and the crude mixture was used without further purification.

4.2.5. Demetallation

For the purpose of iron removal, corresponding conjugates were dissolved in 1 mL H_2O/ACN solvent 50% (v/v) and 1 mL of aqueous Na$_2$EDTA solution (200 mM) was added. The resulting mixtures were stirred for 4 h at ambient temperature followed by preparative RP-HPLC purification to give slightly to intensively pink coloured, iron free FSC-based Tz-conjugates after lyophilisation.

- DAFC-PEG$_5$-Tz (=Tz-monomer): 2.35 mg [1.81 μmol, 78%], gradient B (t_R = 31.1 min); Analytical data: RP-HPLC t_R = 11.5 min; MALDI TOF-MS: m/z [M + H]$^+$ = 1303.95 [$C_{60}H_{89}N_{11}O_{21}$; exact mass: 1300.41 (calculated)]
- MAFC-(PEG$_5$-Tz)$_2$ (=Tz-dimer): 3.65 mg [2.09 μmol, 86%], gradient B (t_R = 35.3 min); Analytical data: RP-HPLC t_R = 12.5 min; MALDI TOF-MS: m/z [M + H]$^+$ = 1748.25 [$C_{81}H_{118}N_{16}O_{27}$; exact mass: 1747.89 (calculated)]
- FSC-(PEG$_5$-Tz)$_3$ (=Tz-trimer): 1.68 mg [0.77 μmol, 60%], gradient B (t_R = 37.9 min); Analytical data: RP-HPLC t_R = 13.2 min; MALDI TOF-MS: m/z [M + H]$^+$ = 2200.20 [$C_{102}H_{147}N_{21}O_{33}$; exact mass: 2195.38 (calculated)]

4.2.6. Modification of Rituximab (RTX)

Rituximab was obtained in solution (Mabthera®, 10 mg/mL, Roche Pharma AG, Grenzach-Wyhlen, Germany) and a PD-10 (GE Healthcare, Vienna, Austria) size exclusion column was used for buffer exchange according to manufacturer's protocol to give RTX in 0.1 M NaHCO$_3$ solution (7 mg/mL). For the conjugation of $trans$-cyclooctene (TCO), 2 mL of the RTX solution were mixed with 20 molar equivalent of TCO-NHS ester dissolved in DMSO and the reaction was stirred for 30 min at ambient temperature followed by incubation overnight at 4 °C under light exclusion. Subsequently, the modified antibody (RTX-TCO) was purified using size exclusion chromatography (PD-10) to give 10 mg of RTX-TCO dissolved in PBS. The antibody was treated following the same procedure as described above without adding TCO-NHS ester, in order to obtain a non-modified RTX counterpart as negative control.

4.3. Fluorescence Activated Cell-Sorting (FACS)

The humanoid lymphoblast-like CD20-expressing B-lymphocyte cells (Raji cells) were purchased from American Type Culture Collection (ATCC, Manassas, VA, USA). Flow cytometric analysis of CD20 expression was evaluated on (Raji cells) adjusted to 5×10^5 cells/sample in DMEM (including 10% FCS, 1% Pen/Strep). Cells were incubated with FC-Block (containing CD16/CD32 (1:200), e-Bioscience, Thermo Fisher Scientific, Vienna, Austria) for 15 min at 4 °C in order to avoid signals from non-specific binding. The following antibodies were used: RTX-TCO and RTX, both at 20 µM (f. c.). As secondary antibody a APC-labelled anti-human IgG Fc (clone: HP6017; BioLedgend, San Diego, CA, USA) at a dilution of 1:100 was used. Antibodies were incubated for at least 15 min at 4 °C. FACS analysis was performed on BD LSRFortessa™ (Cell Analyzer, BD Bioscience, San Jose, CA, USA). As internal control samples unstained or stained with either primary or secondary antibodies were analyzed. FACS-data was analyzed by FlowJo v10 software.

4.4. Radiolabelling of FSC-Based Tz-Conjugates with Gallium-68

Gallium-68 was obtained as [^{68}Ga]GaCl$_3$ (gallium chloride) by fractioned elution of a ^{68}Ge/^{68}Ga-generator (IGG100, nominal activity 1100 MBq, Eckert & Ziegler, Berlin, Germany) with 0.1 M hydrochloric acid (HCl, Rotem Industries Ltd., Beer-Sheva, Israel). Hereafter, 500 µL of eluate (100 MBq) were mixed with 100 µL sodium acetate solution (1.14 M) to give a pH of 4.5 followed by addition of 10 µg (4.55–7.68 nmol) of corresponding FSC-Tz conjugate. After 5 min incubation at RT the radiolabelling solution was analyzed using radio-RP-HPLC.

4.5. In Vitro Characterization.

4.5.1. Distribution Coefficient (LogD)

To determine the distribution of the ^{68}Ga-labelled conjugates between an organic (octanol) and aqueous (PBS) layer, aliquots (50 µL) of the tracers (~5 µM) were diluted in 1 mL of octanol/PBS (1:1, v/v). The mixture was vortexed at 1400 rpm (MS 3 basic vortexer, IKA, Staufen, Germany) for 15 min at RT followed by centrifugation for 2 min at 4500 rpm. Subsequently, aliquots (50 µL) of both layers were collected and measured in the gamma counter (Wizard2 3", Perkin Elmer, Waltham, MA, USA) followed by logD calculation ($n = 3$, six replicates).

4.5.2. Protein Binding

Serum protein binding was determined using Sephadex G-50 (GE Healthcare Vienna, Austria) size exclusion chromatography [38]. Aliquots (50 µL, $n = 3$) of the radioligand solution (~10 µM) were incubated in 450 µL freshly prepared human serum or 450 µL PBS (controls) and were kept at 37 °C. After 1, 2, and 4 h aliquots (25 µL) were directly transferred to the column (MicroSpin G-50, GE Healthcare) and after centrifugation (2 min, 2000 rcf) the column containing the free conjugate and the eluate containing the protein-bound conjugate were measured in the gamma counter. The percent of activity in both fractions was calculated thereafter.

4.5.3. Stability Studies in Human Serum

Stability of the radioligands was evaluated in human serum as described in [38]. Briefly, 50 µL of the radioligand solution (~10 µM, $n = 2$) were mixed with 950 µL freshly prepared serum or 950 µL PBS (controls). The mixtures were then maintained at 37 °C. At designated time points, 1, 2 and 4 h respectively, aliquots (100 µL) were mixed with 0.1% TFA/ACN, centrifuged for 2 min at 14×10^3 rcf. The supernatant was diluted with H$_2$O (1:1, v/v) and analyzed by analytical RP-HPLC for decomposition without filtration prior to injection.

4.5.4. Competitive Binding Assay

Binding on immobilized RTX-TCO was conducted using high protein-binding capacity Nunc MaxiSorp™ 96-well plates (Thermo Fisher Scientific, Vienna, Austria). Coating was performed by adding 20 µg of antibody (RTX or RTX-TCO) dissolved in 100 µL coating buffer (0.1 M NaHCO$_3$, pH 8.5) to each well and after 2 h incubation at RT the plate was left at 4 °C overnight both under the exclusion of light. After removal of the coating solution 200 µL of blocking buffer (1% BSA in PBS) was added, left for 1 h at room temperature and subsequently each well was washed twice with 200 µL binding buffer (0.1% BSA in PBS). Hereafter, the radioligand was mixed with increasing concentrations of the competitor (=non-labelled conjugate), diluted in binding buffer and 100 µL of the mixture was added to each well. After 30 min at RT the supernatant was removed, each well was washed three times with 150 µL binding buffer and the coating film was finally detached with 2 × 150 µL of hot (80 °C) 2 N sodium hydroxide (NaOH). The NaOH fraction was taken for gamma counter measurement to determine the percentage of binding in contrast to the standard followed by non-liner curve fitting using Origin 6.1 software (Origin Inc., Northampton, MA, USA) to calculate the apparent half maximum inhibitory concentration of the competitor ($n = 3$, 4 replicates).

4.5.5. Cell Binding

Raji-cells were seeded in tissue culture flasks (Cellstar; Greiner Bio-One, Kremsmuenster, Austria) using RPMI-1640 medium supplemented with fetal bovine serum (FBS) to a final concentration of 10% (v/v). In order to do studies on cell binding 10×10^6 cells were washed twice with fresh media, diluted with PBS to a final concentration of 1×10^6 cells per mL and 500 µL of cell suspension was transferred to Eppendorf tubes. Hereafter, 50 µL of RTX-TCO or non-modified RTX as negative control (both 0.5 µM) were added and the cell suspension was maintained at 37 °C under gentle shaking. After 1 h the suspension was centrifuged (2 min, 11×10^3 rcf), the supernatant was discarded, the cells were washed twice and finally resuspended with 450 µL PBS. Subsequently, 50 µL of the radioligand solution (22 nM in PBS) was added and the suspension was incubated for 30 min at 37 °C. After centrifugation and two washing steps with 600 µL PBS, the cells were resuspended in 500 µL PBS and transferred to polypropylene vials for gamma counter measurement followed by calculation from cell-associated activity in comparison to the standard ($n = 3$, six replicates).

4.6. In Vivo Characterization

4.6.1. Ethics Statement

All animal experiments were performed in accordance with regulations and guidelines of the Austrian animal protection laws and the Czech Animal Protection Act (No. 246/1992), with approval of the Austrian Ministry of Science (BMWF-66.011/0161-WF/V/3b/2016), the Czech Ministry of Education, Youth, and Sports (MSMT-18724/2016-2), and the institutional Animal Welfare Committee of the Faculty of Medicine and Dentistry of Palacky University in Olomouc.

4.6.2. Biodistribution Studies

Biodistribution of ^{68}Ga-labelled conjugates was conducted in healthy 5-week-old female BALB/c mice (Charles River Laboratories, Sulzfeld, Germany). Animals ($n = 3$) were injected via lateral tail vain with 1 nmol of conjugate and a total activity of approximately 6 MBq. Mice were sacrificed by cervical dislocation 1 h p.i. followed by collection of the main organs and tissue, subsequent gamma counter measurement and calculation of the percentage of injected activity per gram tissue (% IA/g).

4.6.3. Imaging Studies

MicroPET/CT images were acquired with an Albira PET/SPECT/CT small animal imaging system (Bruker Biospin Corporation, Woodbridge, CT, USA). Mice were pre-treated by intramuscular (i.m.) injection of 50 µL of RTX-TCO to the left hind muscle and 50 µL of RTX to the right hind muscle. Pre-treated mice were retro-orbitally (r.o.) injected with radiolabelled tracer in a dose of 5–10 MBq corresponding to 1–2 µg of conjugate per animal 5 h after the pre-treatment. Anaesthetized (2% isoflurane (FORANE, Abbott Laboratories, Abbott Park, IL, USA)) animals were placed in a prone position in the Albira system before the start of imaging. Static PET/CT images were acquired over 30 min starting 90 min p.i. A 10-min PET scan (axial FOV 148 mm) was performed, followed by a double CT scan (axial FOV 65 mm, 45 kVp, 400 µA, at 400 projections). Scans were reconstructed with the Albira software (Bruker Biospin Corporation) using the maximum likelihood expectation maximization (MLEM) and filtered backprojection (FBP) algorithms. After reconstruction, acquired data was viewed and analyzed with PMOD software (PMOD Technologies Ltd., Zurich, Switzerland). 3D volume rendered images were obtained using VolView software (Kitware, Clifton Park, NY, USA).

Supplementary Materials:
Figure S1: ^{1}H-NMR spectrum of DAFC-PEG$_5$-Tz (Tz-monomer), Figure S2: ^{1}H-NMR spectrum of of MAFC-(PEG$_5$-Tz)$_2$ (Tz-dimer), Figure S3: ^{1}H-NMR spectrum of FSC-(PEG$_5$-Tz)$_3$ (Tz-trimer), Figure S4: Representative RP-HPLC chromatograms of mono- and multimeric FSC-Tz conjugates (A, UV/vis chromatograms) and their ^{68}Ga-labelled counterparts (B, radio-chromatograms), Figure S5: Representative radio-RP-HPLC chromatograms of the stability assessment of ^{68}Ga-labelled mono- and multimeric FSC-Tz conjugates incubated with fresh human serum (A) and PBS (B), Figure S6: Fluorescence-activated cell sorting of unstained Raji cells, RTX, RTX-TCO, secondary antibody (APC), RTX + APC and RTX-TCO + APC (order from left to right).

Author Contributions: L.V. carried out the synthesis of FSC-Tz conjugates under guidance of B.M. and both provided the corresponding part of the manuscript; B.M. evaluated the NMR data; D.S. evaluated the protocol for radiolabelling with gallium-68, reviewed the literature, summarized the results and has written the major part of the manuscript; C.R. performed cell culture, animal housing and animal care; S.M. modified the antibody and evaluated the radiolabelled conjugates in vitro as well as in vivo. K.S. provided the Raji cells and carried out FACS analysis of the antibodies. M.P. evaluated the tumour-surrogate model and performed in vivo imaging studies. C.D. was responsible for conceptualization, funding acquisition, project administration and supervision.

Acknowledgments: We gratefully acknowledge Christoph Kreutz from the Institute of Organic Chemistry, (Leopold-Franzens University, Innsbruck, Austria) for performing NMR analysis, the staff from the hospital pharmacy for supplying us with Rituximab, the Austrian Science Foundation (FWF) and the Czech Ministry of Education Youth and Sports for funding.

Abbreviations

ACN	acetonitrile
BSA	bovine serum albumin
CD	cluster of differentiation
DAFC	N,N'-diacetylfusarinine C
DIPEA	N,N-diisopropylamine
DMF	N,N-dimethylformamide
EDTA	ethylenediaminetetraacetic acid
FSC	fusarinine C
IEDDA	inverse electron-demand Diels-Alder
i.m.	intramuscular
mAb	monoclonal antibody
MAFC	N-monoacetylfusarinine C
NHS	N-hydroxysuccinimide
p.i.	post injection
PBS	phosphate buffered saline
PET/CT	positron emission computed tomography
r.o.	retro-orbitally

RP-HPLC   reversed phase high performance liquid chromatography
RT   room temperature
RTX   rituximab
TCO   *trans*-cyclooctene
TFA   trifluoracetic acid
Tz   tetrazine

References

1. Henricks, L.M.; Schellens, J.H.M.; Huitema, A.D.R.; Beijnen, J.H. The use of combinations of monoclonal antibodies in clinical oncology. *Cancer Treat. Rev.* **2015**, *41*, 859–867. [CrossRef] [PubMed]
2. Zhang, H.; Chen, J. Current status and future directions of cancer immunotherapy. *J. Cancer* **2018**, *9*, 1773–1781. [CrossRef] [PubMed]
3. Knowles, S.M.; Wu, A.M. Advances in immuno-positron emission tomography: Antibodies for molecular imaging in oncology. *J. Clin. Oncol.* **2012**, *30*, 3884–3892. [CrossRef] [PubMed]
4. Van De Watering, F.C.J.; Rijpkema, M.; Perk, L.; Brinkmann, U.; Oyen, W.J.G.; Boerman, O.C. Zirconium-89 labeled antibodies: A new tool for molecular imaging in cancer patients. *Biomed. Res. Int.* **2014**, 1–13. [CrossRef] [PubMed]
5. Jauw, Y.W.S.; Menke-van der Houven van Oordt, C.W.; Hoekstra, O.S.; Hendrikse, N.H.; Vugts, D.J.; Zijlstra, J.M.; Huisman, M.C.; van Dongen, G.A.M.S. Immuno-positron emission tomography with zirconium-89-labeled monoclonal antibodies in oncology: What can we learn from initial clinical trials? *Front. Pharmacol.* **2016**, *7*, 1–15. [CrossRef] [PubMed]
6. Patra, M.; Zarschler, K.; Pietzsch, H.-J.; Stephan, H.; Gasser, G. New insights into the pretargeting approach to image and treat tumours. *Chem. Soc. Rev.* **2016**, *45*, 6415–6431. [CrossRef] [PubMed]
7. Bailly, C.; Bodet-Milin, C.; Rousseau, C.; Faivre-Chauvet, A.; Kraeber-Bodéré, F.; Barbet, J. Pretargeting for imaging and therapy in oncological nuclear medicine. *EJNMMI Radiopharm. Chem.* **2017**, *2*, 1–14. [CrossRef] [PubMed]
8. Altai, M.; Membreno, R.; Cook, B.; Tolmachev, V.; Zeglis, B.M. Pretargeted Imaging and Therapy. *J. Nucl. Med.* **2017**, *58*, 1553–1559. [CrossRef] [PubMed]
9. Karver, M.R.; Weissleder, R.; Hilderbrand, S.A. Synthesis and evaluation of a series of 1,2,4,5-tetrazines for bioorthogonal conjugation. *Bioconjug. Chem.* **2011**, *22*, 2263–2270. [CrossRef] [PubMed]
10. Oliveira, B.L.; Guo, Z.; Bernardes, G.J.L. Inverse electron demand Diels–Alder reactions in chemical biology. *Chem. Soc. Rev.* **2017**, *46*, 4895–4950. [CrossRef] [PubMed]
11. Zeglis, B.M.; Sevak, K.K.; Reiner, T.; Mohindra, P.; Carlin, S.D.; Zanzonico, P.; Weissleder, R.; Lewis, J.S. A Pretargeted PET Imaging Strategy Based on Bioorthogonal Diels–Alder Click Chemistry. *J. Nucl. Med.* **2013**, *54*, 1389–1396. [CrossRef] [PubMed]
12. Cook, B.E.; Adumeau, P.; Membreno, R.; Carnazza, K.E.; Brand, C.; Reiner, T.; Agnew, B.J.; Lewis, J.S.; Zeglis, B.M. Pretargeted PET Imaging Using a Site-Specifically Labeled Immunoconjugate. *Bioconjug. Chem.* **2016**, *27*, 1789–1795. [CrossRef] [PubMed]
13. Meyer, J.P.; Houghton, J.L.; Kozlowski, P.; Abdel-Atti, D.; Reiner, T.; Pillarsetty, N.V.K.; Scholz, W.W.; Zeglis, B.M.; Lewis, J.S. ^{18}F-Based Pretargeted PET Imaging Based on Bioorthogonal Diels-Alder Click Chemistry. *Bioconjug. Chem.* **2016**, *27*, 298–301. [CrossRef] [PubMed]
14. Denk, C.; Svatunek, D.; Mairinger, S.; Stanek, J.; Filip, T.; Matscheko, D.; Kuntner, C.; Wanek, T.; Mikula, H. Design, Synthesis, and Evaluation of a Low-Molecular-Weight ^{11}C-Labeled Tetrazine for Pretargeted PET Imaging Applying Bioorthogonal in Vivo Click Chemistry. *Bioconjug. Chem.* **2016**, *27*, 1707–1712. [CrossRef] [PubMed]
15. Zlitni, A.; Yin, M.; Janzen, N.; Chatterjee, S.; Lisok, A.; Gabrielson, K.L.; Nimmagadda, S.; Pomper, M.G.; Foster, F.S.; Valliant, J.F. Development of prostate specific membrane antigen targeted ultrasound microbubbles using bioorthogonal chemistry. *PLoS ONE* **2017**, *12*, e0176958. [CrossRef] [PubMed]
16. Knight, J.C.; Cornelissen, B. Bioorthogonal chemistry: Implications for pretargeted nuclear (PET/SPECT) imaging and therapy. *Am. J. Nucl. Med. Mol. Imaging* **2014**, *4*, 96–113. [PubMed]

17. Rossin, R.; Verkerk, P.R.; Van Den Bosch, S.M.; Vulders, R.C.M.; Verel, I.; Lub, J.; Robillard, M.S. In vivo chemistry for pretargeted tumor imaging in live mice. *Angew. Chem. Int. Ed.* **2010**, *49*, 3375–3378. [CrossRef] [PubMed]

18. Billaud, E.M.F.; Belderbos, S.; Cleeren, F.; Maes, W.; Van De Wouwer, M.; Koole, M.; Verbruggen, A.; Himmelreich, U.; Geukens, N.; Bormans, G. Pretargeted PET Imaging Using a Bioorthogonal ^{18}F-Labeled trans-Cyclooctene in an Ovarian Carcinoma Model. *Bioconjug. Chem.* **2017**, *28*, 2915–2920. [CrossRef] [PubMed]

19. Keinänen, O.; Fung, K.; Pourat, J.; Jallinoja, V.; Vivier, D.; Pillarsetty, N.V.K.; Airaksinen, A.J.; Lewis, J.S.; Zeglis, B.M.; Sarparanta, M. Pretargeting of internalizing trastuzumab and cetuximab with a ^{18}F-tetrazine tracer in xenograft models. *EJNMMI Res.* **2017**, *7*, 1–12. [CrossRef] [PubMed]

20. Houghton, J.L.; Membreno, R.; Abdel-Atti, D.; Cunanan, K.M.; Carlin, S.; Scholz, W.W.; Zanzonico, P.B.; Lewis, J.S.; Zeglis, B.M. Establishment of the in vivo efficacy of pretargeted radioimmunotherapy utilizing inverse electron demand Diels- Alder click chemistry. *Mol. Cancer Ther.* **2017**, *16*, 124–133. [CrossRef] [PubMed]

21. Membreno, R.; Cook, B.E.; Fung, K.; Lewis, J.S.; Zeglis, B.M. Click-Mediated Pretargeted Radioimmunotherapy of Colorectal Carcinoma. *Mol. Pharm.* **2018**, *15*, 1729–1734. [CrossRef] [PubMed]

22. Läppchen, T.; Rossin, R.; van Mourik, T.R.; Gruntz, G.; Hoeben, F.J.M.; Versteegen, R.M.; Janssen, H.M.; Lub, J.; Robillard, M.S. DOTA-tetrazine probes with modified linkers for tumor pretargeting. *Nucl. Med. Biol.* **2017**, *55*, 19–26. [CrossRef] [PubMed]

23. Meyer, J.P.; Kozlowski, P.; Jackson, J.; Cunanan, K.M.; Adumeau, P.; Dilling, T.R.; Zeglis, B.M.; Lewis, J.S. Exploring Structural Parameters for Pretargeting Radioligand Optimization. *J. Med. Chem.* **2017**, *60*, 8201–8217. [CrossRef] [PubMed]

24. Cook, B.E.; Membreno, R.; Zeglis, B.M. A Dendrimer Scaffold for the Amplification of in Vivo Pretargeting Ligations. *Bioconjug. Chem.* **2018**, *29*, 2734–2740. [CrossRef] [PubMed]

25. Devaraj, N.K.; Thurber, G.M.; Keliher, E.J.; Marinelli, B.; Weissleder, R. Reactive polymer enables efficient in vivo bioorthogonal chemistry. *Proc. Natl. Acad. Sci. USA* **2012**, *109*, 4762–4767. [CrossRef] [PubMed]

26. Nichols, B.; Qin, Z.; Yang, J.; Vera, D.R.; Devaraj, N.K. [68]Ga chelating bioorthogonal tetrazine polymers for the multistep labeling of cancer biomarkers. *Chem. Commun.* **2014**, *50*, 5215–5217. [CrossRef] [PubMed]

27. Zhai, C.; Summer, D.; Rangger, C.; Haas, H.; Haubner, R.; Decristoforo, C. Fusarinine C, a novel siderophore-based bifunctional chelator for radiolabeling with Gallium-68. *J. Label. Compd. Radiopharm.* **2015**, *58*, 209–214. [CrossRef] [PubMed]

28. Summer, D.; Garousi, J.; Oroujeni, M.; Mitran, B.; Andersson, K.G.; Vorobyeva, A.; Löfblom, J.; Orlova, A.; Tolmachev, V.; Decristoforo, C. Cyclic versus Noncyclic Chelating Scaffold for [89]Zr-Labeled ZEGFR:2377 Affibody Bioconjugates Targeting Epidermal Growth Factor Receptor Overexpression. *Mol. Pharm.* **2018**, *15*, 175–185. [CrossRef] [PubMed]

29. Knetsch, P.A.; Zhai, C.; Rangger, C.; Blatzer, M.; Haas, H.; Kaeopookum, P.; Haubner, R.; Decristoforo, C. [68Ga]FSC-(RGD)$_3$ a trimeric RGD peptide for imaging $\alpha_v\beta_3$ integrin expression based on a novel siderophore derived chelating scaffold-synthesis and evaluation. *Nucl. Med. Biol.* **2015**, *42*, 115–122. [CrossRef] [PubMed]

30. Zhai, C.; Summer, D.; Rangger, C.; Franssen, G.M.; Laverman, P.; Haas, H.; Petrik, M.; Haubner, R.; Decristoforo, C. Novel Bifunctional Cyclic Chelator for [89]Zr Labeling-Radiolabeling and Targeting Properties of RGD Conjugates. *Mol. Pharm.* **2015**, *12*, 2142–2150. [CrossRef] [PubMed]

31. Summer, D.; Rangger, C.; Klingler, M.; Laverman, P.; Franssen, G.M.; Lechner, B.E.; Orasch, T.; Haas, H.; von Guggenberg, E.; Decristoforo, C. Exploiting the concept of multivalency with [68]Ga- and [89]Zr-labelled Fusarinine C-minigastrin bioconjugates for targeting CCK2R expression. *Contrast Media Mol. Imaging* **2018**, 1–12. [CrossRef] [PubMed]

32. Summer, D.; Kroess, A.; Woerndle, R.; Rangger, C.; Klingler, M.; Haas, H.; Kremser, L.; Lindner, H.H.; Von Guggenberg, E.; Decristoforo, C. Multimerization results in formation of re- bindable metabolites: A proof of concept study with FSC-based minigastrin imaging probes targeting CCK2R expression. *PLoS ONE* **2018**, *13*, e0201224. [CrossRef] [PubMed]

33. Rossin, R.; Lappchen, T.; van den Bosch, S.M.; Laforest, R.; Robillard, M.S. Diels-Alder Reaction for Tumor Pretargeting: In Vivo Chemistry Can Boost Tumor Radiation Dose Compared with Directly Labeled Antibody. *J. Nucl. Med.* **2013**, *54*, 1989–1995. [CrossRef] [PubMed]

34. Meyer, J.P.; Tully, K.M.; Jackson, J.; Dilling, T.R.; Reiner, T.; Lewis, J.S. Bioorthogonal Masking of Circulating Antibody-TCO Groups Using Tetrazine-Functionalized Dextran Polymers. *Bioconjug. Chem.* **2018**, *29*, 538–545. [CrossRef] [PubMed]

35. Rossin, R.; Van Duijnhoven, S.M.J.; Ten Hoeve, W.; Janssen, H.M.; Kleijn, L.H.J.; Hoeben, F.J.M.; Versteegen, R.M.; Robillard, M.S. Triggered Drug Release from an Antibody-Drug Conjugate Using Fast "click-to-Release" Chemistry in Mice. *Bioconjug. Chem.* **2016**, *27*, 1697–1706. [CrossRef] [PubMed]

36. Rossin, R.; Versteegen, R.M.; Wu, J.; Khasanov, A.; Wessels, H.J.; Steenbergen, E.J.; ten Hoeve, W.; Janssen, H.M.; van Onzen, A.H.A.M.; Hudson, P.J.; et al. Chemically triggered drug release from an antibody-drug conjugate leads to potent antitumour activity in mice. *Nat. Commun.* **2018**, *9*, 1484. [CrossRef] [PubMed]

37. Versteegen, R.M.; Wolter, T.; Rossin, R.; De Geus, M.A.; Janssen, H.M.; Robillard, M.S. Click-to-Release from trans-cyclooctenes: Mechanistic insights and expansion of scope from established carbamate to remarkable ether cleavage. *Angew. Chem. Int. Ed.* **2018**, *57*, 10494–10499. [CrossRef] [PubMed]

38. Summer, D.; Grossrubatscher, L.; Petrik, M.; Michalcikova, T.; Novy, Z.; Rangger, C.; Klingler, M.; Haas, H.; Kaeopookum, P.; von Guggenberg, E.; et al. Developing Targeted Hybrid Imaging Probes by Chelator Scaffolding. *Bioconjug. Chem.* **2017**, *28*, 1722–1733. [CrossRef] [PubMed]

12

[^{177}Lu]Lu-PSMA-617 Salivary Gland Uptake Characterized by Quantitative *In Vitro* Autoradiography

Roswitha Tönnesmann [1][ID], **Philipp T. Meyer** [1,2], **Matthias Eder** [1,2] and **Ann-Christin Baranski** [1,2,*]

1   Department of Nuclear Medicine, University Medical Center Freiburg, Faculty of Medicine, University of Freiburg, 79106 Freiburg, Germany; roswitha.toennesmann@uniklinik-freiburg.de (R.T.); philipp.meyer@uniklinik-freiburg.de (P.T.M.); matthias.eder@uniklinik-freiburg.de (M.E.)
2   Division of Radiopharmaceutical Development, German Cancer Consortium (DKTK), partner site Freiburg, and German Cancer Research Center (DKFZ), 69120 Heidelberg, Germany
*   Correspondence: ann-christin.baranski@uniklinik-freiburg.de

Abstract: Irradiation of salivary glands remains the main dose-limiting side effect of therapeutic PSMA-inhibitors, especially when using alpha emitters. Thus, further advances in radiopharmaceutical design and therapy strategies are needed to reduce salivary gland uptake, thereby allowing the administration of higher doses and potentially resulting in improved response rates and better tumor control. As the uptake mechanism remains unknown, this work investigates the salivary gland uptake of [^{177}Lu]Lu-PSMA-617 by autoradiography studies on pig salivary gland tissue and on PSMA-overexpressing LNCaP cell membrane pellets. Displacement studies were performed with non-labeled PSMA-617 and 2-PMPA, respectively. The uptake of [^{177}Lu]Lu-PSMA-617 in glandular areas was determined to be partly PSMA-specific, with a high non-specific uptake fraction. The study emphasizes that [^{177}Lu]Lu-PSMA-617 accumulation in pig salivary glands can be attributed to a combination of both specific and non-specific uptake mechanisms. The observation is of high impact for future design of novel radiopharmaceuticals addressing the dose-limiting salivary gland irradiation of current alpha endoradiotherapy in prostate cancer.

Keywords: PSMA-617; salivary gland uptake; prostate cancer; endoradiotherapy

1. Introduction

The therapy of metastatic, hormone-refractory prostate cancer poses a major clinical challenge. Treatment options are limited, rendering new developments and advances in therapy strategies of high clinical interest. The development of radioactive labeled prostate-specific membrane antigen (PSMA)-inhibitors suitable for endoradiotherapy has enabled a promising new form of therapy for metastatic, hormone-refractory prostate cancer. In particular, PSMA represents an attractive target structure and proved suitable for highly sensitive and specific nuclear medicine imaging and therapy as it is overexpressed in almost all prostate carcinomas with markedly increased levels in metastases [1–5]. Physiological expression has been shown to be significantly lower, and is limited to a few organs [1,6]. Clinical experience with PSMA-targeting positron emission tomography (PET), especially with [^{68}Ga]Ga-PSMA-11 [7–14], in patients with recurrent prostate cancer show that lesions can be detected in almost all patients, in some cases with very low PSA levels. These findings often have a high impact on further therapeutic strategies [11,12].

When used therapeutically, radiation dose to organs with physiological PSMA expression might be dose-limiting and can thus minimize the therapeutic success of radiolabeled PSMA-inhibitors.

In particular, renal and salivary gland uptake can be of concern, which, in the case of a therapeutic application, gives rise to relevant organ doses and possible side effects. With the development of PSMA-617 showing an improved and fast kidney excretion, a highly promising compound is already being clinically investigated for endoradiotherapy of prostate cancer with ^{177}Lu or [225]Ac [15–17]. In a first-in-man study with [[225]Ac]Ac-PSMA-617, two patients with advanced disease showed complete remission as confirmed by drop in PSA below the detection limit and a radiologic response in [^{68}Ga]Ga-PSMA-11-PET. Alpha therapy did not result in hematologic toxicity or renal impairment. Nevertheless, strong accumulation of PSMA ligands in salivary glands was described in numerous papers, leading to considerable side effects. The salivary glands are significantly and partially irreversibly damaged, in particular during alpha therapy with [225]Ac with a mean radiation dose of approximately 2.3 Sv/MBq compared to 0.7 Sv/MBq for kidneys and 0.05 Sv/MBq for bone marrow [18]. The resulting xerostomia leads to a significant impairment of the patients' quality of life and thus represents a dose-limiting side effect for therapeutic use of radiolabeled small molecule PSMA-inhibitors. In contrast, PSMA-targeting antibodies such as J591 labeled with ^{177}Lu show no significant uptake in salivary glands. Unfortunately, myelotoxicity appears caused by longer blood circulation of antibodies, making them unsuitable for PSMA-directed alpha therapy [19,20]. On the other hand, a reduction of the dose-limiting salivary gland uptake of small molecule PSMA-inhibitors has not yet been achieved by specific molecular design. Besides many rather non successful approaches towards reduction of salivary gland uptake such as local cooling or lemon juice [21,22], Baum et al. reported a 64% decrease in [^{68}Ga]Ga-PSMA-11 uptake after multifocal, ultrasound-guided injections of botulinum toxin A in a parotid gland [23]. Although first approaches resulted in reduced salivary gland uptake of PSMA-targeting radioligands, the exact mechanisms of tracer accumulation, especially the ratio of specific to non-specific uptake in salivary glands, are not yet sufficiently understood. Salivary glands are known to physiologically express PSMA, which results in a PSMA-specific uptake of small molecule PSMA-inhibitors [24]. However, the detected strong salivary gland uptake of PSMA-inhibitors in clinical studies does not correlate with the rather low physiological PSMA-expression in that tissue. This is underlined by the fact that other physiologically PSMA-expressing organs like intestine, spleen and kidney show similar or even lower radiation doses after endoradiotherapy compared to salivary glands [18,25,26].

Therefore, the present study investigates the salivary gland uptake of [^{177}Lu]Lu-PSMA-617 by autoradiography enabling visualization and quantification of tissue radioligand distribution. Therefore, specific and non-specific uptake of [^{177}Lu]Lu-PSMA-617 were analyzed on pig salivary gland, as a close human homologue, in comparison to LNCaP membrane pellets expressing human PSMA as a positive control. This study gives a further insight into the salivary gland uptake of small molecule PSMA-inhibitors, which is crucial for the future development of novel PSMA-inhibitors with reduced salivary gland toxicity in endoradiotherapy of prostate cancer.

2. Results

2.1. Radiolabeling of PSMA-617

Radiolabeling of PSMA-617 with ^{177}Lu resulted in high radiochemical yields > 95%. Thus, the output of labeling reactions was directly diluted with the appropriate buffer for further use in subsequent experiments (Radiochemical purity > 95%). The molar activity amounted to 48 GBq/μmol.

2.2. PSMA-Specific Binding and Saturation Analysis of [^{177}Lu]Lu-PSMA-617 on Pig Salivary Gland Tissue and LNCaP Membrane Pellets

The regional distribution of glandular areas could be visualized on 10 μm pig cryosections of salivary gland tissue after H&E staining (Figure 1A). In particular, glandular areas showed a high enrichment of [^{177}Lu]Lu-PSMA-617 (Figure 1B). Additional blocking with 2-PMPA, a highly potent PSMA-inhibitor, resulted in a reduced uptake of radioligand in the glandular areas, whereby a relevant amount of non-specific bound [^{177}Lu]Lu-PSMA-617 was still detectable with autoradiography (Figure 1C).

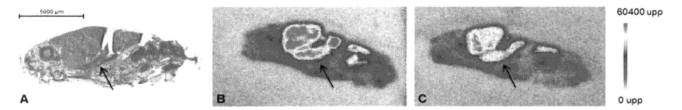

Figure 1. Salivary gland tissue cryosections (pig, 10 μm). Arrows indicate glandular areas. (**A**) H&E staining; autoradiography after incubation for 1.5 h at ambient temperature with 80 nM [^{177}Lu]Lu-PSMA-617 showing total binding (**B**) and additional incubation with 80 μM 2-PMPA (highly potent PSMA-inhibitor) indicating non-specific binding (**C**).

For the saturation binding studies, LNCaP membrane pellets were used as a human PSMA expressing positive control. [^{177}Lu]Lu-PSMA-617 revealed a K_d value in the low nanomolar range to both, pig salivary gland tissue (1.1 ± 0.2 nM) and LNCaP membrane pellets (2.0 ± 0.3 nM) (Figure 2, Table 1).

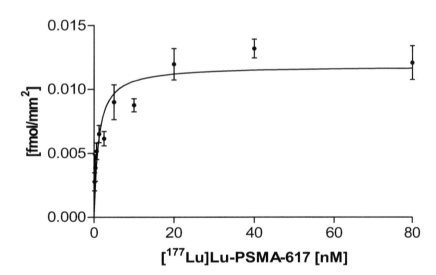

Figure 2. Saturation binding curve (specific binding) of [^{177}Lu]Lu-PSMA-617 to pig salivary gland cryosections. Sections were incubated with 10 different concentrations of [^{177}Lu]Lu-PSMA-617 (0.2–80 nM) for 1.5 h at ambient temperature. Autoradiography was performed with a Cyclone Plus Phosphorimager after an exposure time of 24 h.

Besides the specific binding of [^{177}Lu]Lu-PSMA-617, non-specific uptake in salivary gland tissue accompanied by a reduced B_{max} value of 0.01 ± 0.0006 fmol/mm^2 was notably high as compared to LNCaP membrane pellets (4.9 ± 0.5 fmol/mm^2). Non-specific binding was determined at the presence of a 1000-fold excess of 2-PMPA, indicating a lower PSMA density and higher non-specific uptake in salivary gland tissue in contrast to PSMA overexpressing LNCaP membranes (Table 1).

Table 1. Binding affinity of [^{177}Lu]Lu-PSMA-617 and receptor density of PSMA on LNCaP membrane pellets and pig salivary gland tissue.

Specimen	K_d [nM]	Receptor Density (PSMA) B_{max} [fmol/mm^2]
LNCaP membrane pellets (human, PSMA$^+$)	2.0 ± 0.3	4.9 ± 0.5
Salivary gland tissue (pig)	1.1 ± 0.2	0.01 ± 0.0006

2.3. Competitive Binding Analysis of PSMA-617

In competitive binding studies, PSMA-617 revealed high binding affinities in the low nanomolar range using the non-labeled precursor PSMA-617 as a competitor (Figure 3). The IC_{50} value on LNCaP membrane pellets was determined to be 2.7 ± 0.1 nM and on pig salivary gland tissue 6.0 ± 0.1 nM. Furthermore, a high non-specific uptake fraction in pig salivary gland tissue was detected, whereas LNCaP cell membrane pellets showed only negligible non-specific uptake (Figure 3).

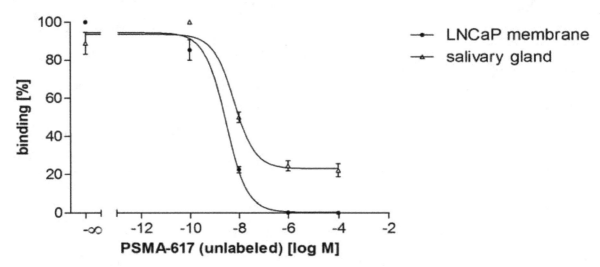

Figure 3. Competitive binding studies of PSMA-617 on LNCaP membrane pellets and pig salivary gland tissue. 6 nM radioligand ([177Lu]Lu-PSMA-617) were incubated with increasing concentrations (0.1 nM–100 μM) of PSMA-617 (unlabeled) as competitor for 1.5 h at ambient room temperature. Autoradiography was performed with a Cyclone Plus Phosphorimager after an exposure time of 48 h.

3. Discussion

Endoradiotherapy of metastatic, hormone-refractory prostate cancer with small molecule PSMA-inhibitors represents a promising approach in the clinical challenging treatment regimen of those patients. In particular, endoradiotherapy with the small molecule PSMA-inhibitor PSMA-617 labeled with alpha emitters was reported to have the potential of complete remission in advanced stage prostate cancer patients [27]. Due to the high linear energy transfer of alpha emitters, critical doses are achieved in accumulating tissue. Besides a highly specific uptake in tumor tissue, rapid excretion of radiopharmaceuticals from non-target tissue is therefore crucial for a successful therapy and to minimize potential dose-limiting side effects. Kratochwil et al. reported the salivary gland toxicity to be the severe and the dose-limiting side effect during endoradiotherapy with 225Ac-labeled PSMA-617 strongly reducing the patient's quality of life and limiting therapy success [18].

Thus, further advances in radiopharmaceutical design and therapy strategies are needed to reduce salivary gland uptake, thereby allowing the administration of higher doses potentially resulting in improved response rates and better tumor control. However, the molecular mechanism underlying the salivary gland accumulation of those radiopharmaceuticals still remains unknown. Several studies indicate that the uptake is potentially caused by a combination of non-specific and PSMA-specific uptake, whereby the exact ratio of specific to non-specific uptake is still undefined [23,28,29]. Therefore, the present study focused on the salivary gland uptake of PSMA-617 analyzed by autoradiography enabling an insight to binding characteristics. Pig salivary gland tissue was chosen as an easily accessible human homologue model representing the healthy organ. Glandular areas could be identified by H&E-staining allowing clear delimitation from surrounding tissue for precise quantification. As a PSMA-positive reference, cell membranes derived from LNCaP cells were analyzed, which are a well-established PSMA-expressing androgen-sensitive human prostate model. Saturation binding studies demonstrated that the uptake of [177Lu]Lu-PSMA-617 on pig salivary gland tissue is

PSMA-specific, although a remarkably high proportion of non-specific uptake was noted. The 2-PMPA blocked uptake increased linear in dependence to the radioligand concentration on pig salivary gland tissue indicating a typical characteristic of non-specific binding. In contrast, LNCaP membrane pellets only showed a negligible non-specific bound fraction. Furthermore, the remarkably low B_{max} value detected in the saturation binding study indicates a low PSMA density on pig salivary gland tissue as compared to tumor cell membranes. This confirms that pig salivary gland tissue as a physiologically PSMA expressing tissue has a low PSMA density. As expected and in line with theoretical considerations, the binding affinity of PSMA-617 is not affected by the differences in PSMA densities. The K_d values of [^{177}Lu]Lu-PSMA-617 were observed to be in the low nanomolar range on both species, matching well with previously published binding affinities of PSMA-617 (K_i: 2.34 ± 2.94 nM on LNCaP cells) [16]. The findings of the saturation binding study were confirmed with a competitive experimental design also revealing high binding affinities for PSMA-617 in the low nanomolar range on both tested species comparable to previously published binding data [16]. The respective competitive binding curves showed differences with regard to the bottom plateau representing non-specific binding. In contrast to LNCaP cell membrane pellets, a high non-specific bound fraction of PSMA-617 was observed again on salivary gland tissue samples. Both experimental set ups confirmed the previously published binding affinities of PSMA-617 on the tested species as well, however they were accompanied by a high non-specific bound fraction on pig salivary gland tissue.

The high amount of non-specific tracer uptake determined in this study might contribute to the phenomenon of strong salivary gland uptake of PSMA-inhibitors in clinical studies, which does not correlate with the rather low physiological PSMA-expression in that tissue [24]. In particular, non-specifically bound PSMA-617 was found to be located in glandular areas. Due to high blood supply, salivary glands are likely to enrich systemically applied pharmaceuticals. Ionic charges and molecular weight might also play an important role in non-specific radiotracer uptake.

Further studies should focus on the rational design of chemically modified derivatives of clinically used PSMA-inhibitors in order to reduce the salivary gland uptake. In that context, concepts related to the non-specific uptake should be taken into account as well to improve the endoradiotherapy of prostate cancer. A more rapid elimination of the radiopharmaceutical from salivary gland tissue would avoid severe side effects and subsequently allow the administration of higher doses to better control the disease.

4. Material and Methods

All commercially obtained chemicals were best grade and purchased from common suppliers. [^{177}Lu]LuCl$_3$ was purchased from ITG (Munich, Germany). PSMA-617 and 2-Phosphonomethyl pentanedioic acid (2-PMPA) were purchased from ABX (Radeberg, Germany). All reagents used in cell culture were purchased from Gibco©.

4.1. Radiolabeling of PSMA-617 with ^{177}Lu

The γ- and β-emitter [^{177}Lu]LuCl$_3$ (ITG, Munich), with a $t_{1/2}$ of 6.7 days was used for the autoradiography studies. Radiolabeling was performed by adding 13 µL [^{177}Lu]LuCl$_3$ (~30–37 MBq) in 0.4 mM HCl, 7 µL of diluted peptide (0.1 mM solution of PSMA-617 in nanopure H$_2$O) to 230 µL ammonium-acetate buffer (0.5 M, pH 5.4). The reaction mixture was incubated at 95°C for 30 min. After quality control by HPLC one equivalent of ^{nat}Lu^{3+} (0.7 µL) was added and the mixture was incubated under the same reaction conditions. The radiochemical yield (RCY) was determined using high performance liquid chromatography (RP-HPLC; Chromolith RP-18e, 100 × 4.6 mm; Merck, Darmstadt, Germany). Analytical HPLC runs were performed using an Agilent 1200 series (Agilent Technologies, Santa Clara, CA, USA) equipped with a γ-detector. HPLC runs were performed using a linear gradient of A (0.1% trifluoroacetic acid (TFA) in water) to B (0.1% TFA in acetonitrile) (gradient: 5% B to 80% B in 15 min) at a flow rate of 2 mL/min.

4.2. Quantitative In Vitro Autoradiography with [^{177}Lu]Lu-PSMA-617

Pig salivary gland tissue was obtained from Prof. Dr. Mehrabi, University Hospital Heidelberg in cooperation with DKFZ, Heidelberg. Tissue was immediately frozen after surgical removal on dry-ice and stored at −80 °C in order to block further biological processes including protein degradation and tissue hardening.

The LNCaP membrane pellets were collected by washing LNCaP cells twice with ice-cold 0.05 M Tris-HCl (pH 7.4) in a first step. Afterwards the cells were scraped into ice-cold 0.05 M Tris-HCl (pH 7.4), collected by centrifugation, and homogenized using a Polytron PT1200E (Kinematica AG, Luzern, Switzerland) in the same buffer. After centrifugation at 120× *g* for 5 min at 4 °C, the supernatant was collected and centrifuged again at 48.000× *g* for 30 min at 4 °C. The resulting pellet was re-suspended in ice-cold Tris-HCl, transferred into a microfuge tube, and centrifuged at 20.000× *g* for 15 min at 4 °C. After withdrawal of the supernatant, the membrane pellet was stored at −80 °C.

Tissue and membrane pellets were embedded in Tissue Tek (Tissue-Tek O.C.T., Sakura Finetek Europe B.V). Cryosections of 10 µm were prepared using a cryomicrotome (CM 1950, Leica Microsystems, Wetzlar, Germany) and mounted onto microscope slides (SuperFrost plus, Langenbrinck, Germany). Afterwards mounted sections were stored at least one day to improve adhesion of the tissue to the slide at −20 °C until quantitative *in vitro* autoradiography.

Autoradiographic images were analyzed with a Cyclone Plus Phosphorimager (Perkin Elmer) and data analysis was performed with OptiQuant data processing software Version 5.0, Microsoft Excel and GraphPad Prism Version 5.01.

4.3. Saturation Binding Assay

For the determination of the dissociation constant (K_d) and maximum binding capacity (B_{max}) cryosections of salivary gland tissue (pig) and LNCaP membrane pellets were prepared for quantitative *in vitro* autoradiography as described above.

Consecutive cryosections (20 per saturation binding assay) were incubated with 10 different concentrations of [^{177}Lu]Lu-PSMA-617, one section to measure total binding and one section for non-specific binding, respectively. Samples were covered with 200 µL incubation solution containing increasing concentrations of [^{177}Lu]Lu-PSMA-617 (0.2–80 nM) in 170 mM Tris-HCl buffer (pH 7.4) with 1% bovine serum albumin (BSA), bacitracin (40 µg/mL) and $MgCl_2$ (5 mM) to inhibit endogenous proteases. Non-specific binding was determined at the presence of 2-PMPA at a final concentration of 80 µM. Sections were incubated for 1.5 h at ambient temperature. Thereafter sections were washed twice for 5 min in ice-cold 170 mM Tris-HCl buffer (pH 7.4) containing 0.25% BSA and once in ice-cold 170 mM Tris-HCl buffer (pH 7.4). Finally, sections were dipped in distilled water to remove buffer salts and dried rapidly under a stream of cool dry air. The sections were placed on a multisensitive storage phosphor screen for exposure in dedicated lead shielded cassettes. Exposure time for sufficient screen saturation was 10 min for LNCaP membrane pellets and 24 h for pig salivary gland tissue with the same experiment conditions. For data analysis the Phosphor Imager software (OptiQuant) expresses the radioactivity signal of the probes in digital light units per square millimeter (DLU/mm^2). The intensity of the light from the retained energy is proportional to the amount of activity in the sample. As a standard, aliquots (2 µL) of the radioligand concentrations were spotted on ITLC paper (Polygram®SilG, Machery-Nagel, Düren, Germany) and co-exposed with the samples. From the known specific activity of the radioligand stock solution, the corresponding relative concentration (fmol/mm^2) of the receptor was calculated. Regions of interests (ROIs) were drawn in the particular experiments to receive DLU/mm^2 values. The dissociation constant (K_d) and maximum binding capacity (B_{max}) were analyzed and calculated by nonlinear regression using GraphPad Prism.

4.4. Competitive Binding Assay

In order to determine the potency (IC_{50}) of PSMA-617 on salivary gland tissue (pig) and LNCaP membranes, a competitive binding assay was performed. Therefore, non-labeled compound PSMA-617 was tested with [^{177}Lu]Lu-PSMA-617 as radioligand. For experiments, five adjacent cryosections were analyzed. Samples were covered with 200 µL incubation solution with increasing concentrations of the competitor ranging from 0.1 nM–1 µM in the presence of 6 nM radioligand. Sections were incubated for 1.5 h at ambient temperature, and were subsequently washed twice for 5 min in ice-cold 170 mM Tris-HCl buffer (pH 7.4) containing 0.25% BSA and once in ice-cold 170 mM Tris-HCl buffer (pH 7.4). Afterwards, sections were dipped in distilled water to remove buffer salts and dried rapidly under a stream of cool dry air. Autoradiography was performed as described in the section above. Exposure time for sufficient screen saturation was 48 h for all samples. Regions of interests (ROIs) were drawn using Phosphor Imager software (OptiQuant), which calculated the intensity units in each region as the fraction of activity in the region with the highest activity. IC_{50} values were analyzed by nonlinear regression using GraphPad Prism.

4.5. Statistical Aspects

All experiments were performed at least in triplicate. Quantitative data were expressed as mean $\pm$ SD.

Author Contributions: Conceptualization, R.T., M.E. and A.C.B.; methodology, R.T. and A.C.B.; writing—original draft preparation, R.T., A.C.B.; writing—review and editing, R.T., P.T.M., M.E., and A.C.B.; visualization, R.T. and A.C.B.; supervision, A.C.B and M.E.; funding acquisition, M.E.

Acknowledgments: The authors gratefully acknowledge the funding by the Research Committee of the Faculty of Medicine, University of Freiburg, Freiburg, Germany (EDE1140/17).

References

1.   Silver, D.A.; Pellicer, I.; Fair, W.R.; Heston, W.D.; Cordon-Cardo, C. Prostate-specific membrane antigen expression in normal and malignant human tissues. *Clin. Cancer Res.* **1997**, *3*, 81–85. [PubMed]

2.   Wright, G.L., Jr.; Haley, C.; Beckett, M.L.; Schellhammer, P.F. Expression of prostate-specific membrane antigen in normal, benign, and malignant prostate tissues. *Urol. Oncol.* **1995**, *1*, 18–28. [CrossRef]

3.   Sweat, S.D.; Pacelli, A.; Murphy, G.P.; Bostwick, D.G. Prostate-specific membrane antigen expression is greatest in prostate adenocarcinoma and lymph node metastases. *Urology* **1998**, *52*, 637–640. [CrossRef]

4.   Mhawech-Fauceglia, P.; Zhang, S.; Terracciano, L.; Sauter, G.; Chadhuri, A.; Herrmann, F.R.; Penetrante, R. Prostate-specific membrane antigen (psma) protein expression in normal and neoplastic tissues and its sensitivity and specificity in prostate adenocarcinoma: An immunohistochemical study using mutiple tumour tissue microarray technique. *Histopathology* **2007**, *50*, 472–483. [CrossRef] [PubMed]

5.   Minner, S.; Wittmer, C.; Graefen, M.; Salomon, G.; Steuber, T.; Haese, A.; Huland, H.; Bokemeyer, C.; Yekebas, E.; Dierlamm, J.; et al. High level psma expression is associated with early psa recurrence in surgically treated prostate cancer. *Prostate* **2011**, *71*, 281–288. [CrossRef] [PubMed]

6.   Ghosh, A.; Heston, W.D. Tumor target prostate specific membrane antigen (psma) and its regulation in prostate cancer. *J. Cell. Biochem.* **2004**, *91*, 528–539. [CrossRef] [PubMed]

7.   Afshar-Oromieh, A.; Holland-Letz, T.; Giesel, F.L.; Kratochwil, C.; Mier, W.; Haufe, S.; Debus, N.; Eder, M.; Eisenhut, M.; Schafer, M.; et al. Diagnostic performance of (68)ga-psma-11 (hbed-cc) pet/ct in patients with recurrent prostate cancer: Evaluation in 1007 patients. *Eur. J. Nucl. Med. Mol. Imaging* **2017**, *44*, 1258–1268. [CrossRef]

8.   Uprimny, C.; Kroiss, A.S.; Decristoforo, C.; Fritz, J.; von Guggenberg, E.; Kendler, D.; Scarpa, L.; di Santo, G.; Roig, L.G.; Maffey-Steffan, J.; et al. (68)ga-psma-11 pet/ct in primary staging of prostate cancer: Psa and gleason score predict the intensity of tracer accumulation in the primary tumour. *Eur. J. Nucl. Med. Mol. Imaging* **2017**, *44*, 941–949. [CrossRef]

9.   Sachpekidis, C.; Kopka, K.; Eder, M.; Hadaschik, B.A.; Freitag, M.T.; Pan, L.; Haberkorn, U.; Dimitrakopoulou-Strauss, A. 68ga-psma-11 dynamic pet/ct imaging in primary prostate cancer. *Clin. Nucl. Med.* **2016**, *41*, e473–e479. [CrossRef]

10. Afshar-Oromieh, A.; Hetzheim, H.; Kubler, W.; Kratochwil, C.; Giesel, F.L.; Hope, T.A.; Eder, M.; Eisenhut, M.; Kopka, K.; Haberkorn, U. Radiation dosimetry of 68ga-psma-11 (hbed-cc) and preliminary evaluation of optimal imaging timing. *Eur. J. Nucl. Med. Mol. Imaging* **2016**, *43*, 1611–1620. [CrossRef]

11. Sterzing, F.; Kratochwil, C.; Fiedler, H.; Katayama, S.; Habl, G.; Kopka, K.; Afshar-Oromieh, A.; Debus, J.; Haberkorn, U.; Giesel, F.L. (68)ga-psma-11 pet/ct: A new technique with high potential for the radiotherapeutic management of prostate cancer patients. *Eur. J. Nucl. Med. Mol. Imaging* **2016**, *43*, 34–41. [CrossRef] [PubMed]

12. Hope, T.A.; Aggarwal, R.; Chee, B.; Tao, D.; Greene, K.L.; Cooperberg, M.R.; Feng, F.; Chang, A.; Ryan, C.J.; Small, E.J.; et al. Impact of (68)ga-psma-11 pet on management in patients with biochemically recurrent prostate cancer. *J. Nucl. Med.* **2017**, *58*, 1956–1961. [CrossRef] [PubMed]

13. Eder, M.; Schafer, M.; Bauder-Wust, U.; Hull, W.E.; Wangler, C.; Mier, W.; Haberkorn, U.; Eisenhut, M. (68)ga-complex lipophilicity and the targeting property of a urea-based psma inhibitor for pet imaging. *Bioconjugate Chem.* **2012**, *23*, 688–697. [CrossRef] [PubMed]

14. Jilg, C.A.; Drendel, V.; Rischke, H.C.; Beck, T.; Vach, W.; Schaal, K.; Wetterauer, U.; Schultze-Seemann, W.; Meyer, P.T. Diagnostic accuracy of ga-68-hbed-cc-psma-ligand-pet/ct before salvage lymph node dissection for recurrent prostate cancer. *Theranostics* **2017**, *7*, 1770–1780. [CrossRef] [PubMed]

15. Benesova, M.; Schafer, M.; Bauder-Wust, U.; Afshar-Oromieh, A.; Kratochwil, C.; Mier, W.; Haberkorn, U.; Kopka, K.; Eder, M. Preclinical evaluation of a tailor-made dota-conjugated psma inhibitor with optimized linker moiety for imaging and endoradiotherapy of prostate cancer. *J. Nucl. Med.* **2015**, *56*, 914–920. [CrossRef] [PubMed]

16. Benesova, M.; Bauder-Wust, U.; Schafer, M.; Klika, K.D.; Mier, W.; Haberkorn, U.; Kopka, K.; Eder, M. Linker modification strategies to control the prostate-specific membrane antigen (psma)-targeting and pharmacokinetic properties of dota-conjugated psma inhibitors. *J. Med. Chem.* **2016**, *59*, 1761–1775. [CrossRef] [PubMed]

17. Rahbar, K.; Ahmadzadehfar, H.; Kratochwil, C.; Haberkorn, U.; Schafers, M.; Essler, M.; Baum, R.P.; Kulkarni, H.R.; Schmidt, M.; Drzezga, A.; et al. German multicenter study investigating 177lu-psma-617 radioligand therapy in advanced prostate cancer patients. *J. Nucl. Med.* **2017**, *58*, 85–90. [CrossRef] [PubMed]

18. Kratochwil, C.; Bruchertseifer, F.; Rathke, H.; Bronzel, M.; Apostolidis, C.; Weichert, W.; Haberkorn, U.; Giesel, F.L.; Morgenstern, A. Targeted alpha-therapy of metastatic castration-resistant prostate cancer with (225)ac-psma-617: Dosimetry estimate and empiric dose finding. *J. Nucl. Med.* **2017**, *58*, 1624–1631. [CrossRef]

19. Bander, N.H.; Milowsky, M.I.; Nanus, D.M.; Kostakoglu, L.; Vallabhajosula, S.; Goldsmith, S.J. Phase i trial of 177lutetium-labeled j591, a monoclonal antibody to prostate-specific membrane antigen, in patients with androgen-independent prostate cancer. *J. Clin. Oncol.* **2005**, *23*, 4591–4601. [CrossRef]

20. Tagawa, S.T.; Milowsky, M.I.; Morris, M.; Vallabhajosula, S.; Christos, P.; Akhtar, N.H.; Osborne, J.; Goldsmith, S.J.; Larson, S.; Taskar, N.P.; et al. Phase ii study of lutetium-177-labeled anti-prostate-specific membrane antigen monoclonal antibody j591 for metastatic castration-resistant prostate cancer. *Clin. Cancer Res.* **2013**, *19*, 5182–5191. [CrossRef]

21. van Kalmthout, L.W.M.; Lam, M.; de Keizer, B.; Krijger, G.C.; Ververs, T.F.T.; de Roos, R.; Braat, A. Impact of external cooling with icepacks on (68)ga-psma uptake in salivary glands. *EJNMMI Res.* **2018**, *8*, 56. [CrossRef]

22. Taieb, D.; Foletti, J.M.; Bardies, M.; Rocchi, P.; Hicks, R.J.; Haberkorn, U. Psma-targeted radionuclide therapy and salivary gland toxicity: Why does it matter? *J. Nucl. Med.* **2018**, *59*, 747–748. [CrossRef] [PubMed]

23. Baum, R.P.; Langbein, T.; Singh, A.; Shahinfar, M.; Schuchardt, C.; Volk, G.F.; Kulkarni, H. Injection of botulinum toxin for preventing salivary gland toxicity after psma radioligand therapy: An empirical proof of a promising concept. *Nucl. Med. Mol. Imaging* **2018**, *52*, 80–81. [CrossRef] [PubMed]

24. Troyer, J.K.; Beckett, M.L.; Wright, G.L., Jr. Detection and characterization of the prostate-specific membrane antigen (psma) in tissue extracts and body fluids. *Int. J. Cancer* **1995**, *62*, 552–558. [PubMed]

25. Herrmann, K.; Bluemel, C.; Weineisen, M.; Schottelius, M.; Wester, H.J.; Czernin, J.; Eberlein, U.; Beykan, S.; Lapa, C.; Riedmiller, H.; et al. Biodistribution and radiation dosimetry for a probe targeting prostate-specific membrane antigen for imaging and therapy. *J. Nucl. Med.* **2015**, *56*, 855–861. [CrossRef]

26. Kratochwil, C.; Giesel, F.L.; Stefanova, M.; Benesova, M.; Bronzel, M.; Afshar-Oromieh, A.; Mier, W.; Eder, M.; Kopka, K.; Haberkorn, U. Psma-targeted radionuclide therapy of metastatic castration-resistant prostate cancer with 177lu-labeled psma-617. *J. Nucl. Med.* **2016**, *57*, 1170–1176. [CrossRef]
27. Kratochwil, C.; Bruchertseifer, F.; Giesel, F.L.; Weis, M.; Verburg, F.A.; Mottaghy, F.; Kopka, K.; Apostolidis, C.; Haberkorn, U.; Morgenstern, A. 225ac-psma-617 for psma-targeted alpha-radiation therapy of metastatic castration-resistant prostate cancer. *J. Nucl. Med.* **2016**, *57*, 1941–1944. [CrossRef] [PubMed]
28. Kratochwil, C.; Giesel, F.L.; Leotta, K.; Eder, M.; Hoppe-Tich, T.; Youssoufian, H.; Kopka, K.; Babich, J.W.; Haberkorn, U. Pmpa for nephroprotection in psma-targeted radionuclide therapy of prostate cancer. *J. Nucl. Med.* **2015**, *56*, 293–298. [CrossRef]
29. Rathke, H.; Kratochwil, C.; Hohenberger, R.; Giesel, F.L.; Bruchertseifer, F.; Flechsig, P.; Morgenstern, A.; Hein, M.; Plinkert, P.; Haberkorn, U.; et al. Initial clinical experience performing sialendoscopy for salivary gland protection in patients undergoing (225)ac-psma-617 rlt. *Eur. J. Nucl. Med. Mol. Imaging* **2019**, *46*, 139–147. [CrossRef] [PubMed]

13

Cholecystokinin-2 Receptor Targeting with Novel C-terminally Stabilized HYNIC-Minigastrin Analogs Radiolabeled with Technetium-99m

Maximilian Klingler[ID], **Christine Rangger, Dominik Summer**[ID], **Piriya Kaeopookum**[ID], **Clemens Decristoforo**[ID] **and Elisabeth von Guggenberg** *[ID]

Department of Nuclear Medicine, Medical University of Innsbruck, Anichstrasse 35, A-6020 Innsbruck, Austria; maximilian.klingler@i-med.ac.at (M.K.); christine.rangger@i-med.ac.at (C.R.); dominik.summer@i-med.ac.at (D.S.); piriya.kaeopookum@student.i-med.ac.at (P.K.); clemens.decristoforo@i-med.ac.at (C.D.)
* Correspondence: elisabeth.von-guggenberg@i-med.ac.at

Abstract: The high overexpression of cholecystokinin-2 receptors (CCK2R) in tumors, such as medullary thyroid carcinoma, allows for highly specific diagnostic and therapeutic targeting with radiolabeled peptide probes derived from natural ligands for the receptor. Based on the ideal imaging characteristics, high availability and low cost of technetium-99m (^{99m}Tc)-labeled radiopharmaceuticals we have developed two hydrazinonicotinic acid (HYNIC) conjugated minigastrin analogs allowing labeling at high specific activity. The CCK2R targeting peptide conjugates show specific amino acid substitutions in the C-terminal receptor-specific sequence with the aim to increase stability and tumor targeting. The CCK2R affinity and the cell uptake of the new radioligands were analyzed using A431 human epidermoid carcinoma cells stably transfected with human CCK2R and mock transfected cells. Metabolic studies in BALB/c mice revealed a high resistance against enzymatic degradation for both radioligands. Biodistribution studies in tumor-xenografted athymic BALB/c nude mice at 1 h and 4 h p.i. showed that the two ^{99m}Tc-labeled compounds showed varying uptake in receptor expressing organs, stomach and pancreas (1.3–10.4% IA/g), as well as kidneys, the main route of excretion (7.8–19.9% IA/g). The tumor uptake in A431-CCK2R xenografts was 24.75 ± 4.38% IA/g for [^{99m}Tc]Tc-HYNIC-MGS5 and 42.48 ± 6.99% IA/g for [^{99m}Tc]Tc-HYNIC-MGS11 at 4 h p.i., whereas the tumor-to-kidney ratio was comparable (2.6–3.3). On demand availability and potential application for radioguided surgery of a ^{99m}Tc-labeled minigastrin analog support the further evaluation of these highly promising new compounds.

Keywords: cholecystokinin-2 receptor; minigastrin; molecular imaging; radiometals; technetium-99m; hydrazinonicotinic acid (HYNIC)

1. Introduction

Regulatory peptides exhibiting high target specificity are suitable lead structures, particularly in the field of oncology, for the development of analogs for radionuclide imaging and therapy [1,2]. Such peptide analogs have the advantage of an easy production via well-established solid phase peptide synthesis (SPPS) allowing the conjugation of a chelator for radiolabeling and the introduction of different modifications into the peptide sequence to optimize pharmacokinetics. Additionally, peptide analogs show low immunogenicity and toxicity and are therefore preferable candidates as new targeting agents [3,4]. A highly promising molecular target to develop radiopeptides for diagnostic imaging and targeted radiotherapy (TRT) of medullary thyroid carcinoma (MTC), small cell lung cancer (SCLC), astrocytoma, stromal ovarian cancer, as well as carcinoids and other tumors of neuroendocrine origin is the cholecystokinin-2 receptor (CCK2R) as an increased level of expression is observed in these malignancies [5,6].

The most promising CCK2R targeting radiopeptides developed so far, are based on the peptide sequence of minigastrin (MG), a naturally occurring ligand for this receptor [7]. MG and its analogs bind to CCK2R with their bioactive C-terminal region (Trp-Met-Asp-Phe-NH_2). In the last 20 years a variety of MG analogs conjugated to different chelators for nuclear medicine procedures have been reported [7–9]. Most of the preclinically [10–16] and clinically [17,18] investigated MG analogs have been conjugated to the bifunctional chelator 1,4,7,10-tetraazacyclododecane-1,4,7,10-tetraacetic acid (DOTA) allowing stable radiolabeling with trivalent radiometals such as Gallium-68, Indium-111 or Lutetium-177 suitable for positron emission tomography (PET), single photon emission computed tomography (SPECT) and TRT. Due to radioprotection issues and regulatory requirements for the in-house production of radiopharmaceuticals, such as the need of hot cells, automated synthesis modules, aseptic processing and trained personnel, the availability of these radiopeptides seems to be restricted to a limited number of clinics.

A cost-effective and broadly available alternative for CCK2R imaging in hospitals without PET would be a kit-based MG analog suitable for ^{99m}Tc-labeling. Such a kit is already available for somatostatin receptor targeting using [^{99m}Tc]Tc-EDDA/HYNIC-Tyr^3-octreotide (Tektrotyd, Polatom, Otwock, Poland). Technetium-99m can be easily eluted from a licensed ^{99}Mo/^{99m}Tc-generator and is used in the major part of nuclear medicine procedures. Due to its ideal physical properties (half-life of 6 h, monoenergetic gamma photons of 140 keV, low radiation burden) Technetium-99m remains the most attractive radionuclide for SPECT applications as well as for gamma probe detection during radioguided surgery [19,20].

Different attempts have been made to develop MG analogs with high tumor accumulation and a biodistribution profile suitable for gastrin receptor scintigraphy [19,21,22]. However, only two ^{99m}Tc-labeled MG analogs have been investigated in clinical studies. [^{99m}Tc]Tc-Demogastrin 2 ([^{99m}Tc]Tc-N$_4$-Gly-dGlu-(Glu)$_5$-Ala-Tyr-Gly-Trp-Met-Asp-Phe-NH_2) contains an open chain tetraamine chelator forming a monocationic complex [23,24]. [^{99m}Tc]Tc-EDDA/HYNIC-MG11 ([^{99m}Tc]Tc-EDDA/HYNIC-dGlu-Ala-Tyr-Gly-Trp-Met-Asp-Phe-NH_2) conjugated to the monodentate ligand hydrazinonicotinic acid (HYNIC) needs additional coligands such as tris(hydroxymethyl)-methylglycine (tricine) or ethylenediamine-N,N'-diacetic acid (EDDA) to complete the coordination sphere [25]. The administration of these two ^{99m}Tc-labeled MG analogs to patients was well tolerated showing no to only mild side effects. With [^{99m}Tc]Tc-Demogastrin 2 all known lesions in nine MTC patients could be visualized. In a comparative study with [^{99m}Tc]Tc-EDDA/HYNIC-MG11 and [^{99m}Tc]Tc-EDDA/HYNIC-TOC the potential additional information which can be obtained in MTC patients using gastrin receptor scintigraphy was pointed out. The same MG analogs conjugated to DOTA showed drawbacks related to high kidney uptake or low in vivo stability, requiring further improvement to develop a CCK2R targeting peptide analog with optimal tumor targeting and biodistribution profile [8].

Various research groups have worked on the development of metabolically stable MG analogs. Different strategies such as cyclization, dimerization and substitutions of amino acids mainly in the N-terminal part of the peptide sequence were investigated [8]. However, due to rapid C-terminal enzymatic degradation the need of alternative stabilization strategies was suggested [26]. Recently we could present different amino acid substitutions introduced into the C-terminal receptorspecific sequence of MG analogs improving the stability against enzymatic degradation and the biodistribution profile [15,16]. After an intense preclinical evaluation of different substitutions, we discovered that most promising results in terms of improved in vivo stability and enhanced tumor targeting could be achieved when substituting methionine (Met) with N-methyl-norleucine ((N-Me)-Nle) and phenylalanine (Phe) with 1-naphtyl-alanine (1-Nal). With the new MG analog DOTA-dGlu-Ala-Tyr-Gly-Trp-(N-Me)Nle-Asp-1-Nal-NH_2 (DOTA-MGS5) radiolabeled with Gallium-68, Indium-111 and Lutetium-177 a very promising targeting profile was achieved [16].

In the present study we have conjugated the clinically well-established HYNIC ligand to MGS5 to develop a ^{99m}Tc-labeled MG analog, suitable for SPECT and radioguided surgery. Furthermore the HYNIC-conjugate dGlu-Ala-Tyr-Gly-Trp-(N-Me)Nle-Asp-(N-Me)1-Nal-NH$_2$ (HYNIC-MGS11) with additional N-methylation of the peptide bond between Asp and 1-Nal was synthesized to evaluate if a further stabilizing effect can be achieved. The two ^{99m}Tc-labeled MG analogs were characterized in vitro and in vivo, including receptor affinity and cell uptake assays, as well as metabolic and biodistribution studies in tumor-xenografted BALB/c nude mice.

2. Results and Discussion

2.1. Peptide Synthesis and Radiolabeling

Following straightforward SPPS HYNIC-MGS5 and HYNIC-MGS11 were synthesized using 30 μmol of resin, 150 μmol of each Fmoc-protected amino acid and 90 μmol of HYNIC. After purification by RP-HPLC and lyophilization the peptide conjugates were obtained in ~10% yield with a chemical purity ≥95% as confirmed by RP-HPLC and MALDI-TOF MS. The amino acid sequences and chemical structures of both MG analogs are presented in Figure 1.

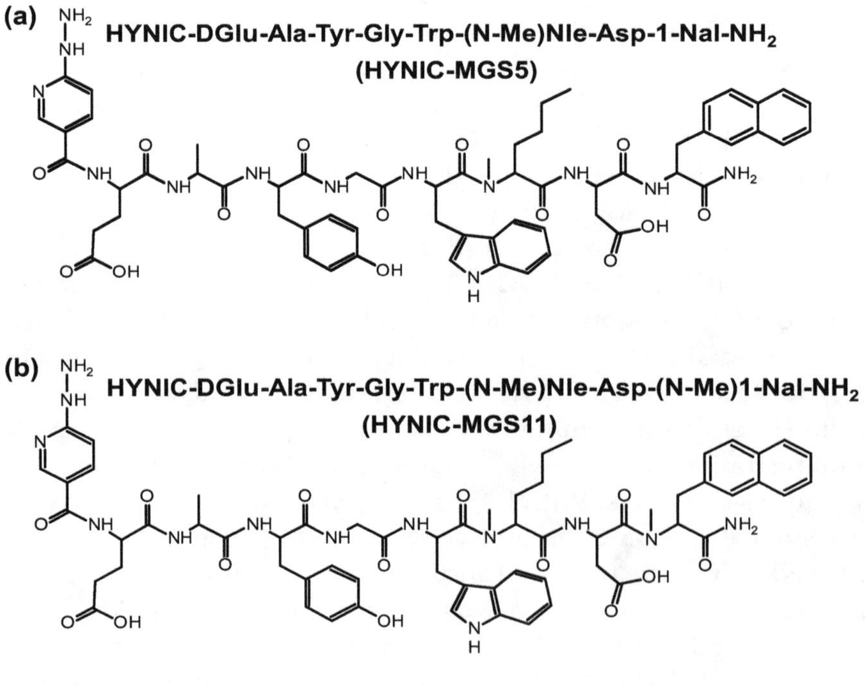

Figure 1. Amino acid sequence and chemical structure of (a) HYNIC-MGS5 and (b) HYNIC-MGS11.

Radiolabeling with technetium-99m using the exchange labeling approach from tricine, used as an intermediate coligand, to EDDA yielded in [^{99m}Tc]Tc-HYNIC-MGS5 and [^{99m}Tc]Tc-HYNIC-MGS11 at high molar activity of 35–40 GBq/μmol comparable to previously published results [22,27]. The main peak occurring in the radio-HPLC chromatogram after labeling indicates complete conversion of the initial tricine complex into the EDDA complex, as already described previously [28,29]. Minor hydrophilic impurities, related to free pertechnetate and ^{99m}Tc-coligands, could be efficiently removed by solid phase extraction (SPE) resulting in labeling with radiochemical purity >95%. Peptide related side products with relative retention of 0.9–1.1 were below 5%. Representative radiochromatograms are displayed in Figure 2.

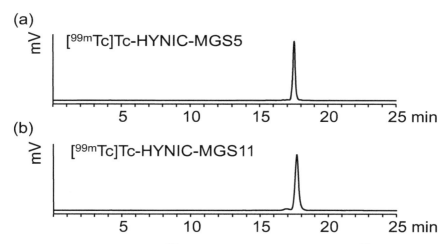

Figure 2. Radiochromatograms of (**a**) [^{99m}Tc]Tc-HYNIC-MGS5 and (**b**) [^{99m}Tc]Tc-HYNIC-MGS11.

2.2. Characterization in Vitro

The stability of the two radiopeptides was analyzed in PBS, confirming a high complex stability obtained by exchange labeling. After 24 h incubation, still a high percentage of intact radiopeptide was present ([^{99m}Tc]Tc-HYNIC-MGS5: 95.1%; [^{99m}Tc]Tc-HYNIC-MGS11: 94.4%). MG analogs missing the penta-Glu motif are generally known for their low in vitro serum stability regardless of whether they are conjugated to DOTA [26] or HYNIC [30]. This can be changed by introducing site-specific amino acid substitutions into their C-terminal peptide sequence [15,16]. For [^{99m}Tc]Tc-HYNIC-MGS5 and [^{99m}Tc]Tc-HYNIC-MGS11 showing such substitutions, a high stability with no evidence of enzymatic degradation was found in human serum (>95% intact radiopeptide after 24 h incubation). These results are in accordance with previous results reported for ^{111}In-, ^{68}Ga- or ^{177}Lu-labeled DOTA-MGS5 (96–98% intact radiopeptide) incubated under the same conditions [16]. From the octanol/PBS distribution a log D value of -2.91 ± 0.06 was calculated for [^{99m}Tc]Tc-HYNIC-MGS5. The additional methyl group in [^{99m}Tc]Tc-HYNIC-MGS11 did not change the hydrophobicity (log D value of -2.84 ± 0.08; $p = 0.07$). Protein binding with values of $36.8 \pm 0.1\%$ for [^{99m}Tc]Tc-HYNIC-MGS5 and $34.5 \pm 2.2\%$ for [^{99m}Tc]Tc-HYNIC-MGS11 after 24 h incubation was in the same range. The results of serum stability and protein binding observed over the incubation period of up to 24 h are summarized in Figure 3.

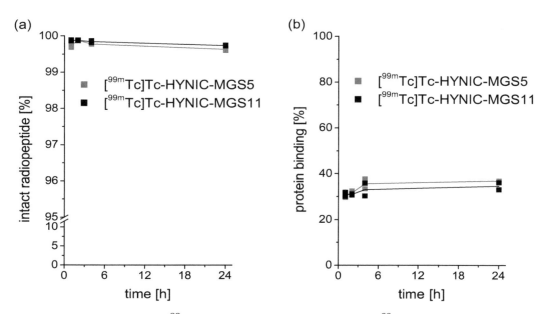

Figure 3. In vitro properties of [^{99m}Tc]Tc-HYNIC-MGS5 (red) and [^{99m}Tc]Tc-HYNIC-MGS11 (blue): (**a**) stability in human serum ($n = 2$), (**b**) protein binding ($n = 2$).

2.3. Receptor Binding and Cell Internalization Studies

Saturation binding experiments on A431-CCK2R cells revealed a high affinity to the human CCK2R. The mean values for the dissociation constant (K_d) calculated by fitting the data from two experiments to a one-site binding model ($r^2 \geq 0.99$) were 13.7 ± 1.1 nM for [^{99m}Tc]Tc-HYNIC-MGS5 and 14.7 ± 1.2 nM for [^{99m}Tc]Tc-HYNIC-MGS11. In Figure 4 a representative saturation binding curve is displayed for both radioligands.

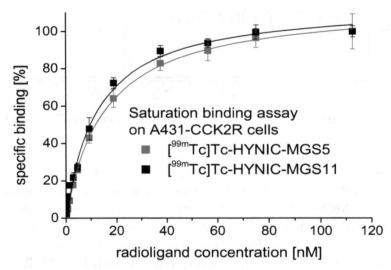

Figure 4. Representative saturation binding curve obtained on A431-CCK2R cells with [^{99m}Tc]Tc-HYNIC-MGS5 (red) and [^{99m}Tc]Tc-HYNIC-MGS11 (blue).

In the internalization assays performed on A431-CCK2R cells a high receptor mediated cell uptake was observed. With [^{99m}Tc]Tc-HYNIC-MGS5 $13.1 \pm 0.4\%$ of the totally added radioactivity was internalized already after 15 min and this value increased over time reaching $62.0 \pm 1.6\%$ after 2 h incubation. Even though [^{99m}Tc]Tc-HYNIC-MGS5 and [^{99m}Tc]Tc-HYNIC-MGS11 showed very similar K_d values, the cell uptake of [^{99m}Tc]Tc-HYNIC-MGS11 was distinctly lower. After 15 min $4.0 \pm 0.7\%$ of the radioactivity was internalized and this value increased to $24.4 \pm 1.9\%$ after 2 h incubation. These unexpected differences between the two MG analogs indicate a possible different binding mode to human CCK2R of MGS5. Also for DOTA-conjugated MGS5 labeled with different radiometals a similarly enhanced cell uptake was found [16]. The results of the internalization experiments are displayed in Figure 5.

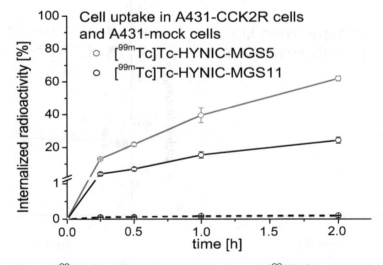

Figure 5. Cell uptake of [^{99m}Tc]Tc-HYNIC-MGS5 (red) and [^{99m}Tc]Tc-HYNIC-MGS11 (blue) into A431-CCK2R (solid line) and A431-mock (dashed line) cells for up to 2 h incubation.

In A431-mock cells lacking CCK2R expression a low and comparable non-specific uptake of radioactivity ($\leq$0.1%) was observed for both radiopeptides at each time point. The receptor specificity of the uptake in A431-CCK2R cells could be confirmed by additional blocking studies with 1 μM pentagastrin showing a clear blockage of the CCK2R mediated uptake to values $\leq$1.0% after 2 h incubation for both radiopeptides (data not shown).

2.4. In Vivo Stability in BALB/c Mice

Metabolic studies in BALB/c mice were performed to further evaluate the enzymatic stability of the radiopeptides. In these studies differences in the stability against enzymatic degradation could be observed between the two radiopeptides. For [^{99m}Tc]Tc-HYNIC-MGS5 >65% intact radiopeptide was found in the blood and liver of BALB/c mice at 10 min after injection. Interestingly, the stability against metabolic degradation was further increased for [^{99m}Tc]Tc-HYNIC-MGS11. The values of intact radiopeptide at 10 min p.i. were 96.0 $\pm$ 1.4% in blood and 95.2 $\pm$ 0.7% in liver. A faster degradation was observed in the excretory system. Much lower levels of intact radiopeptide were detectable in kidneys ([^{99m}Tc]Tc-HYNIC-MGS5: 13.9 $\pm$ 0.5%; [^{99m}Tc]Tc-HYNIC-MGS11: 40.0 $\pm$ 2.0%) and urine ([^{99m}Tc]Tc-HYNIC-MGS5: 3.0 $\pm$ 1.6%; [^{99m}Tc]Tc-HYNIC-MGS11: 9.8 $\pm$ 2.2%). Peptide related impurities already present after radiolabeling and with a relative retention of 0.9–1.1 were not considered as metabolites formed during digestion. Representative radio-HPLC profiles of the different analyzed samples are presented in Figure 6. For [^{99m}Tc]Tc-HYNIC-MGS5 two main metabolites were observed in blood and liver, an early eluting hydrophilic metabolite with retention time (t_R) of ~3.5 min and a second more hydrophobic metabolite eluting at t_R ~15.7 min. For [^{99m}Tc]Tc-HYNIC-MGS11 only the metabolite with t_R ~3.5 min was detected whereas the second metabolite was missing. This indicates that additional methylation of the peptide bond between Asp and 1-Nal prevents the formation of this metabolite during systemic circulation. No further investigations have been performed yet to identify the metabolite found for [^{99m}Tc]Tc-HYNIC-MGS5. From the shift in retention time between [^{99m}Tc]Tc-HYNIC-MGS5 (t_R = ~17.5 min) and the formed metabolite (t_R = ~15.7 min) as well as from data available on the literature cleavage at two different positions, namely between (N-Me)Nle-Asp or Asp-1-Nal, seems possible.

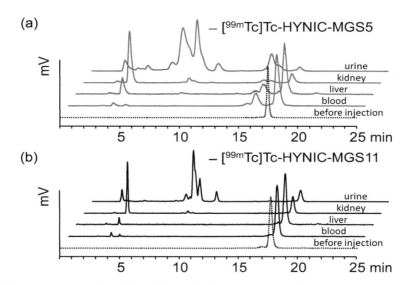

Figure 6. Radiochromatograms for blood, liver, kidney and urine from metabolite studies in BALB/c mice injected with (**a**) [^{99m}Tc]Tc-HYNIC-MGS5 (red) and (**b**) [^{99m}Tc]Tc-HYNIC-MGS11 (blue) as analyzed 10 min p.i.; dashed line showing the radiochromatogram of the radiopeptide before injection.

Ocak et al. have suggested a common enzymatic cleavage site of different MG analogs between Asp and Phe-NH2 when incubated in human serum [26]. Recently, Sauter et al. studied the stability of three ^{177}Lu-labeled MG analogs in different human proteases finding that substitution of Met with

Nle had a stabilizing effect and only cleavage between Nle and Asp occured [18]. In kidney and urine a much higher degree of enzymatic degradation was observed for [99mTc]Tc-HYNIC-MGS5 and [99mTc]Tc-HYNIC-MGS11. In kidneys mainly the hydrophilic metabolite with t_R ~3.5 min not corresponding to pertechnetate eluting at t_R 2.6 min was observed, whereas in urine a variety of additional metabolites with t_R < 15 min was detected.

2.5. Biodistribution in Tumor-xenografted BALB/c Nude Mice

The results of the biodistribution studies in the A431-CCK2R/A431-mock tumor-xenograft model at 1 h and 4 h p.i. evaluating the tumor targeting and tissue uptake are displayed in Figure 7a. For selected organs additional autoradiography studies were performed at 1 h p.i. (see Figure 7b). The uptake values calculated for the tumors and different dissected tissues are summarized in the supplementary material (Table S1). Rapid clearance from the body mainly through the kidneys resulted in low non-specific uptake in most tissues and organs for [99mTc]Tc-HYNIC-MGS5 as well as for [99mTc]Tc-HYNIC-MGS11. The uptake of both radiopeptides significantly decreased in most tissues from 1 h to 4 h p.i. ($p < 0.05$) except for stomach ($p = 0.07$), intestine ($p = 0.14$) and bone ($p = 0.18$) in mice injected with [99mTc]Tc-HYNIC-MGS5 as well as pancreas ($p = 0.12$) and kidneys ($p = 0.18$) in mice injected with [99mTc]Tc-HYNIC-MGS11. [99mTc]Tc-HYNIC-MGS5 showed a significantly lower uptake in blood at 1 h in comparison with [99mTc]Tc-HYNIC-MGS11 ($p < 0.01$), however both radiopeptides showed a similar hydrophobicity and protein binding. At 4 h p.i. a similar trend was observed in blood, but this was not significant ($p = 0.06$). Also the non-specific uptake in lung, heart, spleen and liver was higher for [99mTc]Tc-HYNIC-MGS11 at 1 h and 4 h p.i. ($p < 0.05$). In mouse CCK2R are primarily localized in brain and stomach and at lower expression levels also in colon, pancreas, kidney and ovary [31]. Due to the overall negative charge the two radioligands are unable to cross the blood-brain barrier, but we found a considerable uptake in stomach and pancreas, which was significantly higher for [99mTc]Tc-HYNIC-MGS5 at both time points. For [99mTc]Tc-HYNIC-MGS5 at 4 h p.i. a stomach uptake of 12.89 ± 2.91% IA/g and a pancreas uptake of 6.64 ± 2.21% IA/g was found, whereas [99mTc]Tc-HYNIC-MGS11 displayed much lower values of 3.95 ± 0.15% IA/g in stomach ($p = 0.0009$) and 1.30 ± 0.42% IA/g in pancreas ($p = 0.003$) at the same time point. Also the intestinal uptake of [99mTc]Tc-HYNIC-MGS11 with values of 0.82 ± 0.14% IA/g versus 1.39 ± 0.34% IA/g for [99mTc]Tc-HYNIC-MGS5 at 4 h p.i. was significantly lower ($p = 0.02$). In line with the high CCK2R expression level confirmed for A431-CCK2R cells [32], an impressively high CCK2R mediated tumor uptake was observed in A431-CCK2R xenografts, whereas the uptake in A431-mock xenografts remained at very low levels (<1% IA/g). Tumor weights as determined after sacrifice were 0.17 ± 0.06 g for A431-CCK2R xenografts ($n = 16$) and 0.16 ± 0.12 g for A431-mock xenografts ($n = 15$). One mouse did not develop the A431-mock tumor. In A431-CCK2R xenografts, [99mTc]Tc-HYNIC-MGS5 showed a high and persistent uptake with values of 25.09 ± 2.39% IA/g at 1 h and 24.75 ± 4.38% IA/g at 4 h p.i. The uptake values of [99mTc]Tc-HYNIC-MGS11 were almost doubled (39.87 ± 7.12% IA/g at 1 h and 42.48 ± 6.99% IA/g at 4 h p.i.; $p < 0.01$). This improvement was rather surprising given the lower cell uptake observed in vitro (24.4 ± 1.9% for [99mTc]Tc-HYNIC-MGS11 versus 62.0 ± 1.6% for [99mTc]Tc-HYNIC-MGS5 after 2 h incubation). Receptor specificity was only tested by blocking studies *in vitro*, however, the very low uptake values observed in A431-mock tumor-xenografts (0.17–0.93% IA/g) for both radioligands confirmed that the tumor uptake was highly receptor specific. A very low and similar peptide amount of ~15 pmol was injected to the animals studied with both radiopeptides to avoid possible receptor saturating effects. The divergent uptake values observed for mouse stomach and pancreas in comparison with A431-CCK2R tumor-xenografts observed with both radioligands are therefore rather related to interspecies receptor differences between mouse and human CCK2R, than varying receptor expression levels. Even though the mouse and human CCK2R share an amino acid identity of ~90% [31], methylation of the peptide bond between Asp and 1-Nal in [99mTc]Tc-HYNIC-MGS11 seems to affect the uptake into CCK2R-expressing organs in mouse. Interspecies differences between human and rat CCK2R have been reported also for other radiolabeled

MG analogs [15,33]. The observed differences in stomach and pancreas need to be interpreted with caution as a different physiological uptake may occur in humans. However, no further experiments were carried out to investigate the affinity of the two MG analogs for mouse CCK2R.

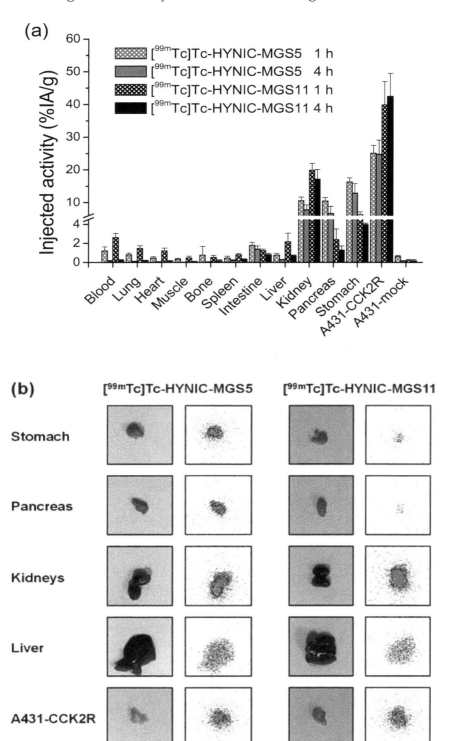

Figure 7. Biodistribution of [^{99m}Tc]Tc-HYNIC-MGS5 (red) and [^{99m}Tc]Tc-HYNIC-MGS11 (blue) in the A431-CCK2R/A431-mock xenograft model: (**a**) tissue distribution and tumor uptake at 1 h and 4 h p.i. with values expressed as % IA/g (mean ± SD, n = 4); (**b**) autoradiography performed for selected organs at 1 h p.i. (color scale, pixel intensity: min 9 (blue), max 100 (red)).

The structural difference of the two radioligands also had a strong impact on the kidney uptake. The kidney uptake of [99mTc]Tc-HYNIC-MGS11 (19.90 ± 2.09% IA/g at 1 h and 17.17 ± 2.93% IA/g at 4 h p.i.) was two times higher in comparison with [99mTc]Tc-HYNIC-MGS5 (10.56 ± 1.15% IA/g at 1 h and 7.80 ± 1.47% IA/g at 4 h p.i.). Despite CCK2R-related uptake, reabsorption and retention of radiolabeled peptides in kidneys is mainly driven by multiple transport mechanisms, involving megalin and cubulin [34]. In megalin-deficient mice a significantly reduced renal reabsorption was confirmed for a radiolabeled minigastrin analog, with renal uptake values reduced to 37–49% when compared to wild-type mice [35]. It has been shown for different radiolabeled MG analogs that the uptake in stomach and CCK2R-expressing tumor-xenografts can be efficiently blocked by co-injection of a 1000-fold molar excess of unlabeled peptide, whereas no considerable effect occurs in kidneys [36]. In this study no additional blocking studies were performed in vivo to confirm the receptor-specific uptake in the different organs.

The tumor targeting profile of [99mTc]Tc-HYNIC-MGS5 well compares with previous results obtained with [111In]In-DOTA-MGS5, showing a similar tumor uptake of 19.53 ± 5.42% IA/g and 23.49 ± 1.25% IA/g at 1 h and 4 h p.i., respectively [15]. This high and persistent tumor uptake is clearly superior when compared to other 99mTc-labeled MG analogs previously studied [37]. For [99mTc]Tc-Demogastrin-2 evaluated in A431-CCK2R xenografted SCID mice at a similar injected peptide amount of 10 pmol a tumor uptake of 12.89 ± 4.69% ID/g at 4 h p.i. was reported, which was however, connected with a very high kidney uptake (58.62 ± 8.98% ID/g). The metabolic stability of this compound (60% intact radiopeptide at 5 min p.i.) was comparable to [99mTc]Tc-HYNIC-MGS5 [37]. In our previous studies with radiolabeled DOTA-MGS5 we concluded that a combination of increased protein binding and stabilization against enzymatic degradation might be responsible for the highly improved targeting profile. The enhanced protection against metabolic degradation of [99mTc]Tc-HYNIC-MGS11 led to a further doubling in tumor uptake. Such an improvement could not be achieved by enzymatic stabilization alone, as exemplified by the co-injection of protease inhibitors [37]. [99mTc]Tc-Demogastrin-2 coinjected with 300 µg phosphoramidon showed a similar enzymatic stability in vivo (85% intact radiopeptide at 5 min p.i.) as compared to [99mTc]Tc-HYNIC-MGS11, but the tumor uptake was clearly inferior (18.21 ± 5.97% ID/g at 4 h p.i.). When comparing the tumor-to-organ activity ratios of [99mTc]Tc-HYNIC-MGS5 and [99mTc]Tc-HYNIC-MGS11, somewhat lower tumor-to-blood ratios were observed for [99mTc]Tc-HYNIC-MGS11. Thus, [99mTc]Tc-HYNIC-MGS11 also showed increased non-specific uptake in most organs at both investigated time points. Due to the concomitant increase of the uptake in A431-CCK2R xenografts and kidneys observed for [99mTc]Tc-HYNIC-MGS11, a similar tumor-to-kidney ratio was found for both radiopeptides (2.4–3.3 for [99mTc]Tc-HYNIC-MGS5 and 2.0–2.6 for [99mTc]Tc-HYNIC-MGS11). The respective tumor-to-organ activity ratios calculated for blood, kidney, intestine, pancreas and stomach for both radioligands at different time points are displayed in Table 1.

Table 1. Tumor-to-organ activity ratios for A431-CCK2R tumor-xenografts of [99mTc]Tc-HYNIC-MGS5 and [99mTc]Tc-HYNIC-MGS11 (mean ± SD, n = 4).

	[99mTc]Tc-HYNIC-MGS5		[99mTc]Tc-HYNIC-MGS11	
	1 h p.i.	4 h p.i.	1 h p.i.	4 h p.i.
Tumor/blood	21.6 ± 5.1	273 ± 151	15.6 ± 4.5	177 ± 55
Tumor/kidney	2.4 ± 0.3	3.3 ± 1.1	2.0 ± 0.6	2.6 ± 0.8
Tumor/stomach	1.5 ± 0.2	2.0 ± 0.4	6.5 ± 1.9	10.7 ± 1.4
Tumor/pancreas	2.4 ± 0.3	4.2 ± 2.0	20.6 ± 11.7	34.8 ± 9.7
Tumor/intestine	14.2 ± 1.7	19.2 ± 7.5	32.3 ± 5.0	61.1 ± 14.3

To our knowledge this is the first report on 99mTc-labeled CCK2R targeting peptide analogs showing such an astonishingly improved tumor uptake along with clearly reduced kidney uptake.

[^{99m}Tc]Tc-HYNIC-MGS5 showed a very similar targeting profile when compared to DOTA-MGS5 radiolabeled with different radiometals suitable for SPECT, PET and TRT [15]. The tumor uptake of [^{99m}Tc]Tc-HYNIC-MGS11 was further improved, however, connected with a concomitant increase in kidney uptake. Recently, two ^{99m}Tc-labeled non-peptidic radioligands have been described showing high tumor uptake in a mouse tumor model based on human epithelial cells transfected with CCK2R, however, tumor-to-kidney ratio was clearly inferior [38,39].

These developments give high promise that in the near future a kit for ^{99m}Tc-labeling will be available allowing the localization and staging of CCK2R expressing tumors. Gastrin receptor scintigraphy might show a lower sensitivity when compared to PET imaging with a ^{68}Ga-labeled CCK2R targeting MG analog, but additionally allows for radioguided surgery. The concept of surgical guidance with conventional gamma probes for intraoperative identification and removal of metastatic lesions has already been successfully introduced into clinical practice by the use of ^{99m}Tc-labeled somatostatin analogs in patients with neuroendocrine tumors [40] as well as ^{99m}Tc-labeled ligands targeting prostate specific membrane antigen in patients with prostate cancer [41]. Due to its high tumor uptake and tumor retention combined with high clearance from other tissues [^{99m}Tc]Tc-HYNIC-MGS11 might be favorable for imaging and radioguided surgery. [^{99m}Tc]Tc-HYNIC-MGS5 well compares with DOTA-MGS5 and shows the advantage of using the same peptide for different applications, [^{68}Ga]Ga-DOTA-MGS5 for PET, [^{99m}Tc]Tc-HYNIC-MGS5 for SPECT and radioguided surgery, as well as [^{177}Lu]Lu-DOTA-MGS5 for TRT.

3. Materials and Methods

3.1. Materials

All commercially obtained chemicals were of analytical grade and used without further purification. Na[^{99m}Tc]TcO$_4$ was obtained from a commercial ^{99}Mo/^{99m}Tc-generator (Ultratechnekow, Mallinckrodt, Petten, The Netherlands) eluted with physiological saline. The A431 human epidermoid carcinoma cell line stably transfected with the plasmid pCR3.1 containing the full coding sequence for the human CCK2R (A431-CCK2R) as well as the same cell line transfected with the empty vector alone (A431-mock) were kindly provided by Dr. Luigi Aloj [42]. Both cell lines were cultured in Dulbecco's Modified Eagle Medium (DMEM) supplemented with 10% (v/v) fetal bovine serum and 5 mL of a $100\times$ penicillin-streptomycin-glutamine mixture at 37 °C in a humidified 95% air/5% CO$_2$ atmosphere. Media and supplements were purchased from Invitrogen Corporation (Lofer, Austria).

3.2. Peptide Synthesis

HYNIC-dGlu-Ala-Tyr-Gly-Trp-(N-Me)Nle-Asp-1-Nal-NH$_2$ (HYNIC-MGS5) and HYNIC-dGlu-Ala-Tyr-Gly-Trp-(N-Me)Nle-Asp-(N-Me)1-Nal-NH$_2$ (HYNIC-MGS11) were synthesized using 9-fluorenylmethoxycarbonyl (Fmoc) chemistry. The peptides were assembled on 60 mg Rink Amide MBHA resin with capacity 0.5 mmol/g resin (Novabiochem, Hohenbrunn, Germany). The reactive side chains of the amino acids were masked with the following protection groups: tert-butyl ester for Asp and dGlu, tert-butyl ether for Tyr, and tertbutyloxycarbonyl (BOC) for Trp. All coupling reactions were performed using a 5-fold excess of Fmoc-protected amino acids, 1-hydroxy-7-aza-benzotriazole (HOAt) and O-(7-Azabenzotriazole-1-yl)-N, N,N'N'-tetramethyluronium hexa-fluorophosphate (HATU) in N-Methyl-2-pyrrolidone (NMP) pH adjusted to 8-9 with N,N'-diisopropylethylamine. Coupling of the Fmoc-protected amino acids following (N-Me)Nle or (N-Me)1-Nal was repeated twice. For the coupling of HYNIC a 3-fold molar excess of BOC-HYNIC, HOAt and HATU was used. The introduction of an additional methyl group into the peptide bound between Asp and 1-Nal in HYNIC-MGS11 was performed by direct N-methylation of 1-Nal during the peptide synthesis on the solid resin as described by Chatterjee et al. [43]. Cleavage of the peptides from the resin with concomitant removal of acid-labile protecting groups was achieved by treatment with a mixture of trifluoroacetic acid (TFA), triisopropylsilane, and water in a ratio 95/2.5/2.5 $v/v/v$. The crude peptides were precipitated and washed with ether before HPLC purification and characterized by analytical HPLC and MALDI-TOF MS. The lyophilized peptide derivatives were stored at $-20\,°C$.

3.3. Analytical Systems and Methods

For preparative HPLC purification a Gilson 322 chromatography system (Gilson International, Limburg, Germany) with Gilson UV/VIS-155 multi-wavelength detector, equipped with an Eurosil Bioselect Vertex Plus C18A precolumn (300 Å, 5 μm, 30 × 8 mm) and a Eurosil Bioselect Vertex Plus C18A column (300 Å 5 μm 300 × 8 mm) (Knauer, Berlin, Germany) was used with a gradient system starting from 80% solvent A (water containing 0.1% TFA) and increasing concentrations of solvent B (acetonitrile (ACN) containing 0.1% TFA) with a flow rate 2 mL/min: 0–4 min 20% B, 4–24 min 20–60% B, 24–26 min 60% B, 26–27 min 60–80% B, 27–28 min 80% B, 28–29 min 80–20% B, 29–37 min 20% B.

Analytical HPLC was performed using an UltiMate 3000 chromatography system (Dionex, Germering, Germany) consisting of a HPLC pump, a variable UV-detector (UV-VIS at $\lambda = 280$ nm), an autosampler, a radiodetector (GabiStar, Raytest, Straubenhardt, Germany), equipped with a Phenomenex Jupiter 4 μm Proteo C12 90 Å 250 × 4.6 mm column (Phenomenex Ltd., Aschaffenburg, Germany) using a flow rate of 1 mL/min together with the following gradient system: 0–3 min 10% B, 3–18 min 10–55% B, 18–20 min 80% B, 20–21 min 80–10% B, 21–25 min 10% B.

For Matrix Assisted Laser Desorption Ionization Time-of-Flight Mass Spectrometry (MALDI-TOF MS) a Bruker microflex benchtop MALDI-TOF MS (Bruker Daltonics, Bremen, Germany) was used in reflector acquisition mode with a positive ion source and 200 shots per spot. MALDI samples were prepared on a α-cyano-4-hydroxycinnamic acid (HCCA) matrix using dried droplet procedure. Flex Analysis 2.4 software was used to analyze the recorded data.

3.4. ^{99m}Tc-Radiolabeling Using the Tricine/EDDA Exchange Method

^{99m}Tc-labeling was performed using a previously described exchange labeling approach with tricine and EDDA [27]. For this purpose 10–20 μg of the corresponding HYNIC-conjugated peptide analog (dissolved in EtOH/H$_2$O 30/70 v/v at a concentration of 0.5 μg/μL) together with 250 μL of EDDA solution (20 mg/mL in 0.1 M NaOH), 250 μL tricine solution (40 mg/mL in 0.2 M PBS pH 6), 500 μL of Na[^{99m}Tc]TcO$_4$ ($\leq$750 MBq) and 20 μl of tin(II) chloride solution (20 mg of SnCl$_2$ * 2 H$_2$O in 10 mL 0.1 N HCl), were incubated in a sealed glass vial at 100 °C for 15–20 min. Radiochemical purity of [^{99m}Tc]Tc-HYNIC-MGS5 and [^{99m}Tc]Tc-HYNIC-MGS11 was determined by analytical HPLC. For in vivo assays the radiolabeled peptides were purified by SPE. For this purpose, the labeling mixture was passed through a C18-SepPak-Light cartridge (Waters, Milford, MA, USA), followed by 5 mL saline, and the radiolabeled peptide was eluted with EtOH/H$_2$O 65/35 v/v and diluted with PBS.

3.5. Evaluation of the in Vitro Properties

The resistance against degradation of [^{99m}Tc]Tc-HYNIC-MGS5 and [^{99m}Tc]Tc-HYNIC-MGS11 (1000 pmol/mL, $n = 2$) in human serum was studied for up to 24 h. Furthermore, the radiopeptides were incubated in PBS (1000 pmol/mL, $n = 1$). At each time point of 1, 2, 4 and 24 h after incubation the intact radiopeptide was assessed by analytical HPLC. Serum samples were precipitated with ACN and centrifuged to collect the supernatant and diluted with water prior to radio-HPLC. For the determination of the distribution coefficient (log D), 500 μL of the radiopeptide solutions (50 pmol/mL in PBS) were added to 500 μL octanol (1:1) vigorously vortexed ($n = 8$) for 15 min and centrifuged to separate the two phases. From each phase a 75 μL sample was taken, the radioactivity measured in a 2480 Wizard^2 automatic gamma-counter (PerkinElmer Life Sciences and Analytical Sciences,

Wallac Oy, Turku, Finland) and the distribution of the radiopeptides calculated. The protein binding in human serum (500 pmol/mL, $n = 2$) was assessed by Sephadex G-50 size-exclusion chromatography (GE Healthcare Illustra, Little Chalfont, UK) for up to 24 h.

3.6. Receptor Binding and Cell Internalization Studies

The receptor affinity of the radioligands prepared using the above described labeling protocol was evaluated in saturation studies on A431-CCK2R cells. For the assay, 96-well filter plates (MultiScreen$_{HTS}$-FB, Merck Group, Darmstadt, Germany) were pretreated with 10 mM TRIS/139 mM NaCl buffer, pH 7.4 (TRIS-buffer) (2×250 µL) and 400,000 A431-CCK2R cells per well were added in 35 mM HEPES buffer, pH 7.4, containing 10 mM MgCl$_2$, 14 µM bacitracin, and 0.5% bovine serum albumin (BSA), a hypotonic solution disturbing the integrity of the cell membranes. Thereafter, increasing concentrations of the radiolabeled peptide conjugates (0.1–112 nM) were added in triplicate reaching a total volume of 200 µL. In parallel, non-specific binding was determined by co-incubation with 1 µM pentagastrin. After 1 h incubation at room temperature, the medium was removed by filtration followed by two rapid rinses with ice-cold TRIS buffer (200 µL). The filters were collected and counted in a gamma-counter. The K_d value was calculated fitting the data with Origin software (Origin 6.1, OriginLab Corporation, Northampton, MA, USA) to a one-site binding model using the formula $y = B_{max} \times x/(K_d + x)$.

For internalization experiments, A431-CCK2R and A431-mock cells were seeded at a density of 1.0×10^6 cells per well in 6-well plates and grown to confluence for 48 h. At the day of the experiment, cells were washed twice with ice-cold internalization medium supplemented with 1% (v/v) fetal bovine serum and supplied with fresh medium before incubation with [^{99m}Tc]Tc-HYNIC-MGS5 and [^{99m}Tc]Tc-HYNIC-MGS11 at a final peptide concentration of 0.4 nM in a total volume of 1.5 mL in triplicates. At different time points for up to 2 h incubation the cell uptake was interrupted by removal of the medium and rapid rinsing with ice-cold internalization medium (two times). Thereafter, the cells were incubated twice at ambient temperature in acid wash buffer (50 mM glycine buffer pH 2.8, 0.1 M NaCl) for 5 min, to remove the membrane-bound radioligand. Finally, the cells were lyzed by treatment in 1 M NaOH and collected (internalized radioligand fraction). All collected fractions (supernatant, surface wash, lyzed cells) were measured together with a standard in the gamma counter. The radioactivity of the lyzed cells was expressed as percentage of the total radioactivity added (% of internalized radioactivity). Non-specific binding was evaluated in A431-mock cells and in additional blocking studies with 1 µM pentagastrin.

3.7. Evaluation of the in Vivo Stability and Biodistribution

All animal experiments were conducted in compliance with the Austrian animal protection laws and with the approval of the Austrian Ministry of Science (BMWFW-66.011/0075-WF/V/3b/2016).

3.7.1. Metabolic Stability in BALB/c Mice

Metabolic stability studies in vivo with [^{99m}Tc]Tc-HYNIC-MGS5 and [^{99m}Tc]Tc-HYNIC-MGS11 were performed in 5–6 week-old female BALB/c mice (Charles River, Sulzfeld, Germany; $n = 2$). Mice were injected intravenously via a lateral tail vain with 37–74 MBq of the ^{99m}Tc-labeled HYNIC-analogs (corresponding to 2 nmol total peptide). Ten minutes post injection (p.i.) mice were euthanized and a sample of blood and urine was collected together with the liver and kidneys. Liver and kidneys were rapidly homogenized in 0.5 mL of a 20 mM HEPES buffer pH 7.3 with an Ultra-Turrax T8 homogenator (IKA-Werke, Staufen, Germany) for 1 min at RT. Before determining the percentage of intact radiopeptide by analytical radio-HPLC samples were precipitated with ACN, centrifuged and diluted with H$_2$O (1:1).

3.7.2. Biodistribution in Tumor-xenografted BALB/c Nude Mice

Biodistribution studies evaluating the tumor uptake of [^{99m}Tc]Tc-HYNIC-MGS5 and [^{99m}Tc]Tc-HYNIC-MGS11 were performed in 7 week-old female athymic BALB/c nude mice (Charles River, Sulzfeld, Germany). To induce tumor-xenografts, mice were injected subcutaneously with 2×10^6 A431-CCK2R (right flank) and A431-mock cells (left flank). The tumor-xenografts were allowed to grow for 11–12 days reaching medium tumor weights of ~0.2 g. Mice were randomly divided into groups of four and injected intravenously via a lateral tail vein with 0.3 MBq of the ^{99m}Tc-labeled HYNIC-analogs (corresponding to ~15 pmol total peptide). The groups of animals were sacrificed at 1 h and 4 h p.i., tumors and other tissues (blood, lung, heart, muscle, bone, spleen, intestine, liver, kidney, stomach and pancreas) were removed, weighed, and the radioactivity measured together with a standard in the gamma counter. Results were expressed as percentage of injected activity per gram tissue (% IA/g) and tumor-to-organ activity ratios were calculated for selected tissues. Statistical analysis was performed using independent two population t-test (significance level $p = 0.05$) with Origin software. The radioactivity in selected organs (stomach, pancreas, liver, kidneys, A431-CCK2R and A431-mock xenograft) was additionally visualized by autoradiography using a phosphorimager (Cyclone Plus, PerkinElmer Life Sciences and Analytical Sciences, Downers Grove, Il, USA). After dissection, the organs were exposed to a multisensitive storage phosphor screen for 40 min and image analysis was performed using OptiQuant^{TM} software (OptiQuant 5.0, PerkinElmer Life Sciences and Analytical Sciences, Downers Grove, Il, USA).

Author Contributions: Conceptualization, Supervision, Project Administration and Funding Acquisition, E.v.G.; Methodology and Investigation, M.K., D.S., P.K., E.v.G., C.D. and C.R.; Writing-Original Draft Preparation: M.K., D.S.; Writing-Review & Editing, E.v.G., C.R. and C.D.

Acknowledgments: Technical assistance of Sedigheh Rezaeianpour in stability assays and of Joachim Pfister in biodistribution studies is greatly acknowledged.

References

1. Laverman, P.; Sosabowski, J.K.; Boerman, O.C.; Oyen, W.J.G. Radiolabelled peptides for oncological diagnosis. *Eur. J. Nucl. Med. Mol. Imaging* **2012**, *39*, 78–92. [CrossRef] [PubMed]
2. Fani, M.; Maecke, H.R. Radiopharmaceutical development of radiolabelled peptides. *Eur. J. Nucl. Med. Mol. Imaging* **2012**, *39*, S11–S30. [CrossRef] [PubMed]
3. Fani, M.; Maecke, H.R.; Okarvi, S.M. Radiolabeled peptides: Valuable tools for the detection and treatment of cancer. *Theranostics* **2012**, *2*, 481–501. [CrossRef] [PubMed]
4. Koopmans, K.P.; Glaudemans, A.W.J.M. Rationale for the use of radiolabelled peptides in diagnosis and therapy. *Eur. J. Nucl. Med. Mol. Imaging* **2012**, *39*, 4–10. [CrossRef] [PubMed]
5. Reubi, J.C.; Schaer, J.C.; Waser, B. Cholecystokinin(CCK)-A and CCK-B/gastrin receptors in human tumors. *Cancer Res.* **1997**, *57*, 1377–1386. [PubMed]
6. Reubi, J.C. Targeting CCK receptors in human cancers. *Curr. Top. Med. Chem.* **2007**, *7*, 1239–1242. [CrossRef] [PubMed]
7. Kaloudi, A.; Nock, B.A.; Krenning, E.P.; Maina, T.; De Jong, M. Radiolabeled gastrin/CCK analogs in tumor diagnosis: Towards higher stability and improved tumor targeting. *Q. J. Nucl. Med. Mol. Imaging* **2015**, *59*, 287–302. [PubMed]
8. Roosenburg, S.; Laverman, P.; van Delft, F.L.; Boerman, O.C. Radiolabeled CCK/gastrin peptides for imaging and therapy of CCK2 receptor-expressing tumors. *Amino Acids* **2011**, *41*, 1049–1058. [CrossRef]
9. Fani, M.; Peitl, P.; Velikyan, I. Current status of radiopharmaceuticals for the theranostics of neuroendocrine neoplasms. *Pharmaceuticals* **2017**, *10*, 30. [CrossRef] [PubMed]
10. Krošelj, M.; Mansi, R.; Reubi, J.C.; Maecke, H.R.; Kolenc Peitl, P. Comparison of DOTA-coupled minigastrin analogues and corresponding Nle congeners. *Eur. J. Nuclear Med. Mol. Imaging* **2012**, *39*, S533–S534. [CrossRef]

11. Kaloudi, A.; Nock, B.A.; Lymperis, E.; Krenning, E.P.; de Jong, M.; Maina, T. Improving the In Vivo Profile of Minigastrin Radiotracers: A Comparative Study Involving the Neutral Endopeptidase Inhibitor Phosphoramidon. *Cancer Biother. Radiopharm.* **2016**, *31*, 20–28. [CrossRef] [PubMed]

12. Pawlak, D.; Rangger, C.; Kolenc Peitl, P.; Garnuszek, P.; Maurin, M.; Ihli, L.; Kroselj, M.; Maina, T.; Maecke, H.; Erba, P.; et al. From preclinical development to clinical application: Kit formulation for radiolabelling the minigastrin analogue CP04 with In-111 for a first-in-human clinical trial. *Eur. J. Pharm. Sci.* **2016**, *85*, 1–9. [CrossRef] [PubMed]

13. Grob, N.M.; Behe, M.; von Guggenberg, E.; Schibli, R.; Mindt, T.L. Methoxinine—An alternative stable amino acid substitute for oxidation-sensitive methionine in radiolabelled peptide conjugates. *J. Pept. Sci.* **2017**, *23*, 38–44. [CrossRef] [PubMed]

14. Rangger, C.; Klingler, M.; Balogh, L.; Pöstényi, Z.; Polyak, A.; Pawlak, D.; Mikołajczak, R.; von Guggenberg, E. ^{177}Lu Labeled Cyclic Minigastrin Analogues with Therapeutic Activity in CCK2R Expressing Tumors: Preclinical Evaluation of a Kit Formulation. *Mol. Pharm.* **2017**, *14*, 3045–3058. [CrossRef] [PubMed]

15. Klingler, M.; Decristoforo, C.; Rangger, C.; Summer, D.; Foster, J.; Sosabowski, J.K.; von Guggenberg, E. Site-specific stabilization of minigastrin analogs against enzymatic degradation for enhanced cholecystokinin-2 receptor targeting. *Theranostics* **2018**, *8*, 2896–2908. [CrossRef] [PubMed]

16. Klingler, M.; Summer, D.; Rangger, C.; Haubner, R.; Foster, J.; Sosabowski, J.; Decristoforo, C.; Virgolini, I.; von Guggenberg, E. DOTA-MGS5, a new cholecystokinin-2 receptor targeting peptide analog with optimized targeting profile for theranostic use. *J. Nucl. Med.* **2018**. [CrossRef] [PubMed]

17. Konijnenberg, M.; Erba, P.A.; Mikolajczak, R.; Decristoforo, C.; Maecke, H.; Maina-Nock, T.; Zaletel, K.; Kolenc-Peitl, P.; Virgolini, I.; Przybylik-Mazurek, E.; et al. First biosafety, biodistribution and dosimetry study of the gastrin analogue ^{111}In-CP04 in medullary thyroid cancer. Phase I clinical trial, GRANT-T-MTC. *Eur. J. Nucl. Med. Mol. Imaging* **2017**, *44*, S258.

18. Sauter, A.W.; Mansi, R.; Hassiepen, U.; Muller, L.; Panigada, T.; Wiehr, S.; Wild, A.-M.; Geistlich, S.; Béhé, M.; Rottenburger, C.; et al. Targeting of the cholecystokinin-2 receptor with the minigastrin analog ^{177}Lu-DOTA-PP-F11N: Does the use of protease inhibitors further improve in vivo distribution? *J. Nucl. Med.* **2018**. [CrossRef]

19. Nock, B.; Maina, T. Tetraamine-coupled peptides and resulting ^{99m}Tc-radioligands: An effective route for receptor-targeted diagnostic imaging of human tumors. *Curr. Top. Med. Chem.* **2012**, *12*, 2655–2667. [CrossRef]

20. Povoski, S.R.; Neff, R.L.; Mojzisik, C.M.; O'Malley, D.M.; Hinkle, G.H.; Hall, N.C.; Murrey, D.A.; Knopp, M.V.; Martin, E.W. A comprehensive overview of radioguided surgery using gamma detection probe technology. *World J. Surg. Oncol.* **2009**, *7*, 11. [CrossRef]

21. Von Guggenberg, E.; Dietrich, H.; Skvortsova, I.; Gabriel, M.; Virgolini, I.J.; Decristoforo, C. ^{99m}Tc-labelled HYNIC-minigastrin with reduced kidney uptake for targeting of CCK-2 receptor-positive tumours. *Eur. J. Nucl. Med. Mol. Imaging* **2007**, *34*, 1209–1218. [CrossRef] [PubMed]

22. Von Guggenberg, E.; Sallegger, W.; Helbok, A.; Ocak, M.; King, R.; Mather, S.J.; Decristoforo, C. Cyclic minigastrin analogues for gastrin receptor scintigraphy with technetium-99m: Preclinical evaluation. *J. Med. Chem.* **2009**, *52*, 4786–4793. [CrossRef] [PubMed]

23. Breeman, W.A.P.; Fröberg, A.C.; de Blois, E.; van Gameren, A.; Melis, M.; de Jong, M.; Maina, T.; Nock, B.A.; Erion, J.L.; Mäcke, H.R.; et al. Optimised labeling, preclinical and initial clinical aspects of CCK-2 receptor-targeting with 3 radiolabeled peptides. *Nucl. Med. Biol.* **2008**, *35*, 839–849. [CrossRef] [PubMed]

24. Fröberg, A.C.; De Jong, M.; Nock, B.A.; Breeman, W.A.P.; Erion, J.L.; Maina, T.; Verdijsseldonck, M.; De Herder, W.W.; Van Der Lugt, A.; Kooij, P.P.M.; et al. Comparison of three radiolabelled peptide analogues for CCK-2 receptor scintigraphy in medullary thyroid carcinoma. *Eur. J. Nucl. Med. Mol. Imaging* **2009**, *36*, 1265–1272. [CrossRef] [PubMed]

25. Kosowicz, J.; Mikołajczak, R.; Czepczyński, R.; Ziemnicka, K.; Gryczyńska, M.; Sowiński, J. Two Peptide Receptor Ligands ^{99m}Tc-EDDA/HYNIC-Tyr^3-Octreotide and ^{99m}Tc-EDDA/HYNIC-$_D$ Glu-Octagastrin for Scintigraphy of Medullary Thyroid Carcinoma. *Cancer Biother. Radiopharm.* **2007**, *22*, 613–628. [CrossRef] [PubMed]

26. Ocak, M.; Helbok, A.; Rangger, C.; Peitl, P.K.; Nock, B.A.; Morelli, G.; Eek, A.; Sosabowski, J.K.; Breeman, W.A.P.; Reubi, J.C.; et al. Comparison of biological stability and metabolism of CCK2 receptor

targeting peptides, a collaborative project under COST BM0607. *Eur. J. Nucl. Med. Mol. Imaging* **2011**, *38*, 1426–1435. [CrossRef] [PubMed]

27. Von Guggenberg, E.; Behe, M.; Behr, T.M.; Saurer, M.; Seppi, T.; Decristoforo, C. ^{99m}Tc-labeling and in vitro and in vivo evaluation of HYNIC- and (Nalpha-His)acetic acid-modified [D-Glu[1]]-minigastrin. *Bioconjug. Chem.* **2004**, *15*, 864–871. [CrossRef]

28. Von Guggenberg, E.; Sarg, B.; Lindner, H.; Melendez Alafort, L.; Mather, S.J.; Moncayo, R.; Decristoforo, C. Preparation via coligand exchange and characterization of [^{99m}Tc-EDDA-HYNIC-D-Phe[1],Tyr[3]]Octreotide (^{99m}Tc-EDDA/HYNIC-TOC). *J. Label. Compd. Radiopharm.* **2003**, *46*, 307–318. [CrossRef]

29. Surfraz, M.B.; King, R.; Mather, S.J.; Biagini, S.C.G.; Blower, P.J. Trifluoroacetyl-HYNIC Peptides: Synthesis and [99m]Tc Radiolabeling. *J. Med. Chem.* **2007**, *50*, 1418–1422. [CrossRef] [PubMed]

30. King, R.C.; Surfraz, M.B.; Biagini, S.C.G.; Blower, P.J.; Mather, S.J. How do HYNIC-conjugated peptides bind technetium? Insights from LC-MS and stability studies. *Dalton Trans.* **2007**, 4998–5007. [CrossRef]

31. Lay, J.M.; Jenkins, C.; Friis-Hansen, L.; Samuelson, L.C. Structure and developmental expression of the mouse CCK-B receptor gene. *Biochem. Biophys. Res. Commun.* **2000**, *272*, 837–842. [CrossRef] [PubMed]

32. Kossatz, S.; Béhé, M.; Mansi, R.; Saur, D.; Czerney, P.; Kaiser, W.A.; Hilger, I. Multifactorial diagnostic NIR imaging of CCK2R expressing tumors. *Biomaterials* **2013**, *34*, 5172–5180. [CrossRef] [PubMed]

33. Aloj, L.; Aurilio, M.; Rinaldi, V.; D'ambrosio, L.; Tesauro, D.; Peitl, P.K.; Maina, T.; Mansi, R.; von Guggenberg, E.; Joosten, L.; et al. Comparison of the binding and internalization properties of 12 DOTA-coupled and ^{111}In-labelled CCK2/gastrin receptor binding peptides: A collaborative project under COST Action BM0607. *Eur. J. Nucl. Med. Mol. Imaging.* **2011**, *38*, 1417–1425. [CrossRef] [PubMed]

34. Vegt, E.; de Jong, M.; Wetzels, J.F.; Masereeuw, R.; Melis, M.; Oyen, W.J.; Gotthardt, M.; Boerman, O.C. Renal toxicity of radiolabeled peptides and antibody fragments: Mechanisms, impact on radionuclide therapy, and strategies for prevention. *J. Nucl. Med.* **2010**, *51*, 1049–1058. [CrossRef] [PubMed]

35. Vegt, E.; Melis, M.; Eek, A.; de Visser, M.; Brom, M.; Oyen, W.J.; Gotthardt, M.; de Jong, M.; Boerman, O.C. Renal uptake of different radiolabelled peptides is mediated by megalin: SPECT and biodistribution studies in megalin-deficient mice. *Eur. J. Nucl. Med. Mol. Imaging* **2011**, *38*, 623–632. [CrossRef] [PubMed]

36. Laverman, P.; Joosten, L.; Eek, A.; Roosenburg, S.; Kolenc Peitl, P.; Maina, T.; Mäcke, H.; Aloj, L.; von Guggenberg, E.; Sosabowski, J.K.; et al. Comparative biodistribution of 12 ^{111}In-labelled gastrin/CCK2 receptor-targeting peptides. *Eur. J. Nucl. Mol. Imaging* **2011**, *38*, 1410–1416. [CrossRef] [PubMed]

37. Kaloudi, A.; Nock, B.A.; Lymperis, E.; Krenning, E.P.; de Jong, M.; Maina, T. ^{99m}Tc-labeled gastrins of varying peptide chain length: Distinct impact of NEP/ACE-inhibition on stability and tumor uptake in mice. *Nucl. Med. Biol.* **2016**, *43*, 347–354. [CrossRef] [PubMed]

38. Maina, T.; Kaloudi, A.; Nock, B.A. ^{99m}Tc-DGA1, a new radiotracer derived from a non-peptidic CCK2R-antagonist, showing excellent prospects for diagnostic imaging of CCK2R-positive human tumors with SPECT. *Nucl. Med. Biol.* in press.

39. Wayua, C.; Low, P.S. Evaluation of a nonpeptidic ligand for imaging of cholecystokinin 2 receptor-expressing cancers. *J. Nucl. Med.* **2015**, *56*, 113–119. [CrossRef]

40. Hubalewska-Dydejczyk, A.; Kulig, J.; Szybinski, P.; Mikolajczak, R.; Pach, D.; Sowa-Staszczak, A.; Fröss-Baron, K.; Huszno, B. Radio-guided surgery with the use of [^{99m}Tc-EDDA/HYNIC]octreotate in intra-operative detection of neuroendocrine tumours of the gastrointestinal tract. *Eur. J. Nucl. Med. Mol. Imaging* **2007**, *34*, 1545–1555. [CrossRef]

41. Robu, S.; Schottelius, M.; Eiber, M.; Maurer, T.; Gschwend, J.; Schwaiger, M.; Wester, H.-J. Preclinical Evaluation and First Patient Application of ^{99m}Tc-PSMA-I&S for SPECT Imaging and Radioguided Surgery in Prostate Cancer. *J. Nucl. Med.* **2017**, *58*, 235–242. [CrossRef] [PubMed]

42. Aloj, L.; Caracò, C.; Panico, M.; Zannetti, A.; Del Vecchio, S.; Tesauro, D.; De Luca, S.; Arra, C.; Pedone, C.; Morelli, G.; et al. In vitro and in vivo evaluation of ^{111}In-DTPAGlu-G-CCK8 for cholecystokinin-B receptor imaging. *J Nucl. Med.* **2004**, *45*, 485–494. [PubMed]

43. Chatterjee, J.; Gilon, C.; Hoffman, A.; Kessler, H. N-methylation of peptides: A new perspective in medicinal chemistry. *Acc. Chem. Res.* **2008**, *41*, 1331–1342. [CrossRef] [PubMed]

14

Development of [^{131}I]I-EOE-TPZ and [^{131}I]I-EOE-TPZMO: Novel Tirapazamine (TPZ)-Based Radioiodinated Pharmaceuticals for Application in Theranostic Management of Hypoxia

Hassan Elsaidi [1,2], **Fatemeh Ahmadi** [3], **Leonard I. Wiebe** [1,4] and **Piyush Kumar** [1,*]

[1]   Department of Oncology, Cross Cancer Institute, Faculty of Medicine and Dentistry, University of Alberta, 11560 University Avenue, Edmonton, AB T6G 1Z2, Canada; elsaidi@ualberta.ca (H.E.); leonard.wiebe@ualberta.ca (L.I.W.)

[2]   Department of Pharmaceutical Chemistry, Faculty of Pharmacy, University of Alexandria, El Sultan Hussein St. Azarita, Alexandria 21521, Egypt

[3]   Current address: Centre for Probe Development and Commercialization, 1280 Main Street West, Hamilton, ON L8S 4K1, Canada; fahmadi@ualberta.ca

[4]   Joint Appointment to Faculty of Pharmacy and Pharmaceutical Sciences, University of Alberta, Edmonton, AB T6G 2E1, Canada

*   Correspondence: pkumar@ualberta.ca

Abstract: *Introduction*: Benzotriazine-1,4-dioxides (BTDOs) such as tirapazamine (TPZ) and its derivatives act as radiosensitizers of hypoxic tissues. The benzotriazine-1-monoxide (BTMO) metabolite (SR 4317, TPZMO) of TPZ also has radiosensitizing properties, and via unknown mechanisms, is a potent enhancer of the radiosensitizing effects of TPZ. Unlike their 2-nitroimidazole radiosensitizer counterparts, radiolabeled benzotriazine oxides have not been used as radiopharmaceuticals for diagnostic imaging or molecular radiotherapy (MRT) of hypoxia. The radioiodination chemistry for preparing model radioiodinated BTDOs and BTMOs is now reported. *Hypothesis*: Radioiodinated 3-(2-iodoethoxyethyl)-amino-1,2,4- benzotriazine-1,4-dioxide (I-EOE-TPZ), a novel bioisosteric analogue of TPZ, and 3-(2-iodoethoxyethyl)-amino-1,2,4-benzotriazine-1-oxide (I-EOE-TPZMO), its monoxide analogue, are candidates for in vivo and in vitro investigations of biochemical mechanisms in pathologies that develop hypoxic microenvironments. In theory, both radiotracers can be prepared from the same precursors. *Methods*: Radioiodination procedures were based on classical nucleophilic [^{131}I]iodide substitution on Tos-EOE-TPZ (P1) and by [^{131}I]iodide exchange on I-EOE-TPZ (P2). Reaction parameters, including temperature, reaction time, solvent and the influence of pivalic acid on products' formation and the corresponding radiochemical yields (RCY) were investigated. *Results*: The [^{131}I]iodide labeling reactions invariably led to the synthesis of both products, but with careful manipulation of conditions the preferred product could be recovered as the major product. Radioiodide exchange on P2 in ACN at $80 \pm 5\ °C$ for 30 min afforded the highest RCY, 89%, of [^{131}I]I-EOE-TPZ, which upon solid phase purification on an alumina cartridge gave 60% yield of the product with over 97% of radiochemical purity. Similarly, radioiodide exchange on P2 in ACN at $50 \pm 5\ °C$ for 30 min with pivalic acid afforded the highest yield, 92%, of [^{131}I]I-EOE-TPZMO exclusively with no trace of [^{131}I]I-EOE-TPZ. In both cases, extended reaction times and/or elevated temperatures resulted in the formation of at least two additional radioactive reaction products. *Conclusions*: Radioiodination of P1 and P2 with [^{131}I]iodide leads to the facile formation of [^{131}I]I-EOE-TPZMO. At 80 °C and short reaction times, the facile reduction of the N-4-oxide moiety was minimized to afford acceptable radiochemical yields of [^{131}I]I-EOE-TPZ from either precursor. Regeneration of [^{131}I]I-EOE-TPZ from [^{131}I]I-EOE-TPZMO is impractical after reaction work-up.

Keywords: hypoxia; radiosensitizer; benzotriazine-1,4-dioxide (BTDO), benzotriazine-1-monoxide (BTMO), tirapazamine (TPZ), SR 4317; radioiodination

---

1. Introduction

Solid tumors frequently demonstrate rapid growth and aberrant vasculature, leading to microenvironmental deficiencies of oxygen (hypoxia), nutrients and therapeutic drugs. Tumor hypoxia is an early event and an independent risk factor for progression of all types of cancers. Hypoxic tumors are relatively more resistant than oxygenated tumors to killing by ionizing radiation during conventional radiotherapy, and recurrent cancers may be metastatically aggressive. Clearly, identification of hypoxic microenvironments and more effective cancer management based on assessments of their hypoxic stature is central to effective treatment [1–5]. In vivo imaging offers insights into the detection and management of tumor hypoxia [6–10] and, of the imaging modalities available, nuclear imaging is both effective and widely available. Radiolabeled azomycin (2-nitroimidazole) derivatives are the most studied and used radiopharmaceuticals for hypoxia imaging [11–13].

Like the nitroimidazoles, 1,2,4-benzotriazines (BTDOs such as 1,2,4-benzotriazine-3-amino-1,4-dioxide (tirapazamine, TPZ) and its derivatives are bioactivated via a single electron reduction that is reversible in the presence of oxygen [14]. TPZ was synthesized as a potential antimicrobial agent in 1957 [15,16], and the rediscovery of TPZ and its monoxide homologue (TPZMO; SR 4317) as radiosensitizers [17,18] opened the door to hypoxic radiosensitization by bioreductively-activated BTDOs that offer an alternative mechanism to that of the nitroimidazoles [19–22]. Radiolabeled BTDOs and BTMOs for hypoxia imaging or radiotherapy appear unreported to date.

A recent publication on the synthesis of 3-(2-iodoethoxyethyl)-amino-1,2,4-benzotriazine-1,4-dioxide (I-EOE-TPZ) and 3-(2-iodoethoxyethyl)-amino-1,2,4-benzotriazine-1-monoxide (I-EOE-TPZMO) reports that the in vitro toxicity and radiosensitizing potency of I-EOE-TPZ were similar to that of TPZ [23]. These investigations into the radiosyntheses of [131I]I-EOE-TPZ and its monoxide homologue, [131I]I-EOE-TPZMO, represent the next step in the evaluation of these compounds as radiotheranostic pharmaceuticals. The chemical structures of TPZ, Tos-EOE-TPZ, the precursor for nucleophilic radioiodination (P1), and I-EOE-TPZ, the precursor for isotope exchange radiolabeling (P2), and I-EOE-TPZMO are depicted in Figure 1.

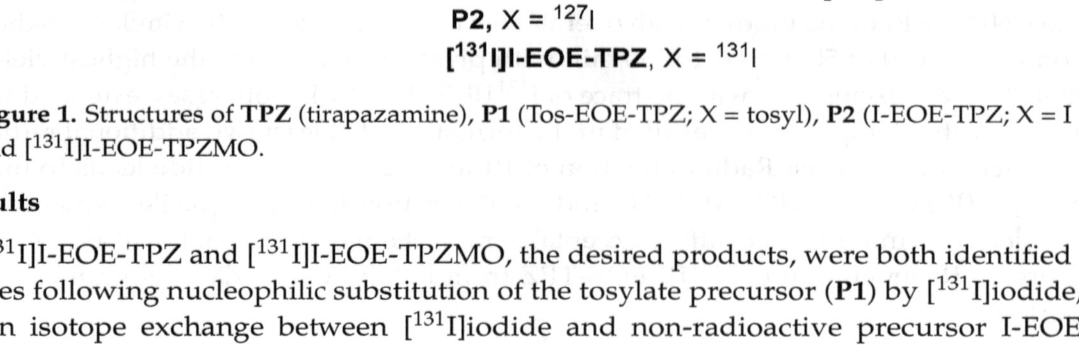

TPZ

P1, X = OTs
P2, X = ^{127}I
[^{131}I]I-EOE-TPZ, X = ^{131}I

[^{131}I]I-EOE-TPZMO

Figure 1. Structures of **TPZ** (tirapazamine), **P1** (Tos-EOE-TPZ; X = tosyl), **P2** (I-EOE-TPZ; X = I = ^{127}I), and [^{131}I]I-EOE-TPZMO.

2. Results

[^{131}I]I-EOE-TPZ and [^{131}I]I-EOE-TPZMO, the desired products, were both identified in reaction mixtures following nucleophilic substitution of the tosylate precursor (**P1**) by [^{131}I]iodide, and upon halogen isotope exchange between [^{131}I]iodide and non-radioactive precursor I-EOE-TPZ (**P2**). Radiochemical yields were strongly dependent upon reaction conditions.

2.1. Nucleophilic Radioiodination of P1

Nucleophilic reactions on P1, irrespective of reaction duration, in either DMF or ACN at 22 °C and at 60 °C demonstrated no formation of either [131I]I-EOE-TPZ or [131I]I-EOE-TPZMO, with only unreacted [131I]iodide detected by RTLC (Table 1). However, reaction for 60 min at higher temperatures (80 °C and 100 °C) in ACN afforded both products. Using DMF as a solvent at these (higher) temperatures also led to the formation of *I-EOE-TPZ, albeit in lower yields. Radioiodination at 80 °C for 60 min in ACN appeared to be the best condition for synthesizing [131I]I-EOE-TPZ (RCY 48.5%; entry 3 Table 1) via nucleophilic substitution of precursor P1; at 100 °C, this reaction favored production of [131I]I-EOE-TPZMO (RCY 50.2%; entry 4 Table 1). Reaction conditions and product yields are given in Table 1 and typical radiochromatograms for 80 and 100 °C are shown in Figure 2 (A and B).

Table 1. Radioiodination of precursor Tos-EOE-TPZ (**P1**) via nucleophilic substitution of tosyl by [131I]iodide.

Solvent	Temp (°C)	Time (min)	[131I]I-EOE-TPZ % of Total [131I]	[131I]I-EOE-TPZMO % of Total [131I]
ACN	22	30 and 60	0, 0	0, 0
ACN	60	30 and 60	0, 0	17.2, 31.2
ACN	80	60	48.5	20.7
ACN	100	60	10.1	50.2
DMF	22	30 and 90	0, 0	0, 0
DMF	60	30 and 60	0, 0	0, 0
DMF	80	60	24.6	16.7
DMF	100	60	7.8	34.2

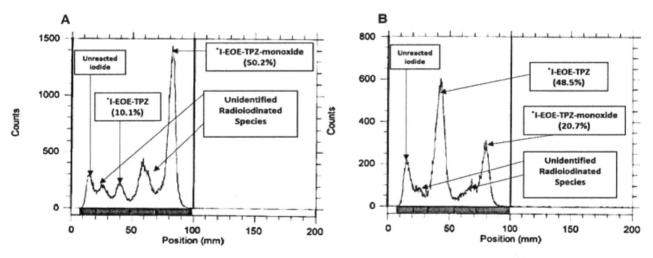

Figure 2. RTLC of the reaction mixture post-nucleophilic radioiodination of **P1** by [131I]iodide in ACN after 60 min at 100 °C (**A**) and at 80 °C (**B**).

2.2. Isotope Exchange Radioiodination of P2

Radioiodination of I-EOE-TPZ (**P2**) by [131I]iodide was monitored under a range of reaction conditions. The first attempt, using the conditions applied to nucleophilic labelling (**P1**) in DMF at 22 °C, showed a high yield of [131I]I-EOE-TPZMO and no [131I]I-EOE-TPZ at 30 min, and a small yield of [131I]I-EOE-TPZ (18%) at 1 h; both radiochromatograms revealed a complex mixture of the desired products, radioiodide and at least two unknown radioiodinated by-products (Figure 3 and Table 2).

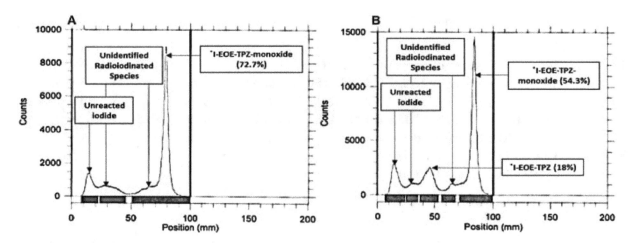

Figure 3. RTLC of the reaction mixture following [^{131}I]iodide exchange on **P2** at 22 °C. [^{131}I]I-EOE-TPZMO is the main product by 30 min (**A**), [^{131}I]I-EOE-TPZ is evident in low radiochemical yield (18%) at 60 min (**B**).

Table 2. Radioiodination conditions and product yields for [^{131}I]iodide exchange on **P2**.

Solvent	Temp (°C)	Time (min)	Pivalic Acid (mg)	[^{131}I]I-EOE-TPZ % of Total [^{131}I]	[^{131}I]I-EOE-TPZMO % of Total [^{131}I]
DMF	22	30, 60	0	0, 18	72.7, 54.3
ACN	22	30, 60	0	0, 0	34.7, 7.5
ACN	80	30	0	89	6.9
ACN	50	30, 60	3.5	0, 7.7	**92.4**, 66
ACN	22	30, 60, 90	3.5	3.2, 3.5, 3	54, 50, 48.7
EtOH/ACN	22	30, 60, 90	3.5	0, 0, 0	43, 42.4, 42.2

Exchange radioiodination of P2 was conducted in ACN at 50 °C in the presence of pivalic acid for 30 min. Under these conditions, RTLC showed the highest yield, 92.4%, of [^{131}I]I-EOE-TPZMO but with no [^{131}I]I-EOE-TPZ (Figure 4A). At 60 min, a third radioactive compound at R_f 0.75, running just behind [^{131}I]I-EOE-TPZMO, was apparent in the RTLC as well as a trace evidence, 7.7%, of [^{131}I]I-EOE-TPZ (Figure 4B).

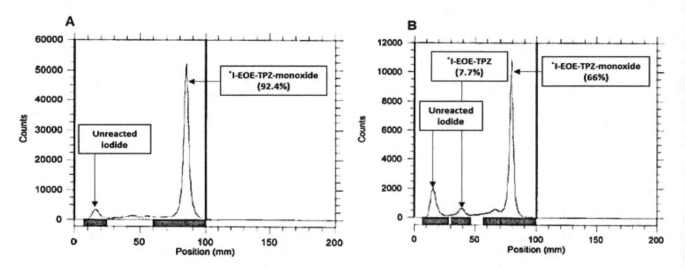

Figure 4. RTLC of the post-labelling exchange reaction mixture using precursor **P2** in ACN and pivalic acid after 30 min (**A**) and 60 min (**B**) at 50 °C.

To determine if pivalic acid was responsible for promoting the formation of the peak at R_f 0.75 at the higher temperature (i.e., 50 °C), radioiodination was performed at a room temperature (22 °C) after

30, 60 and 90 min in ACN. The RTLCs showed an increased appearance in by-products at R_f 0.35 and 0.75 (Figure 5). A room temperature experiment using pivalic acid in a protic solvent (ACN/ETOH mixture) yielded similar (no improvement) results, but with lower peak resolution (not shown).

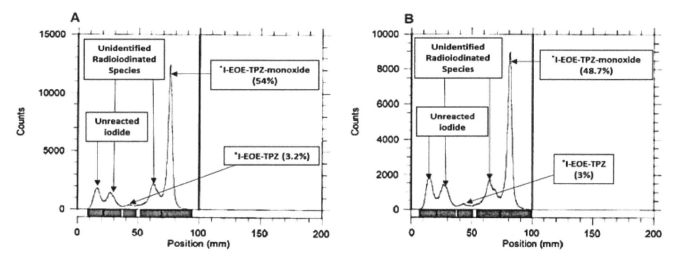

Figure 5. RTLC of the exchange reaction mixture using precursor **P2** and pivalic acid in ACN after 30 min (**A**) and 90 min (**B**) at 22 °C.

Radioiodine exchange on precursor P2 in ACN at 80 °C for 30 min provided the highest radiochemical yield of [131I]I-EOE-TPZ (89%; Table 2). Subsequent solid phase purification on an alumina cartilage afforded [131I]I-EOE-TPZ in radiochemical yields of 60% with over 97% radiochemical purity and a trace of [131I]I-EOE-TPZMO (Figure 6).

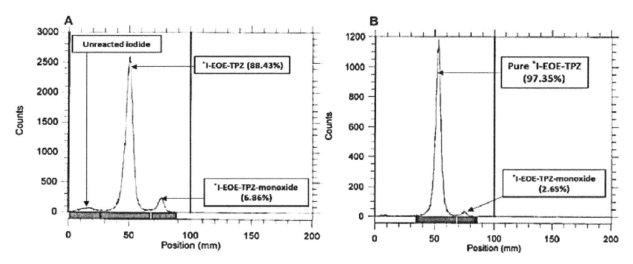

Figure 6. (**A**) The RTLC of the exchange-labeled [131I]I-EOE-TPZ (**P2**) reaction mixture in ACN, 30 min after reacting at 80 °C with sodium [131I]iodide. (**B**) The RTLC of (**A**) after purification through a neutral alumina cartridge.

3. Discussion

The radiosynthesis of [131I]I-EOE-TPZ by nucleophilic radioiodination of the corresponding tosylate, Tos-EOE-TPZ, was associated with the production of a second hypoxia-selective radiosensitizer, [131I]I-EOE-TPZMO. In fact, minimizing the production of this radiolabeled 1-monoxide was a major challenge to preparing the radiolabeled, fully oxidized, 1,4-dioxide, analogue. There is precedence to the formation of the 1-monoxide in the literature, both as SR 4317, an analogue of TPZ [16,24], and as a product of TPZ metabolism [25,26]. The synthetic chemistry of the

X-EOE-TPZ series similarly involved the production of the corresponding X-EOE-TPZMO 1-oxides [23]. Unfortunately, up-oxidation of the monoxides to their 1,4-dioxides was difficult or even unachievable, thereby squelching the idea of simply using the highly efficient production of [^{131}I]I-EOE-TPZMO (by either halogen exchange or nucleophilic substitution) and then simply oxidizing the monoxide to [^{131}I]I-EOE-TPZ.

The unanticipated, but facile reduction of I-EOE-TPZ by (radio)iodide in both exchange labelling and nucleophilic substitution procedures appears to lie in the ease of oxidizing iodide to iodonium species. Iodide may first serve as the single electron donor, giving rise to the BTDO radical intermediate, and also provide the second electron to form the monoxide. Examples of functional group reductions via iodide salts include amine N-oxides [27], isoxazolodines [28], sulfoxides [29] and graphene oxide [30] and others [31] Plausible mechanisms have been proffered for the bioreduction of TPZ [24–26] to its 1-monoxide, and these may apply when iodide is the initial electron donor.

Although it seems unlikely that pivalic acid directly affects the initial single electron reduction in this scheme, facilitation of radioiodide/halogen exchange radiolabeling by pivalic acid is well established in the radiopharmaceutical literature [32] In the current case, it is possible that pivalic acid skews the equilibrium between the protonated and non-protonated radical in the aprotic solvent, an effect that may not influence formation of the reduced monoxide, but that leads to the formation of other reductive intermediates as well. The latter postulate is supported by the prominence of two new radioactive by-products in the pivalic acid isotope exchange reactions, products that are also prominent in the nucleophilic substitution reactions at 100 °C and when the reaction is carried out in a protic (ACN-ethanol) solvent. A plausible mechanism for the facile conversion of I-EOE-TPZ and Tos-EOE-TPZ to [^{131}I]I-EOE-TPZMO, is presented in Scheme 1.

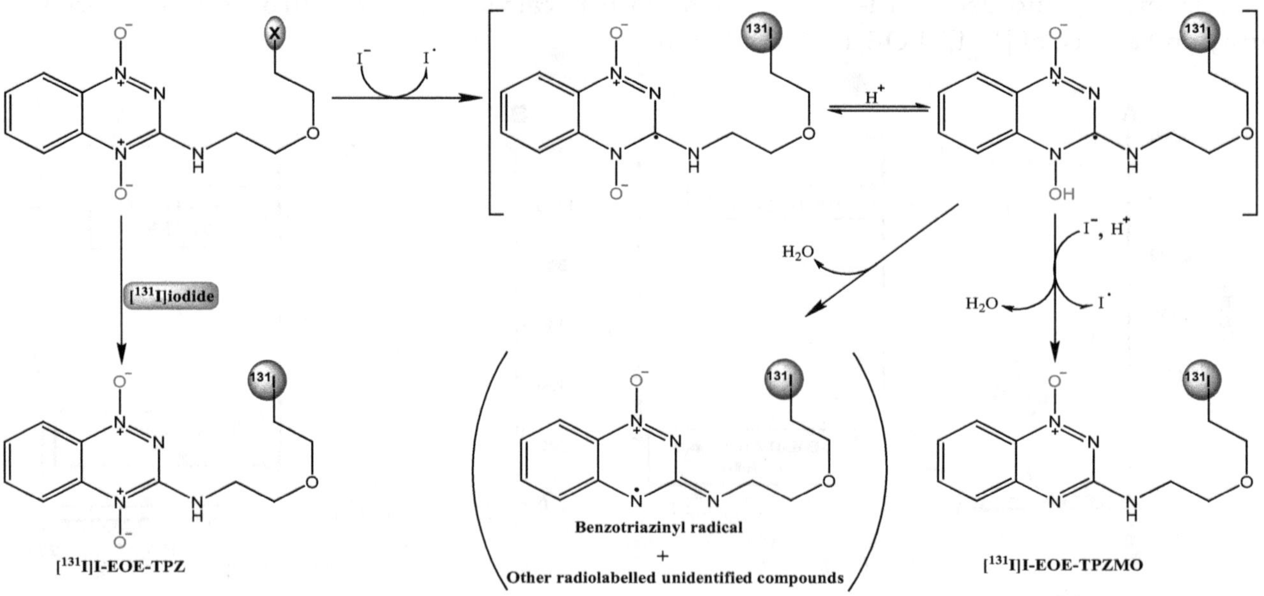

Scheme 1. A proposed model for the formation of [^{131}I]I-EOE-TPZMO by [^{131}I]iodide during isotope exchange with I-EOE-TPZ and nucleophilic substitution on Tos-EOE-TPZ. This model is based in part on a model proposed by Siim et al. for TPZ metabolism [26].

4. Experimental

4.1. Materials

Precursors P1 and P2 were synthesized as reported [23] Anhydrous EtOH, sterile water for injection (SWFI) and 0.9% bacteriostatic saline were purchased from commercial suppliers. All solvents (ethyl acetate [EtOAc], acetonitrile [ACN] and dimethylformamide [DMF] were reagent grade, purchased from commercial suppliers, and used without further purification. Sodium [^{131}I]iodide was purchased by the Edmonton Radiopharmacy Center from NTP Radioisotopes (Pretoria, South Africa), and was provided to us at no cost for experimental development. Reacti-V-vials (4 mL; reactivial) were purchased from Wheaton, Millville, NJ, USA, while disposable sterile items (syringes and needles of various size, vent needles, product vials [Hollister, 20 mL], GS filters [22 μm pore; Millipore, Cork, Ireland], neutral alumina cartridges [Waters, Milford, MS, USA]) were purchased from respective suppliers. Progress of reactions, and radiochemical purity of final products were monitored on silica gel pre-coated glass TLC plates (2.5 × 7.5 cm; Whatman). RadioTLC (RTLC) plates were scanned using a Bioscan TLC scanner (Eckert & Ziegler, Berlin, Germany). Specific quality control tests that included confirming radionuclidic identity by determining the half-life by counting a sample of purified product (from optimized synthesis batch) in a counting well and checking pH of purified product solution using pH test strips. The authentic reference standards, I-EOE-TPZ and I-EOE-TPZMO monoxide that were co-spotted, were visible as red (R_f 0.45 ± 0.05) and yellow (R_f 0.85± 0.05) spots, respectively.

4.2. Methods

4.2.1. Nucleophilic Radioiodination of Tos-EOE-TPZ (Precursor P1)

It started by mixing a solution of P1 (100 μg/100 μL) in the selected solvent and adding this to the reactivial containing [131I]iodide (nominally 37 kBq). After radiometry, the vial was placed on a pre-heated block and radioiodination was performed for the specified time. The reaction vial was removed, cooled to room temperature, and then aliquots were taken for RTLC. Data are presented in Table 1.

4.2.2. Halogen Isotope Exchange Radioiodination of I-EOE-TPZ (Precursor P2)

The procedure was based on the procedure used for synthesizing P2.[23] P2 (100 μg), pre-dissolved in an appropriate reaction solvent (100 μL), was added to the reaction v-vial containing sodium [131I]iodide (nominally 37 kBq). The vial was capped and the radioactivity measured. Reaction vials that required heating were placed on a heating block (50 or 80 °C). Progress of reactions was monitored using radioTLC and co-chromatography with authentic reference standards. Reaction times, temperatures and product yields for exchange radiolabeling are given in Table 2. In reactions where pivalic acid was used, a solution of P2 (100 μg) in acetonitrile (100 μL) was added to pivalic acid (3.5 mg), the solution was gently swirled and then transferred to a reactivial containing [131I]iodide.

4.3. Cartridge-Based Purification

Once the labeling process was complete, the reaction vial was cooled in an ice-bath. Acetonitrile (10 μL) was added to the reaction vial, the vial was gently swirled to dissolve the mixture and the contents were diluted with additional SWFI (10 mL) and then the entire solution was withdrawn into a 20 mL syringe. After removing the syringe needle, the syringe barrel was attached to a Waters alumina cartridge (preconditioned by USP-grade ethanol [10 mL], followed by sterile water [10 mL]) fitted with a filter (Millex GS, Millipore, Cork, Ireland) and needle assembly that was connected to a vented 20 mL sterile product vial. Contents of the needle were slowly pushed through the cartridge to recover the purified products.

5. Conclusions

Two approaches to radiolabel I-EOE-TPZ are reported. Both methods, isotope exchange and nucleophilic substitution, produce two compounds of interest, [131I]I-EOE-TPZ and [131I]I-EOE-TPZMO, their relative proportions being dependent on reaction conditions. [131I]I-EOE-TPZMO was obtained almost exclusively in high yield from P2 via isotope radioiodination in ACN and pivalic acid after 30 min at 50 °C. Whereas the highest yield of [131I]I-EOE-TPZ was obtained from P1 via halogen isotope exchange radioiodination in ACN and no pivalic acid after 60 min at 80 °C. A simple solid phase extraction process, a methodology that is preferred in clinical settings, was developed and used to purify and isolate [^{131}I]I-EOE-TPZ in 45%–60% radiochemical yield and >97% purity.

This is the first report of developing bioreductively-activated, radiohalogenated BTDO and BTMO molecules for assessing focal hypoxia. Preclinical evaluations of these radiotracers are in progress in animal models of tumor hypoxia.

Author Contributions: Conceptualization, P.K. and L.W.; Formal analysis, L.W., H.E. and P.K.; Funding acquisition, P.K.; Methodology, H.E. and F.A.; Supervision, P.K.; Validation, F.A.; Writing—original draft, H.E.; Writing—review & editing, L.W., P.K. and H.E.

Acknowledgments: The authors acknowledge Alberta Innovates for a CRIO Program grant (award #2012164) (PK). The Edmonton Radiopharmacy Center is also sincerely thanked for generously providing [^{131}I]iodide, radioiodination supplies, and access to their manufacturing facility.

References

1.   Vaupel, P.; Mayer, A. Hypoxia in cancer: Significance and impact on clinical outcome. *Cancer Metast. Rev.* **2007**, *26*, 225–239. [CrossRef] [PubMed]

2.   Lee, C.T.; Boss, M.K.; Dewhirst, M.W. Imaging tumor hypoxia to advance radiation oncology. *Antioxid. Redox Signal.* **2014**, *21*, 313–337. [CrossRef] [PubMed]

3.   Challapalli, A.; Carroll, L.; Aboagye, E.O. Molecular mechanisms of hypoxia in cancer. *Clin. Transl. Imaging* **2017**, *5*, 225–253. [CrossRef] [PubMed]

4.   Kim, J.Y.; Lee, J.Y. Targeting tumor adaption to chronic hypoxia: Implications for drug resistance, and how it can be overcome. *Int. J. Mol. Sci.* **2017**, *18*, 1854.

5.   Fleming, I.N.; Manavaki, R.; Blower, P.J.; West, C.; Williams, K.J.; Harris, A.L.; Domarkas, J.; Lord, S.; Baldry, C.; Gilbert, F.J. Imaging tumor hypoxia with positron emission tomography. *Br. J. Cancer* **2015**, *112*, 238–250. [CrossRef] [PubMed]

6.   Wilson, W.R.W.; Hay, M.P.M. Targeting hypoxia in cancer therapy. *Nat. Rev. Cancer* **2011**, *11*, 393–410. [CrossRef] [PubMed]

7.   Epel, B.; Halpern, H.J. In Vivo pO2 Imaging of tumors: Oxymetry with very low-frequency electron paramagnetic resonance. *Methods Enzymol.* **2015**, *564*, 501–527. [PubMed]

8.   Bernsen, M.R.; Kooiman, K.; Segbers, M.; van Leeuwen, F.W.; de Jong, M. Biomarkers in preclinical cancer imaging. *Eur. J. Nucl. Med. Mol. Imaging* **2015**, *42*, 579–596. [CrossRef] [PubMed]

9.   Martelli, C.; Lo Dico, A.; Diceglie, C.; Lucignani, G.; Ottobrini, L. Optical imaging probes in oncology. *Oncotarget* **2016**, *7*, 48753–48787. [CrossRef] [PubMed]

10.   Winfield, J.M.; Payne, G.S.; Weller, A.; deSouza, N.M. DCE-MRI, DW-MRI, and MRS in cancer: Challenges and advantages of implementing qualitative and quantitative multi-parametric imaging in the clinic. *Top. Magn. Reson. Imaging* **2016**, *25*, 245–254. [CrossRef]

11.   Cabral, P.; Cerecetto, H. Radiopharmaceuticals in tumor hypoxia imaging: A review focused on medicinal chemistry aspects. *Anticancer Agents Med. Chem.* **2017**, *17*, 318–332. [CrossRef] [PubMed]

12.   Kumar, P.; Bacchu, V.; Wiebe, L.I. The chemistry and radiochemistry of hypoxia-specific, radiohalogenated nitroaromatic imaging probes. *Semin. Nucl. Med.* **2015**, *45*, 122–135. [CrossRef] [PubMed]

13.   Ricardo, C.L.; Kumar, P.; Wiebe, L.I. Bifunctional metal-nitroimidazole complexes for hypoxia theranosis in cancer. *J. Diagn. Imaging Ther.* **2015**, *2*, 103–158. [CrossRef]

14.   Brown, J.M. SR 4233 (Tirapazamine): A new anticancer drug exploiting hypoxia in solid tumors. *Br. J. Cancer* **1993**, *67*, 1163–1170. [CrossRef] [PubMed]

15.   Robbins, R.F.; Schofield, K. Polyazabicyclic compounds. Part II. Further derivatives of benzo-1:2:4-triazine. *J. Chem. Soc.* **1957**. [CrossRef]

16.   Mason, J.C.; Tennant, G. Heterocyclic *N*-oxides. Part VI. Synthesis and nuclear magnetic resonance spectra of 3-aminobenzo-1,2,4-triazines and their mono- and di-*N*-oxides. *J. Chem. Soc. B* **1970**, 911–916. [CrossRef]

17. Zeman, E.M.; Brown, J.M.; Lemmon, M.J.; Hirst, V.K.; Lee, W.W. SR 4233: A new bioreductive agent with high selective toxicity for hypoxic mammalian cells. *Int. J. Radiat. Oncol. Biol. Phys.* **1986**, *12*, 1239–1242. [CrossRef]

18. Zeman, E.M.; Hirst, V.K.; Lemmon, M.J.; Brown, J.M. Enhancement of radiation-induced tumor cell killing by the hypoxic cell toxin SR 4233. *Radiother. Oncol.* **1988**, *12*, 209–218. [CrossRef]

19. Chopra, S.; Koolpe, G.A.; Tambo-Ong, A.A.; Matsuyama, K.N.; Ryan, K.J.; Tran, T.B.; Doppalapudi, R.S.; Riccio, E.S.; Iyer, L.V.; Green, C.E.; et al. Discovery and optimization of benzotriazine di-N-oxides targeting replicating and nonreplicating *Mycobacterium tuberculosis*. *J. Med. Chem.* **2012**, *55*, 6047–6060. [CrossRef]

20. Xia, Q.; Zhang, L.; Zhang, J.; Sheng, R.; Yang, B.; He, Q.; Hu, Y. Synthesis, hypoxia-selective cytotoxicity of new 3-amino-1,2,4-benzotriazine-1,4-dioxide derivatives. *Eur. J. Med. Chem.* **2011**, *46*, 919–926. [CrossRef]

21. Hay, M.P.; Hicks, K.O.; Pchalek, K.; Lee, H.H.; Blaser, A.; Pruijn, F.B.; Anderson, A.F.; Shinde, S.S.; Wilson, W.R.; Denny, W.A. Tricyclic [1,2,4]Triazine 1,4-Dioxides as hypoxia selective cytotoxins. *J. Med. Chem.* **2008**, *51*, 6853–6865. [CrossRef] [PubMed]

22. Hay, M.P.; Gamage, S.A.; Kovacs, M.S.; Pruijn, F.B.; Anderson, R.F.; Patterson, A.V.; Wilson, W.R.; Brown, M.; Denny, W.A. Structure—activity relationships of 1,2,4-benzotriazine 1,4-dioxides as hypoxia-selective analogues of tirapazamine. *J. Med. Chem.* **2003**, *46*, 169–182. [CrossRef] [PubMed]

23. Elsaidi, H.R.H.; Yang, X.-H.; Ahmadi, F.; Weinfeld, M.; Wiebe, L.I.; Kumar, P. Putative electron-affinic radiosensitizers and markers of hypoxic tissue: Synthesis and preliminary in vitro biological characterization of C3-amino-substituted benzotriazine dioxides. *Eur. J. Med. Chem.* **2018**. submitted.

24. Yin, J.; Glaser, R.; Gates, K.S. On the reaction mechanism of tirapazamine reduction chemistry: Unimolecular N–OH homolysis, stepwise dehydration, or triazene ring-opening. *Chem. Res. Toxicol.* **2012**, *25*, 634–645. [CrossRef] [PubMed]

25. Anderson, R.F.; Shinde, S.S.; Hay, M.P.; Gamage, S.A.; Denny, W.A. Activation of 3-amino-1,2,4-benzotriazine 1,4-dioxide antitumor agents to oxidizing species following their one-electron reduction. *J. Am. Chem. Soc.* **2003**, *125*, 748–756. [CrossRef]

26. Siim, B.G.; Pruijn, F.B.; Sturman, J.R.; Hogg, A.; Hay, M.P.; Brown, J.M.; Wilson, W.R. Selective potentiation of the hypoxic cytotoxicity of tirapazamine by its 1-N-oxide metabolite SR 4317. *Cancer Res.* **2004**, *64*, 736–742. [CrossRef]

27. Yoo, B.W.; Park, M.C. Mild and efficient deoxygenation of amine-N-oxides with MoCl$_5$/NaI system. *Synth. Commun.* **2008**, *38*, 1646–1650. [CrossRef]

28. Revuelta, J.; Cicchi, S.; Brandi, A. Samarium(II) iodide reduction of isoxazolidines. *Tetrahedron Lett.* **2004**, *45*, 8375–8377. [CrossRef]

29. Singh, D.; Singh, V.; Rai, B.P. An efficient method for the reduction of cephalosporin sulfoxide. *Asian J. Chem.* **2007**, *19*, 5787–5789.

30. Das, A.K.; Srivastav, M.; Layek, R.K.; Uddin, M.E.; Jung, D.; Kim, N.H.; Lee, J.H. Iodide-mediated room temperature reduction of graphene oxide: A rapid chemical route for the synthesis of a bifunctional electrocatalyst. *J. Mater. Chem. A* **2014**, *2*, 1332–1340. [CrossRef]

31. Zhang, Y.; Lin, R. Some deoxygenation and reduction reactions with samarium diiodide. *Synth. Commun.* **1987**, *17*, 329–332. [CrossRef]

32. Weichert, J.P.; Van Dort, M.E.; Groziak, M.P.; Counsell, R.E. Radioiodination via isotope exchange in pivalic acid. *Int. J. Rad. Appl. Instrum. A* **1986**, *37*, 907–913. [CrossRef]

15

Localization of ^{99m}Tc-GRP Analogs in GRPR-Expressing Tumors: Effects of Peptide Length and Neprilysin Inhibition on Biological Responses

Aikaterini Kaloudi [1], Emmanouil Lymperis [1], Panagiotis Kanellopoulos [1], Beatrice Waser [2]●, Marion de Jong [3], Eric P. Krenning [4], Jean Claude Reubi [2], Berthold A. Nock [1]● and Theodosia Maina [1,*]●

[1] Molecular Radiopharmacy, INRASTES, NCSR "Demokritos", 15310 Athens, Greece; katerinakaloudi@yahoo.gr (A.K.); mlymperis@hotmail.com (E.L.); kanelospan@gmail.com (P.K.); nock_berthold.a@hotmail.com (B.A.N.)

[2] Cell Biology and Experimental Cancer Research, Institute of Pathology, University of Berne, CH-3010 Berne, Switzerland; waserpatho@rubigen.ch (B.W.); jean.reubi@pathology.unibe.ch (J.C.R.)

[3] Department of Radiology & Nuclear Medicine Erasmus MC, 3015 CN Rotterdam, The Netherlands; m.hendriks-dejong@erasmusmc.nl

[4] Cytrotron Rotterdam BV, Erasmus MC, 3015 CN Rotterdam, The Netherlands; erickrenning@gmail.com

*   Correspondence: maina_thea@hotmail.com

Abstract: The overexpression of gastrin-releasing peptide receptors (GRPRs) in frequently occurring human tumors has provided the opportunity to use bombesin (BBN) analogs as radionuclide carriers to cancer sites for diagnostic and therapeutic purposes. We have been alternatively exploring human GRP motifs of higher GRPR selectivity compared to frog BBN sequences aiming to improve pharmacokinetic profiles. In the present study, we compared two differently truncated human endogenous GRP motifs: GRP(14–27) and GRP(18–27). An acyclic tetraamine was coupled at the N-terminus to allow for stable binding of the SPECT radionuclide ^{99m}Tc. Their biological profiles were compared in PC-3 cells and in mice without or with coinjection of phosphoramidon (PA) to induce transient neprilysin (NEP) inhibition in vivo. The two ^{99m}Tc-N$_4$-GRP(14/18–27) radioligands displayed similar biological behavior in mice. Coinjection of PA exerted a profound effect on in vivo stability and translated into notably improved radiolabel localization in PC-3 experimental tumors. Hence, this study has shown that promising ^{99m}Tc-radiotracers for SPECT imaging may indeed derive from human GRP sequences. Radiotracer bioavailability was found to be of major significance. It could be improved during in situ NEP inhibition resulting in drastically enhanced uptake in GRPR-expressing lesions.

Keywords: bombesin; gastrin-releasing peptide; gastrin-releasing peptide receptor; tumor targeting; ^{99m}Tc-radioligand; metabolic stability; neprilysin-inhibition; phosphoramidon

1. Introduction

Gastrin-releasing peptide receptors (GRPRs) are overexpressed in several human malignancies such as prostate cancer, mammary carcinoma, and lung cancer [1–10]. Consequently, they have attracted considerable attention as potential biomolecular targets for diagnosis and therapy with radionuclide carriers directed to GRPR-positive cancer lesions [11,12]. Originally, the frog tetradecapeptide bombesin (BBN, Pyr-Gln-Arg-Tyr-Gly-Asn-Gln-Trp-Ala-Val-Gly-His-Leu-Met-NH$_2$) and its truncated C-terminal octapeptide fragment BBN(7–14) have served as motifs for the development of GRPR-targeting radioligands. However, BBN-like analogs bind with comparable affinity not only to GRPR (BB$_2$R), but also to the neuromedin B (NMBR, BB$_1$R), another member of the three mammalian bombesin receptor subtypes [1,2]. The above two subtypes are pharmacologically distinguished by their selectivity for different endogenous human homologs of amphibian BBN. Thus, the 27-mer GRP (H-Val-Pro-Leu-Pro-Ala-Gly-Gly-Gly-Thr-Val-Leu-Thr-Lys-Met-Tyr-Pro-Arg-Gly-Asn-His-Trp-Ala-Val-Gly-His-Leu-Met-NH$_2$), the 14-mer GRP(14–27), and the C-terminal decapeptide GRP(18–27) fragments strongly bind to the GRPR, whereas neuromedin B (NMB, H-Gly-Asn-Leu-Trp-Ala-Thr-Gly-His-Phe-Met-NH$_2$) exhibits high affinity for the NMBR [13]. The two GRPR and NMBR subtypes are physiologically expressed in the human brain and the gut, especially in stomach, pancreas, and gastrointestinal tract, and they are also implicated in cancer [14–16]. It is reasonable to assume, that radiolabeled BBN agonists of poor GRPR selectivity will show increased levels of background radioactivity by virtue of their binding to both GRPR and NMBR populations distributed in the body, especially in the abdomen. Furthermore, additive GRPR- and NMBR-mediated effects in the gastrointestinal tract, such as abdominal smooth muscle contraction and stimulation of gastrointestinal hormone secretion, are to be expected after intravenous injection of BBN-like agonist radioligands [17–22].

In contrast to amphibian BBN-like motifs, the respective human homologs have surprisingly remained unexploited as radionuclide carriers for targeting GRPR-positive cancer [13]. Motivated by this gap in the inventory of GRPR-directed radioligands we have expanded our research efforts to native human GRP sequences in order to explore their applicability in GRPR-targeted tumor diagnosis and therapy. First, we introduced a small library of tetraamine derivatized GRP(18–27) analogs labeled with the SPECT radionuclide ^{99m}Tc [23,24]. Compared to previously reported ^{99m}Tc-radiopeptides, which are based on the full-length BBN or its truncated BBN(7–14) octapeptide fragment [25], the ^{99m}Tc-N$_4$-GRP(18–27) showed high GRPR selectivity and superior in vivo characteristics in tumor-bearing mice, such as faster renal clearance and improved tumor to background ratios. On the other hand, single or double amino acid substitutions in the decapeptide backbone exerted pronounced effects on several biological properties, eventually affecting tumor targeting capabilities and pharmacokinetics. In a following study, a series of differently truncated GRP sequences were coupled to the universal chelator DOTA (1,4,7,10- tetraazacyclododecane-1,4,7,10-tetraacetic acid) and labeled with ^{111}In. Receptor affinity, internalization efficiency and tumor uptake of these analogs were favored both by longer peptide chain and by the presence of basic amino acids Lys^{13} and Arg^{17} in the native GRP sequence [26].

Following this line of research, we herein introduced ^{99m}Tc-N$_4$-GRP(14–27) and compared its biological profile in PC-3 cells and mice models with ^{99m}Tc-N$_4$-GRP(18–27) (Figure 1). It should be noted that basic positions Lys^{13} and Arg^{17} in the native GRP sequence are now occupied by the positively charged N$_4^{+x}$/[^{99m}Tc(O)$_2$(N$_4$)]$^{+1}$-moiety and not by the negatively charged DOTA. This arrangement allows for comparisons with the DOTA-derivatized analogs and further studying the influence of positive/negative charges in 13 and 17 positions of the GRP chain [26]. Next, the selectivity of N$_4$-GRP(14–27) for each of the three mammalian bombesin receptor subtypes was investigated applying receptor autoradiography in human excised biopsy samples, expressing one of the GRPR, NMBR, and bombesin subtype 3 (BB$_3$R) receptors. Finally, the impact of in vivo stability of ^{99m}Tc-N$_4$-GRP(14–27) and ^{99m}Tc-N$_4$-GRP(18–27) on tumor targeting and pharmacokinetics was compared in mice. The role of neprilysin (NEP) [27] on the in vivo degradation of the two human GRP-based sequences was monitored by HPLC analysis of blood samples collected without or with coinjection of the NEP-inhibitor phosphoramidon (PA) [28,29], as previously described for BBN-like radioligands [30–34]. The enhancement of radiotracer localization in experimental GRPR-positive PC-3 tumors in mice during transient NEP inhibition induced by PA was assessed.

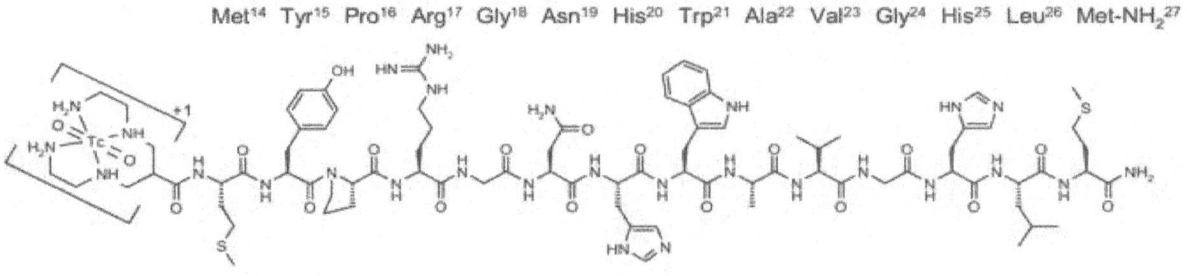

Met¹⁴ Tyr¹⁵ Pro¹⁶ Arg¹⁷ Gly¹⁸ Asn¹⁹ His²⁰ Trp²¹ Ala²² Val²³ Gly²⁴ His²⁵ Leu²⁶ Met-NH₂²⁷

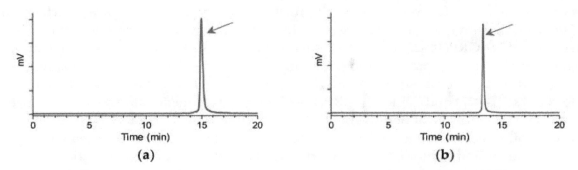

(a)

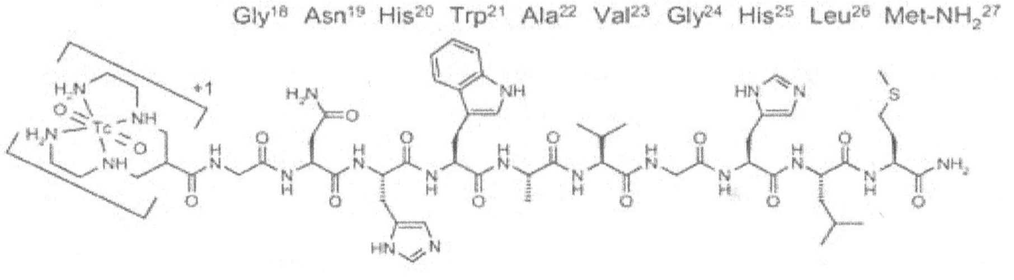

Gly¹⁸ Asn¹⁹ His²⁰ Trp²¹ Ala²² Val²³ Gly²⁴ His²⁵ Leu²⁶ Met-NH₂²⁷

(b)

Figure 1. Chemical structure of (**a**) ^{99m}Tc-N$_4$-GRP(14–27) (red) and (**b**) ^{99m}Tc-N$_4$-GRP(18–27) (blue).

2. Results

2.1. Peptides and Radioligands

The bifunctional acyclic tetraamine chelator (6-(carboxy)-1,4,8,11-tetraazaundecane) was covalently coupled by its carboxy functionality at the N-terminal Met^{14} of GRP(14–27) or the Gly^{18} of GRP(18–27) via an amide bond [24], generating two different length GRP analogs amenable for labeling with the preeminent SPECT radionuclide ^{99m}Tc. Labeling was typically proceeded by a brief incubation with ^{99m}TcO$_4^-$ generator eluate, SnCl$_2$ as reducing agent, and citrate anions as transfer ligand in alkaline pH at ambient temperature at molar activities of 20 to 40 MBq ^{99m}Tc/nmol peptide. Quality control of the radiolabeled products combined HPLC and ITLC analysis. The total radiochemical impurities, comprising ^{99m}TcO$_4^-$, [^{99m}Tc] citrate, and ^{99m}TcO$_2 \times$ H$_2$O, did not exceed 2%, while a single radiopeptide species was detected by RP-HPLC. In view of labeling yields >98% and >99% radiochemical purity of the resultant ^{99m}Tc-N$_4$-GRP(14–27) and ^{99m}Tc-N$_4$-GRP(18–27), the radioligands were used without further purification in all subsequent experiments. Representative radiochromatograms of HPLC analysis of ^{99m}Tc-N$_4$-GRP(14–27) and ^{99m}Tc-N$_4$-GRP(18–27) are included in Figure 2a,b, respectively.

(a)   **(b)**

Figure 2. Representative radiochromatograms of the radiolabeling reaction mixture of (**a**) ^{99m}Tc-N$_4$-GRP(14–27) (red) and (**b**) ^{99m}Tc-N$_4$-GRP(18–27) (blue), confirming the quantitative formation of high purity radioligands at t_R = 14.9 min and t_R = 13.3 min, respectively (HPLC system 1).

2.2. In Vitro Assays

2.2.1. Receptor Autoradiography in Human Tumor Samples

The selective affinities of N_4-GRP(14–27) for each of the three bombesin receptor subtypes found in mammals were studied during in vitro competition binding assays against the universal radioligand ^{125}I-[DTyr^6,βAla^{11},Phe^{13},Nle^{14}]BBN(6–14) [6]. Receptor autoradiography was applied in cryostat sections of well characterized human cancers, preferentially expressing one of the subtypes. As summarized in Table 1, N_4-GRP(14–27) showed high affinity for the GRPR expressed in resected prostate carcinoma specimens (IC$_{50}$ = 4.2 ± 1.0 nM, n = 3, vs. IC$_{50}$ = 2.4 ± 1.0 nM, n = 3 for N_4-GRP(18–27) [23]), very low affinity for NMBR present in ileal carcinoid biopsy samples (IC$_{50}$ = 72 ± 7.6 nM, n = 3, vs. IC$_{50}$ = 106 ± 13 nM; n = 2 for N_4-GRP(18–27) [23]), and no affinity for the BB$_3$R expressed in bronchial carcinoid samples (IC$_{50}$ > 1000 nM, n = 3, identical to N_4-GRP(18–27) [23]). Thus, N_4-GRP(14–27) similarly to N_4-GRP(18–27), displayed good selectivity for the GRPR. Hence, the GRP-based analogs turned out to be more GRPR-preferring compared to BBN-based radioligands, like Demobesin 3 (N_4-[Pro^1,Tyr^4]BBN) [25] or [DTyr^6,βAla^{11},Phe^{13},Nle^{14}]BBN(6–14) (Table 1).

Table 1. Affinities for the three human bombesin receptor subtypes.

Peptide Conjugate	IC$_{50}$s in nM		
	GRPR [1]	NMBR [2]	BB$_3$R [3]
Universal ligand [4]	1.5 ± 0.1 (3)	1.5 ± 0.2 (3)	3.5 ± 0.7 (3)
N_4-GRP(14–27)	4.2 ± 1.0 (3)	72 ± 7.6 (3)	>1000 (3)
N_4-GRP(18–27)	2.4 ± 1.0 (3)	106 ± 13 (2)	>1000 (3)
Demobesin 3	0.5 (2)	1.6 (2)	>100 (3)

The data represents the mean (±SEM; n = 3) for the cold universal ligand and for the two N_4-GRP(14/18–27) analogs and the mean (n = 2) for Demobesin 3. ^{125}I[DTyr^6,βAla^{11}, Phe^{13},Nle^{14}]BBN(6–14) was used as radioligand in all experiments; [1] expressed in human prostate cancer, [2] in human ileal carcinoids and [3] in human lung carcinoids, [4][DTyr^6,βAla^{11},Phe^{13},Nle^{14}]BBN(6–14) was used as cold universal ligand.

2.2.2. Binding Affinity for the Human GRPR

As shown in Figure 3a, N_4-GRP(14–27) and N_4-GRP(18–27) as well as the respective GRP(14–27) and GRP(18–27) parent peptide references displaced [^{125}I-Tyr^4]BBN from GRPR-sites on PC-3 cell membranes in a monophasic and dose-dependent manner. The respective half-maximal inhibitory concentration (IC$_{50}$) values differed, yielding the following rank of decreasing receptor affinity: N_4-GRP(14–27) (IC$_{50}$ 0.32 ± 0.03 nM) > GRP(14–27) (IC$_{50}$ 0.45 ± 0.02 nM) > N_4-GRP(18–27) (IC$_{50}$ 0.63 ± 0.06 nM) > GRP(18–27) (IC$_{50}$ 1.66 ± 0.20 nM). We observe that the longer-chain peptides consistently showed higher binding affinity to GRPR than their shorter chain counterparts. Moreover, coupling of the positively charged acyclic tetraamine unit in the N-terminus of parent GRP(14/18–27) references improved the affinity of resulting analogs to the GRPR, as previously reported for similarly modified peptide analogs [35].

2.2.3. Internalization of ^{99m}Tc-N_4-GRP(14–27) and ^{99m}Tc-N_4-GRP(18–27) in PC-3 Cells

During incubation at 37 °C in PC-3 cells, both ^{99m}Tc-N_4-GRP(14–27) and ^{99m}Tc-N_4-GRP(18–27) were taken up by the cells via a GRPR-mediated process, as demonstrated by the lack of internalization observed in the presence of excess [Tyr^4]BBN. In both cases the bulk of cell-associated radioactivity was found in the cells with ^{99m}Tc-N_4-GRP(14–27) internalizing much faster in PC-3 cells compared to ^{99m}Tc-N_4-GRP(18–27) at all time intervals (Figure 3b). For example, at 1 h, 12.7 ± 0.7% of total added ^{99m}Tc-N_4-GRP(14–27) specifically internalized in the cells vs. 5.0 ± 0.3% of ^{99m}Tc-N_4-GRP(18–27), whereas at 2 h these values increased to 19.5 ± 1.4% and 6.9 ± 1.5%, respectively.

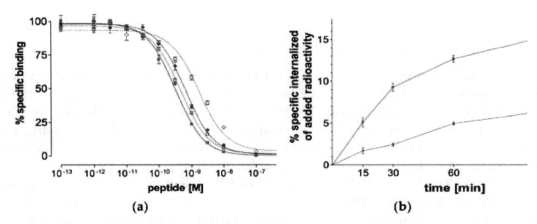

(a)   (b)

Figure 3. (a) [^{125}I-Tyr^4]BBN displacement curves from gastrin-releasing peptide receptor (GRPR)-sites on PC-3 cells after 1-h incubation at 22 °C by N$_4$-GRP(14–27) (red solid line—IC$_{50}$ 0.32±0.03 nM), GRP(14–27) (red dashed line—IC$_{50}$ 0.45 ± 0.02 nM), N$_4$-GRP(18–27) (blue solid line—IC$_{50}$ 0.63±0.06 nM) and GRP(18–27) (blue dashed line—IC$_{50}$ 1.66 ± 0.20 nM). (b) GRPR-specific internalization of ^{99m}Tc-N$_4$-GRP(14–27) (red solid line) and ^{99m}Tc-N$_4$-GRP(18–27) (blue solid line) in PC-3 cells during incubation at 37 °C at 15, 30, 60, and 120 min. Results represent average of cell internalized activity ± sd, n = 3; data is corrected for nonspecific internalization in the presence of 1 μM [Tyr^4]BBN.

2.3. In Vivo Comparison of ^{99m}Tc-N$_4$-GRP(14–27) and ^{99m}Tc-N$_4$-GRP(18–27)

2.3.1. Stability of ^{99m}Tc-N$_4$-GRP(14–27) and ^{99m}Tc-N$_4$-GRP(18–27) in Mice

The two ^{99m}Tc-N$_4$-GRP(14–27) and ^{99m}Tc-N$_4$-GRP(18–27) radiotracers exhibited distinct resistance to degrading proteases after injection in mice. As revealed by HPLC analysis of blood samples collected at 5 min postinjection (pi), ^{99m}Tc-N$_4$-GRP(14–27) was found less stable (20.1 ± 4.5% intact, n = 3) than the shorter chain ^{99m}Tc-N$_4$-GRP(18–27) (31.0 ± 0.9% intact, n = 3). Representative radiochromatograms are shown in Figure 4a,b, respectively.

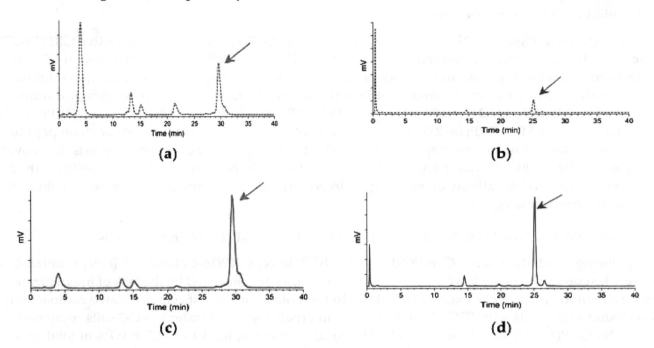

Figure 4. Representative radiochromatograms of HPLC analysis of mouse blood samples collected 5 min pi of (a) ^{99m}Tc-N$_4$-GRP(14–27) (25.2% intact radiotracer; red dashed line) or (b) ^{99m}Tc-N$_4$-GRP(18–27) (31.8% intact radiotracer; blue dashed line) without PA coinjection; the respective radiochromatograms of

(c) ^{99m}Tc-N$_4$-GRP(14–27) (63.1% intact radiotracer; t_R = 29.6 min; red solid line) or (d) ^{99m}Tc-N$_4$-GRP(18–27) (68.1% intact radiotracer; t_R = 25.1 min; blue solid line) with PA coinjection are also included; the t_R of parent radiopeptide was determined by coinjection with the respective radioligand sample in the column (HPLC system 2) and is indicated here by the arrow.

It should be noted that coinjection of the NEP-inhibitor PA remarkably enhanced the in vivo stability of ^{99m}Tc-N$_4$-GRP(14–27) (66.5 ± 4.8% intact, n = 3) and ^{99m}Tc-N$_4$-GRP(18–27) (70.8 ± 5.4% intact, n = 3) in the circulation, revealing NEP as a major degrading protease for both radiotracers in mice. Representative radiochromatograms are included in Figure 4c,d, respectively.

2.3.2. Biodistribution in PC-3 Xenograft-Bearing Mice

The biodistribution of ^{99m}Tc-N$_4$-GRP(14–27) and ^{99m}Tc-N$_4$-GRP(18–27) was studied in severe combined immune deficiency (SCID) mice bearing human PC-3 xenografts expressing the human GRPR. Subcutaneous tumors of suitable size developed in the flanks of mice about four weeks after inoculation of a suspension of prostate adenocarcinoma PC-3 cells and biodistribution was conducted.

Cumulative biodistribution results for ^{99m}Tc-N$_4$-GRP(14–27) at the 1-, 4-, and 24-h pi intervals are summarized in Table 2, and are expressed as mean % injected dose per gram (%ID/g) values ± sd, n = 4. The radiotracer washed rapidly from the blood and the background tissues predominantly via the kidneys and the urinary system. High uptake was observed in the PC-3 tumor at 1-h pi (10.20 ± 0.72%ID/g) that remained at comparably high levels at 4-h pi (8.41 ± 4.16%ID/g; p > 0.05), declining by ~50% at 24-h pi (4.50 ± 0.69%ID/g). Tumor uptake at 4-h pi was significantly lower in the animals treated with excess [Tyr^4]BBN (0.62 ± 0.24%ID/g; p < 0.001), suggestive of a GRPR-mediated process. Likewise, ^{99m}Tc-N$_4$-GRP(14–27) highly localized in the GRPR-rich mouse pancreas via a GRPR-specific process, as demonstrated by the lack of pancreatic uptake during GRPR-blockade by coinjection of excess [Tyr^4]BBN (35.24 ± 4.70%ID/g vs. 0.83 ± 0.24%ID/g in block; p < 0.001).

Table 2. Biodistribution data for ^{99m}Tc-N$_4$-GRP(14–27), expressed as %ID/g mean ± sd, n = 4, in PC-3 xenograft-bearing SCID mice at 1-h, 4-h block, 4-h, and 24-h pi.

Tissue	1 h [1]	4 h [1]	24 h [1]	4 h block [2]
Blood	1.54 ± 0.17	0.10 ± 0.03	0.07 ± 0.01	0.08 ± 0.02
Liver	5.02 ± 0.46	3.75 ± 1.11	3.23 ± 0.78	6.12 ± 2.89
Heart	0.70 ± 0.07	0.11 ± 0.04	0.07 ± 0.01	0.28 ± 0.13
Kidneys	14.82 ± 2.22	4.83 ± 2.12	3.10 ± 0.73	4.85 ± 2.66
Stomach	1.02 ± 0.29	1.42 ± 0.93	0.78 ± 0.33	0.43 ± 0.18
Intestines	7.21 ± 0.52	7.61 ± 2.23	1.73 ± 0.23	1.45 ± 0.44
Muscle	0.29 ± 0.02	0.03 ± 0.01	0.06 ± 0.01	0.05 ± 0.02
Lungs	1.96 ± 0.33	0.49 ± 0.30	0.18 ± 0.04	0.65 ± 0.22
Pancreas	37.85 ± 1.95	35.24 ± 4.70	13.41 ± 0.77	0.83 ± 0.24
Tumor	10.20 ± 0.72	8.41 ± 4.16	4.50 ± 0.69	0.62 ± 0.24

[1] Animal groups injected with 180–370 kBq/10 pmol peptide; [2] block mice group coinjected with 40 nmol [Tyr^4] BBN for in vivo GRPR blockade.

Comparative biodistribution results for ^{99m}Tc-N$_4$-GRP(14–27) and ^{99m}Tc-N$_4$-GRP(18–27) at the 4-h pi interval are included in Table 3. Data from additional 4-h pi animal groups coinjected with the NEP-inhibitor PA (300 µg) is also included in the Table. The radiotracers displayed similar tissue distribution patterns. The observed higher tumor and pancreatic uptake of ^{99m}Tc-N$_4$-GRP(14–27) did not however differ significantly to that of ^{99m}Tc-N$_4$-GRP(18–27) (p > 0.05) [24]. Treatment with PA induced a drastic increase in tumor values for both radiotracers with ^{99m}Tc-N$_4$-GRP(14–27) showing superior tumor values than the shorter chain ^{99m}Tc-N$_4$-GRP(18–27) (38.19 ± 4.79%ID/g vs. 28.37 ± 8.05%ID/g, respectively; p < 0.01). Pancreatic values increased by >3-fold for both radiotracers as well. Thus, in agreement with previous studies on BBN-based analogs [31–34], NEP inhibition likewise resulted in significant stabilization of GRP(14/18–27)-based radioligands in peripheral mouse blood and notable improvement of localization in GRPR-expressing lesions in mice.

Table 3. Comparative biodistribution data for ^{99m}Tc-N$_4$-GRP(14–27) and ^{99m}Tc-N$_4$-GRP(18–27), expressed as %ID/g mean $\pm$ sd, n = 4, in PC-3 xenograft-bearing SCID mice at 4-h pi (controls) and 4-h pi after coinjection of PA.

Tissue	^{99m}Tc-N$_4$-GRP(14–27)		^{99m}Tc-N$_4$-GRP(18–27)	
	4 h [1]	4 h PA [1,2]	4 h[1]	4 h PA [1,2]
Blood	0.10 ± 0.03	0.23 ± 0.08	0.13 ± 0.04	0.21 ± 0.04
Liver	3.75 ± 1.11	4.99 ± 1.53	1.02 ± 0.17	2.13 ± 0.37
Heart	0.11 ± 0.04	0.89 ± 0.06	0.14 ± 0.10	0.47 ± 0.27
Kidneys	4.83 ± 2.12	11.68 ± 1.61	6.01 ± 1.38	7.66 ± 1.39
Stomach	1.42 ± 0.93	3.82 ± 1.10	1.12 ± 0.75	4.02 ± 0.66
Intestines	7.61 ± 2.23	21.35 ± 1.68	7.28 ± 0.60	16.23 ± 3.90
Muscle	0.03 ± 0.01	0.06 ± 0.02	0.03 ± 0.01	0.06 ± 0.01
Lungs	0.49 ± 0.30	1.06 ± 0.19	0.28 ± 0.09	0.84 ± 0.26
Pancreas	35.24 ± 4.70	110.32 ± 8.76	32.18 ± 5.91	95.39 ± 20.34
Tumor	8.41 ± 4.16	38.19 ± 4.79	7.08 ± 1.29	28.37 ± 8.05

[1] Animal groups injected with 180–370 kBq/10 pmol peptide; [2] PA mice groups with animals coinjected with 300 μg PA to in situ inhibit NEP.

3. Discussion

A considerable number of radiolabeled analogs of frog BBN have been developed for potential application in the diagnosis and therapy of GRPR-expressing tumors in *Homo sapiens* [11,12]. This pursuit is based on the overexpression of GRPRs on the surface of malignant cells serving as easily accessible biomolecular targets on cancer lesions [3–10]. Joining this effort, we have previously introduced a series of BBN-like analogs, generated by covalently coupling of an acyclic tetraamine at the N-terminus, Demobesin 3–6 [25]. Like native BBN, these peptide ligands displayed indistinguishable binding affinities for the human bombesin receptor subtypes GRPR and NMBR, but no affinity for the BB$_3$R. The respective radiotracers [^{99m}Tc] Demobesin 3–6 specifically localized in GRPR-expressing human PC-3 xenografts in mice. Moreover, one of the analogs, [^{99m}Tc] Demobesin 4, was able to visualize malignant lesions in a small number of prostate cancer patients with SPECT/CT [36].

We have recently expanded our search toward radioligands based on human endogenous GRP sequences [23,24,26]. The latter are reported for higher GRPR selectivity compared to their frog homolog BBN [13]. This approach has surprisingly remained unexplored up to now, although it offers two major advantages. First, radioactivity levels in abdominal tissues physiologically expressing both GRPR and NMBR subtypes would favorably decrease when GRPR-selective radioligands are used [14–16]. Second, injection of GRPR-selective agonists will not activate the NMBR subtype populations in the gut and is hence associated with less adverse effects [17–22]. Promising GRPR-selective radioligands based on receptor antagonists have been developed and evaluated in animals and in human, showing excellent tumor targeting and pharmacokinetic profiles [37,38]. Yet, the suitability and efficacy of noninternalizing GRPR antagonists for therapy with low-range beta, alpha, or Auger emitters of high LET has not been established thus far [39,40]. Therefore, the study of radiolabeled GRPR-selective agonists is warranted and may provide an alternative platform for the development of radioligands exhibiting new combinations of biological features particularly suited for cancer theranostics.

As a part of this effort we herein introduced two analogs of endogenous truncated fragments of human GRP carrying an acyclic tetraamine at their terminus, one based on the tetradecapeptide GRP(14–27), and the other on a shorter decapeptide GRP(18–27) chain identical to human neuromedin C (NMC) (Figure 1). As revealed during receptor autoradiography studies in excised biopsy samples of well characterized human tumors expressing each of the GRPR, NMBR, and BB$_3$R subtypes using the universal ^{125}I-[DTyr^6,βAla^{11},Phe^{13},Nle^{14}]BBN(6–14) radioligand, both N$_4$-GRP(14–27) and N$_4$-GRP(18–27) analogs showed good selectivity for the GRPR subtype (Table 1). This finding is in agreement with previous reports documenting the preference of human GRP and its C-terminal native fragments for GRPR [13]. In contrast, the tetraamine derivatized BBN-like analogs Demobesin 3–6 do not distinguish between GRPR and NMBR, instead behaving like the native frog BBN [25]. The His^{20} of GRP corresponding to Gln^7 of BBN seems to have significant impact on subtype selectivity, followed by the Met^{14}-Tyr^{13}-Pro^{12}-Arg^{11}-tetrapeptide in GRP(14–27) corresponding to the Pyr^1-Gln^2-Arg^3-Leu^4-counterpart in native BBN.

Both N$_4$-GRP(14–27) and N$_4$-GRP(18–27) analogs displayed sub-nM affinities for the GRPR during competition assays against [^{125}I-Tyr^4]BBN in PC-3 cell membranes, which were found to be increased compared to unmodified GRP(14/18–27) lead structures (Figure 3a). It is interesting to note that the presence of the positively charged N$_4$$^{+x}$-moiety at positions 13 and 17 of the native GRP chain occupy the two basic amino acids Lys^{13} and Arg^{17}. When these positions were taken up by negatively charged DOTA instead, a drastic drop in binding affinity was observed (IC50 DOTA-GRP(14–27) = 6.6 ± 0.9 nM and IC50 DOTA-GRP(18–27) = 112 ± 16 nM) [26]. In all cases, longer chain GRP(14–27) analogs consistently displayed higher GRPR-affinity compared to their C-terminal decapeptide counterparts. In agreement with this observation, the internalization rate of ^{99m}Tc-N$_4$-GRP(14–27) in PC-3 cells was clearly superior to that of ^{99m}Tc-N$_4$-GRP(18–27) (Figure 3b).

A crucial feature for efficient tumor targeting is metabolic stability that will ensure sufficient radioligand supply to tumor sites after injection in the living organism [31]. Recent studies have revealed the significance of in vivo stability assessment of BBN-like radiotracers vs. in vitro determinations in serum or tissue homogenate incubates to more accurately predict the actual protease(s) encountered by the radioligand after entering the circulation. These studies have demonstrated NEP as a major degrading protease of BBN and its radiolabeled analogs [41,42]. In a recently proposed approach, NEP-inhibitors, like PA [28,29], coinjected with the BBN-based radioligand drastically increased metabolic stability leading to notable enhancement of tumor uptake in animal models [31–34]. Following this rationale, we have tested the in vivo stability of the two ^{99m}Tc-N$_4$-GRP(14–27) and ^{99m}Tc-N$_4$-GRP(18–27) radiotracers in peripheral mouse blood collected 5 min pi by radioanalytical HPLC (Figure 4). The longer chain ^{99m}Tc-N$_4$-GRP(14–27) displayed somewhat poorer stability (20.1 ± 4.5% intact, n = 3) compared to shorter chain ^{99m}Tc-N$_4$-GRP(18–27) (31.0 ± 0.9% intact, n = 3). Thus, the presence of additional amide bonds in the longer peptide chain offered further degradation sites for attacking proteases. It is interesting to note, that coinjection of PA drastically increased the stability of both analogs in the circulation, indicating NEP as a major protease in the catabolism of GRP sequences as well.

Aiming to explore the effects of peptide chain as well as NEP inhibition on the pharmacokinetics and tumor targeting capabilities of the two tracers, we have conducted biodistribution experiments in immunosuppressed mice bearing human GRPR-expressing xenografts. Interestingly, the biodistribution patterns of the two radiotracers did not clearly differ (Table 3). Compared to the previously reported ^{111}In-DOTA analogs [26], ^{99m}Tc-N$_4$-GRP(14–27) showed higher tumor uptake. Comparable in vivo tumor targeting was obtained only by ^{111}In-DOTA-GRP(13–27), carrying basic Lys at position 13. However, kidney clearance was notably faster for the ^{99m}Tc-radiotracer (4.83 ± 2.12%/g at 4 h pi) than for the ^{111}In-DOTA-Lys^{13}-analog (46.02 ± 3.73%/g at 4 h pi) [26]. Treatment of mice with PA exerted a profound effect on the in vivo profile of both ^{99m}Tc-N$_4$-GRP(14–27) and ^{99m}Tc-N$_4$-GRP(18–27) (Table 2), is in agreement with previous findings for other BBN-like radioligands. The longer chain ^{99m}Tc-N$_4$-GRP(14–27) exhibited the highest uptake in the experimental tumor, as a combined result of higher internalization rate and pronounced in vivo stabilization induced by PA.

The present study has shown that GRP motifs of different chain length may provide new opportunities for the development of promising GRPR-selective radioligands. The latter may prove to be a useful asset in the arsenal of anti-GRPR radioactive drugs, by internalizing in cancer cells while evading binding to and activation of bombesin receptor subtypes other than the GRPR in the gut.

Furthermore, it has shown the impact of in vivo metabolic stability in maximizing tumor localization. Structural modifications in peptide lead-structures to improve the stability of radiopeptides, such as amino acid replacements, cyclization, or changes of cleavable peptide bonds, may deteriorate other important biological features, as for example receptor affinity, cell uptake, tumor targeting, and overall pharmacokinetics. On the other hand, transient in situ inhibition of NEP represents a smart method to accomplish this goal and warrants further efforts for translation in the clinic. Despite challenges related to biosafety, regulatory and financial hurdles, once established in a proof-of-principal study, this strategy is expected to boost the development and clinical application of other NEP-catabolized radioligands, considerably saving costs and resources [31–34].

4. Materials and Methods

4.1. Peptides and Reagents

The N_4-GRP(14–27) and N_4-GRP(18–27) peptide conjugates were synthesized on the solid support following a published method [24] and were provided by PiChem (Graz, Austria). The [Tyr^4]BBN (Tyr^4-bombesin, Pyr-Gln-Arg-Tyr-Gly-Asn-Gln-Trp-Ala-Val-Gly-His-Leu-Met-NH$_2$) and GRP(14–27) (H-Met-Tyr-Pro-Arg-Gly-Asn-His-Trp-Ala-Val-Gly-His-Leu-Met-NH$_2$) references were purchased from PSL GmbH (Heidelberg, Germany), whereas GRP(18–27) (H-Gly-Asn-His-Trp-Ala-Val-Gly-His-Leu-Met-NH$_2$) was provided by PeptaNova GmbH (Sandhousen, Germany). Phosphoramidon disodium dehydrate (N-(α-rhamnopyranosyloxyhydro xyphosphinyl) -L-leucyl-L-tryptophan × 2Na × 2H$_2$O; PA) was purchased from PeptaNova GmbH (Sandhousen, Germany).

Preparation and Quality Control of ^{99m}Tc-N_4-GRP(14–27) and ^{99m}Tc-N_4-GRP(18–27)

Lyophilized N_4-GRP(14–27) and N_4-GRP(18–27) were dissolved in bidistilled water to a final 1 mM concentration and bulk solutions were distributed in 50 μL aliquots in Eppendorf vials (Protein LoBind Tube 1.5 mL; Eppendorf AG, Hamburg, Germany) and stored at −20 °C. For ^{99m}Tc labeling, the following solutions were added into an Eppendorf tube containing 0.5 M phosphate buffer pH 11.5 (25 μL): 0.1 M sodium citrate (3 μL), [^{99m}Tc]NaTcO$_4$ (210 μL, 150–300 MBq) eluted from a commercial ^{99}Mo/^{99m}Tc generator (Ultratechnekow, Tyco Healthcare, Petten, The Netherlands), N_4-GRP(14–27) or N_4-GRP(18–27) stock solution (7.5 μL, 7.5 nmol), and finally, fresh SnCl$_2$ solution in EtOH (5 μg, 5 μL). After 30 min incubation at ambient temperature the reaction mixture was neutralized by addition of 1 M HCl (4 μL) and EtOH was added (25 μL).

Quality control of the radiolabeled products comprised radioanalytical HPLC and instant thin-layer chromatography (ITLC). HPLC analyses were performed on a Waters Chromatograph coupled to a 2998 photodiode array UV detector (Waters, Vienna, Austria) and a Gabi gamma detector (Raytest RSM Analytische Instrumente GmbH, Germany). For analysis, a Waters Symmetry Shield RP-18 cartridge column (5 μm, 3.9 mm × 20 mm) was eluted at a 1.0 mL/min flow rate with the following gradient, 0% B to 40% B in 20 min, where A = 0.1% aq. trifluoroacetic acid (TFA), B = MeCN (System 1). Under these conditions ^{99m}TcO$_4^-$ eluted at 1.8 min and ^{99m}Tc-N_4-GRP(14–27) and ^{99m}Tc-N_4-GRP(18–27) with a t_R > 12 min. For the detection of reduced hydrolyzed technetium (^{99m}TcO$_2$· × H$_2$O) ITLC was conducted on ITLC-SG strips (Pall Corporation, New York, NY, USA), as previously described. The resultant ^{99m}Tc-N_4-GRP(14–27) and ^{99m}Tc-N_4-GRP(18–27) radioligands were used without further purification in all subsequent experiments.

Radioiodination of [Tyr^4]BBN was performed using ^{125}I ([^{125}I]NaI in 0.1 N NaOH (pH 12–14) provided by MDS Nordion, Ottawa, ON, Canada) according to the chloramine-T methodology, as previously described [34]. Methionine was added to the purified radioligand solution to prevent reoxidation of Met^{14} to the corresponding sulfoxide and the resulting stock solution in 0.1% BSA-PBS was kept at −20 °C; aliquots thereof were used in competition binding assays (molar activity of 81.4 GBq/μmol).

4.2. In Vitro Assays

4.2.1. Cell Lines and Culture

Human androgen-independent prostate adenocarcinoma PC-3 cells endogenously expressing the human GRPR (LGC Promochem, Teddington, UK) were used in the present study [43]. Cells were cultured in Roswell Park Memorial Institute (RPMI)-1640 medium, supplemented with 10% heat-inactivated fetal bovine serum (FBS), 100 U/mL penicillin, and 100 μg/mL streptomycin, and kept in a controlled humidified atmosphere containing 5% CO_2 at 37 °C. Passages were performed weekly using a trypsin/EDTA (0.05%/0.02% w/v) solution. All culture media were purchased from Gibco BRL, Life Technologies and supplements were provided by Biochrom KG Seromed.

4.2.2. Receptor Autoradiography

Binding affinities of N_4-GRP(14–27) were determined by in vitro receptor autoradiography performed on cryostat sections of well characterized human tumor tissues, prostate carcinomas for GRPR, ileal carcinoids for NMBR and bronchial carcinoids for BB_3R, as previously described [23]. The universal radioligand ^{125}I-[DTyr^6,βAla^{11},Phe^{13},Nle^{14}]BBN(6–14) (2 Ci/mol; ANAWA, Wangen Switzerland) was used as tracer known to identify all three bombesin receptor subtypes [6]. IC_{50} values are given in nM $\pm$ SEM.

4.2.3. Competition Binding in PC-3 Cell-Membranes

Competition binding experiments against [^{125}I-Tyr^4] BBN were performed with N_4-GRP(14–27) and N_4-GRP(18–27), or with the unmodified parent peptide references GRP(14–27) and GRP(18–27) in PC-3 cell membranes. For the assay, triplicates per concentration point (concentration range: 10^{-13}–10^{-6} M) of each test peptide were incubated together with the radioligand (~40,000 cpm per assay tube at a 50 pM concentration) in PC-3 cell-membrane homogenates in a total volume of 300 μL binding buffer (BB, 50 mM HEPES pH 7.4, 1% BSA, 5.5 mM $MgCl_2$, 35 μM bacitracin) for 1 h at 22 °C in an Incubator-Orbital Shaker (MPM Instr. SrI, Bernareggio, Italy). Binding was interrupted by ice-cold washing buffer (WB, 10 mM HEPES pH 7.4, 150 mM NaCl) and rapid filtration (Whatman GF/B filters presoaked in BB) on a Brandel Cell Harvester (Adi Hassel Ing. Büro, Munich, Germany). Filters were washed with ice-cold WB and counted in an automatic well-type gamma counter (NaI(Tl) 3'-crystal, Cobra Packard Auto-Gamma 5000 series instrument). The IC_{50} values were calculated using nonlinear regression according to a one-site model applying the PRISM 2 program (Graph Pad Software, San Diego, CA, USA).

4.2.4. Internalization Assay in PC-3 Cells

The internalization rates of ^{99m}Tc-N_4-GRP(14–27) and ^{99m}Tc-N_4-GRP(18–27) were compared in PC-3 cells. Briefly, PC-3 cells were seeded in six-well plates (~1×10^6 cells per well) 24 h before the experiment. Approximately 50,000 cpm of either ^{99m}Tc-N_4-GRP(14–27) or ^{99m}Tc-N_4-GRP(18–27) (corresponding to 250 fmol total peptide in 150 μL of 0.5% BSA/PBS) was added alone (total) or in the presence of 1 μM [Tyr^4]BBN (nonspecific). Cells were incubated at 37 °C for 15, 30, 60, and 120 min and incubation was interrupted each time by placing the plates on ice, removing the supernatants and rapid rinsing with ice-cold 0.5% BSA/PBS. Cells were then treated 2 × 5 min with acid wash buffer (2 × 0.6 mL, 50 mM glycine buffer pH 2.8, 0.1 M NaCl) at room temperature and supernatants were collected (membrane-bound fraction). After rinsing with 1 mL chilled 0.5% BSA/PBS, cells were lysed by treatment with 1 N NaOH (2 × 0.6 mL) and lysates were collected (internalized fraction). Sample radioactivity was measured in the γ-counter and percent internalized radioactivity was determined vs. total added activity. Results represent the average values $\pm$ sd of three experiments performed in triplicate.

4.3. Animal Studies

4.3.1. In Vivo Stability Tests

For stability experiments, healthy male Swiss albino mice (30 ± 5 g, NCSR "Demokritos" Animal House Facility) were used. Test radioligand—^{99m}Tc-N$_4$-GRP(14–27) or ^{99m}Tc-N$_4$-GRP(18–27)—was injected as a 100 µL bolus (37–74 MBq, 3 nmol total peptide) in the tail vein together with injection solution (100 µL; control) or with a PA-solution (100 µL injection solution containing 300 µg PA). Animals were euthanized and blood (0.5–1 mL) was directly withdrawn from the heart in an ice-cold syringe and transferred in a prechilled EDTA and methionine-containing Eppendorf tube on ice. Blood samples were centrifuged for 10 min at 2000 g/4 °C and plasma was collected. After addition of an equal volume of ice-cold MeCN the mixture was centrifuged for 10 min at 15,000 g/4 °C. The supernatant was concentrated under a N$_2$-flux at 60 °C to 0.05–0.1 mL, diluted with saline (0.4 mL), filtered through a 0.22 µm Millex GV filter (Millipore, Milford, CT, USA), and analyzed by RP-HPLC. The Symmetry Shield RP18 (5 µm, 3.9 mm × 20 mm) column was eluted at a flow rate of 1.0 mL/min with the following linear gradient (system 2): 0% B at 0 min to 10% B in 10 min and then in 40 min to 30% B; A = 0.1% aq. TFA and B = MeCN. The t_R of the intact radiopeptide was determined by coinjection with the ^{99m}Tc-N$_4$-GRP(14–27) and ^{99m}Tc-N$_4$-GRP(18–27) reference in the HPLC.

4.3.2. Induction of PC-3 Xenografts in SCID Mice

A suspension containing freshly harvested human PC-3 cells (≈150 µL of a ≈1.2 × 10^7 cells) was subcutaneously injected in the flanks of female SCID mice (15 ± 3 g, six weeks of age at the day of arrival, NCSR "Demokritos" Animal House Facility). The animals were kept under aseptic conditions and 4 weeks later developed well-palpable tumors (80–200 mg) at the inoculation sites.

4.3.3. Biodistribution in PC-3 Xenograft-Bearing SCID Mice

For the biodistribution study, animals in groups of 4 received via the tail vein a 100 µL bolus of ^{99m}Tc-N$_4$-GRP(14–27) (180–370 kBq, corresponding to 10 pmol total peptide) coinjected either with injection solution (100 µL; control) or PA-solution (300 µg PA dissolved in 100 µL injection solution; 4 h + PA), or with excess [Tyr^4]BBN (100 µL injection solution containing 50 µg [Tyr^4]BBN for in vivo GRPR-blockade; 4 h block). Animals were euthanized at 1-, 4-, and 24-h pi; in the case of ^{99m}Tc-N$_4$-GRP(18–27) two animal groups were included at the 4-h pi interval, namely the control and PA groups described above. Mice were dissected; samples of blood, tumors, and organs of interest were collected, weighed, and measured for radioactivity in the gamma counter. Intestines and stomach were not emptied of their contents. Data was calculated as percent injected dose per gram tissue (%ID/g) with the aid of standard solutions and represent mean values ± sd, *n* = 4. All animal experiments were performed in compliance with national and European guidelines and approved by national authorities (Prefecture of Athens, EL 25 BIO 021; #1609 and #1610).

Author Contributions: Conceptualization, B.A.N.; Methodology, B.A.N., T.M.N. and J.C.R.; Investigation, A.K., E.L., P.K., B.W., B.A.N., T.M.N. and J.C.R.; Writing—Original Draft Preparation, T.M.N.; Writing—Review and Editing, B.A.N., M.d.J., E.P.K. and J.C.R.

References

1. Kroog, G.S.; Jensen, R.T.; Battey, J.F. Mammalian bombesin receptors. *Med. Res. Rev.* **1995**, *15*, 389–417. [CrossRef]
2. Jensen, R.T.; Battey, J.F.; Spindel, E.R.; Benya, R.V. International union of pharmacology. LXVIII. Mammalian bombesin receptors: Nomenclature, distribution, pharmacology, signaling, and functions in normal and disease states. *Pharmacol. Rev.* **2008**, *60*, 1–42. [CrossRef]

3. Markwalder, R.; Reubi, J.C. Gastrin-releasing peptide receptors in the human prostate: Relation to neoplastic transformation. *Cancer Res.* **1999**, *59*, 1152–1159. [PubMed]

4. Körner, M.; Waser, B.; Rehmann, R.; Reubi, J.C. Early over-expression of GRP receptors in prostatic carcinogenesis. *Prostate* **2014**, *74*, 217–224. [CrossRef] [PubMed]

5. Beer, M.; Montani, M.; Gerhardt, J.; Wild, P.J.; Hany, T.F.; Hermanns, T.; Muntener, M.; Kristiansen, G. Profiling gastrin-releasing peptide receptor in prostate tissues: Clinical implications and molecular correlates. *Prostate* **2012**, *72*, 318–325. [CrossRef] [PubMed]

6. Reubi, J.C.; Wenger, S.; Schmuckli-Maurer, J.; Schaer, J.C.; Gugger, M. Bombesin receptor subtypes in human cancers: Detection with the universal radioligand ^{125}I-[d-Tyr^6,beta-Ala^{11},Phe^{13},Nle^{14}]bombesin(6-14). *Clin. Cancer Res.* **2002**, *8*, 1139–1146.

7. Halmos, G.; Wittliff, J.L.; Schally, A.V. Characterization of bombesin/gastrin-releasing peptide receptors in human breast cancer and their relationship to steroid receptor expression. *Cancer Res.* **1995**, *55*, 280–287. [PubMed]

8. Gugger, M.; Reubi, J.C. Gastrin-releasing peptide receptors in non-neoplastic and neoplastic human breast. *Am. J. Pathol.* **1999**, *155*, 2067–2076. [CrossRef]

9. Mattei, J.; Achcar, R.D.; Cano, C.H.; Macedo, B.R.; Meurer, L.; Batlle, B.S.; Groshong, S.D.; Kulczynski, J.M.; Roesler, R.; Dal Lago, L.; et al. Gastrin-releasing peptide receptor expression in lung cancer. *Arch. Pathol. Lab. Med.* **2014**, *138*, 98–104. [CrossRef]

10. Guinee, D.G., Jr.; Fishback, N.F.; Koss, M.N.; Abbondanzo, S.L.; Travis, W.D. The spectrum of immunohistochemical staining of small-cell lung carcinoma in specimens from transbronchial and open-lung biopsies. *Am. J. Clin. Pathol.* **1994**, *102*, 406–414. [CrossRef] [PubMed]

11. Moreno, P.; Ramos-Alvarez, I.; Moody, T.W.; Jensen, R.T. Bombesin related peptides/receptors and their promising therapeutic roles in cancer imaging, targeting and treatment. *Expert. Opin. Ther. Targets* **2016**, *20*, 1055–1073. [CrossRef] [PubMed]

12. Maina, T.; Nock, B.A. From bench to bed: New gastrin-releasing peptide receptor-directed radioligands and their use in prostate cancer. *PET Clin.* **2017**, *12*, 205–217. [CrossRef] [PubMed]

13. Uehara, H.; Gonzalez, N.; Sancho, V.; Mantey, S.A.; Nuche-Berenguer, B.; Pradhan, T.; Coy, D.H.; Jensen, R.T. Pharmacology and selectivity of various natural and synthetic bombesin related peptide agonists for human and rat bombesin receptors differs. *Peptides* **2011**, *32*, 1685–1699. [CrossRef] [PubMed]

14. Vigna, S.R.; Mantyh, C.R.; Giraud, A.S.; Soll, A.H.; Walsh, J.H.; Mantyh, P.W. Localization of specific binding sites for bombesin in the canine gastrointestinal tract. *Gastroenterology* **1987**, *93*, 1287–1295. [CrossRef]

15. Chave, H.S.; Gough, A.C.; Palmer, K.; Preston, S.R.; Primrose, J.N. Bombesin family receptor and ligand gene expression in human colorectal cancer and normal mucosa. *Br. J. Cancer* **2000**, *82*, 124–130. [CrossRef]

16. Fleischmann, A.; Laderach, U.; Friess, H.; Buechler, M.W.; Reubi, J.C. Bombesin receptors in distinct tissue compartments of human pancreatic diseases. *Lab. Investig.* **2000**, *80*, 1807–1817. [CrossRef] [PubMed]

17. Delle Fave, G.; Annibale, B.; de Magistris, L.; Severi, C.; Bruzzone, R.; Puoti, M.; Melchiorri, P.; Torsoli, A.; Erspamer, V. Bombesin effects on human GI functions. *Peptides* **1985**, *6* (Suppl. 3), 113–116. [CrossRef]

18. Bruzzone, R.; Tamburrano, G.; Lala, A.; Mauceri, M.; Annibale, B.; Severi, C.; de Magistris, L.; Leonetti, F.; Delle Fave, G. Effect of bombesin on plasma insulin, pancreatic glucagon, and gut glucagon in man. *J. Clin. Endocrinol. Metab.* **1983**, *56*, 643–647. [CrossRef]

19. Delle Fave, G.; Kohn, A.; De Magistris, L.; Annibale, B.; Bruzzone, R.; Sparvoli, C.; Severi, C.; Torsoli, A. Effects of bombesin on gastrin and gastric acid secretion in patients with duodenal ulcer. *Gut* **1983**, *24*, 231–235. [CrossRef]

20. Severi, C.; Jensen, R.T.; Erspamer, V.; D'Arpino, L.; Coy, D.H.; Torsoli, A.; Delle Fave, G. Different receptors mediate the action of bombesin-related peptides on gastric smooth muscle cells. *Am. J. Physiol.* **1991**, *260*, G683–G690. [CrossRef]

21. Bitar, K.N.; Zhu, X.X. Expression of bombesin-receptor subtypes and their differential regulation of colonic smooth muscle contraction. *Gastroenterology* **1993**, *105*, 1672–1680. [CrossRef]

22. Falconieri Erspamer, G.; Severini, C.; Erspamer, V.; Melchiorri, P.; Delle Fave, G.; Nakajima, T. Parallel bioassay of 27 bombesin-like peptides on 9 smooth muscle preparations. Structure-activity relationships and bombesin receptor subtypes. *Regul. Pept.* **1988**, *21*, 1–11. [CrossRef]

23. Nock, B.A.; Cescato, R.; Ketani, E.; Waser, B.; Reubi, J.C.; Maina, T. [^{99m}Tc]Demomedin C, a radioligand based on human gastrin releasing peptide(18–27): Synthesis and preclinical evaluation in gastrin releasing peptide receptor-expressing models. *J. Med. Chem.* **2012**, *55*, 8364–8374. [CrossRef] [PubMed]

24. Marsouvanidis, P.J.; Maina, T.; Sallegger, W.; Krenning, E.P.; de Jong, M.; Nock, B.A. ^{99m}Tc Radiotracers based on human GRP(18–27): Synthesis and comparative evaluation. *J. Nucl. Med.* **2013**, *54*, 1797–803. [CrossRef] [PubMed]

25. Nock, B.A.; Nikolopoulou, A.; Galanis, A.; Cordopatis, P.; Waser, B.; Reubi, J.C.; Maina, T. Potent bombesin-like peptides for GRP-receptor targeting of tumors with ^{99m}Tc: A preclinical study. *J. Med. Chem.* **2005**, *48*, 100–110. [CrossRef] [PubMed]

26. Marsouvanidis, P.J.; Maina, T.; Sallegger, W.; Krenning, E.P.; de Jong, M.; Nock, B.A. Tumor diagnosis with new ^{111}In-radioligands based on truncated human gastrin releasing peptide sequences: Synthesis and preclinical comparison. *J. Med. Chem.* **2013**, *56*, 8579–8587. [CrossRef]

27. Roques, B.P.; Noble, F.; Dauge, V.; Fournie-Zaluski, M.C.; Beaumont, A. Neutral endopeptidase 24.11: Structure, inhibition, and experimental and clinical pharmacology. *Pharmacol. Rev.* **1993**, *45*, 87–146. [PubMed]

28. Suda, H.; Aoyagi, T.; Takeuchi, T.; Umezawa, H. Letter: A thermolysin inhibitor produced by actinomycetes: Phosphoramidon. *J. Antibiot. (Tokyo)* **1973**, *26*, 621–623. [CrossRef]

29. Oefner, C.; D'Arcy, A.; Hennig, M.; Winkler, F.K.; Dale, G.E. Structure of human neutral endopeptidase (neprilysin) complexed with phosphoramidon. *J. Mol. Biol.* **2000**, *296*, 341–349. [CrossRef] [PubMed]

30. Marsouvanidis, P.J.; Melis, M.; de Blois, E.; Breeman, W.A.; Krenning, E.P.; Maina, T.; Nock, B.A.; de Jong, M. In vivo enzyme inhibition improves the targeting of [^{177}Lu]DOTA-GRP(13-27) in GRPR-positive tumors in mice. *Cancer Biother. Radiopharm.* **2014**, *29*, 359–367. [CrossRef] [PubMed]

31. Nock, B.A.; Maina, T.; Krenning, E.P.; de Jong, M. "To serve and protect": Enzyme inhibitors as radiopeptide escorts promote tumor targeting. *J. Nucl. Med.* **2014**, *55*, 121–127. [CrossRef]

32. Chatalic, K.L.; Konijnenberg, M.; Nonnekens, J.; de Blois, E.; Hoeben, S.; de Ridder, C.; Brunel, L.; Fehrentz, J.A.; Martinez, J.; van Gent, D.C.; et al. In vivo stabilization of a gastrin-releasing peptide receptor antagonist enhances pet imaging and radionuclide therapy of prostate cancer in preclinical studies. *Theranostics* **2016**, *6*, 104–117. [CrossRef] [PubMed]

33. Maina, T.; Kaloudi, A.; Valverde, I.E.; Mindt, T.L.; Nock, B.A. Amide-to-triazole switch vs. In vivo NEP-inhibition approaches to promote radiopeptide targeting of GRPR-positive tumors. *Nucl. Med. Biol.* **2017**, *52*, 57–62. [CrossRef]

34. Lymperis, E.; Kaloudi, A.; Sallegger, W.; Bakker, I.L.; Krenning, E.P.; de Jong, M.; Maina, T.; Nock, B.A. Radiometal-dependent biological profile of the radiolabeled gastrin-releasing peptide receptor antagonist SB3 in cancer theranostics: Metabolic and biodistribution patterns defined by neprilysin. *Bioconjug. Chem.* **2018**, *29*, 1774–1784. [CrossRef]

35. Nock, B.; Maina, T. Tetraamine-coupled peptides and resulting ^{99m}Tc-radioligands: An effective route for receptor-targeted diagnostic imaging of human tumors. *Curr. Top. Med. Chem.* **2012**, *12*, 2655–2667. [CrossRef] [PubMed]

36. Mather, S.J.; Nock, B.A.; Maina, T.; Gibson, V.; Ellison, D.; Murray, I.; Sobnack, R.; Colebrook, S.; Wan, S.; Halberrt, G.; et al. GRP receptor imaging of prostate cancer using [^{99m}Tc]Demobesin 4: A first-in-man study. *Mol. Imaging Biol.* **2014**, *16*, 888–895. [CrossRef] [PubMed]

37. De Castiglione, R.; Gozzini, L. Bombesin receptor antagonists. *Crit. Rev. Oncol. Hematol.* **1996**, *24*, 117–151. [CrossRef]

38. Maina, T.; Nock, B.A.; Kulkarni, H.; Singh, A.; Baum, R.P. Theranostic prospects of gastrin-releasing peptide receptor-radioantagonists in oncology. *PET Clin.* **2017**, *12*, 297–309. [CrossRef] [PubMed]

39. Kassis, A.I. Therapeutic radionuclides: Biophysical and radiobiologic principles. *Semin. Nucl. Med.* **2008**, *38*, 358–366. [CrossRef]

40. Wild, D.; Frischknecht, M.; Zhang, H.; Morgenstern, A.; Bruchertseifer, F.; Boisclair, J.; Provencher-Bolliger, A.; Reubi, J.C.; Maecke, H.R. Alpha- versus beta-particle radiopeptide therapy in a human prostate cancer model (^{213}Bi-DOTA-Pesin and ^{213}Bi-AMBA versus ^{177}Lu-DOTA-Pesin). *Cancer Res.* **2011**, *71*, 1009–1018. [CrossRef]

41. Linder, K.E.; Metcalfe, E.; Arunachalam, T.; Chen, J.; Eaton, S.M.; Feng, W.; Fan, H.; Raju, N.; Cagnolini, A.; Lantry, L.E.; et al. In vitro and in vivo metabolism of Lu-AMBA, a GRP-receptor binding compound, and the synthesis and characterization of its metabolites. *Bioconjug. Chem.* **2009**, *20*, 1171–1178. [CrossRef] [PubMed]

42. Shipp, M.A.; Tarr, G.E.; Chen, C.Y.; Switzer, S.N.; Hersh, L.B.; Stein, H.; Sunday, M.E.; Reinherz, E.L. CD10/neutral endopeptidase 24.11 hydrolyzes bombesin-like peptides and regulates the growth of small cell carcinomas of the lung. *Proc. Natl. Acad. Sci. USA* **1991**, *88*, 10662–10666. [CrossRef] [PubMed]

43. Reile, H.; Armatis, P.E.; Schally, A.V. Characterization of high-affinity receptors for bombesin/gastrin releasing peptide on the human prostate cancer cell lines PC-3 and DU-145: Internalization of receptor bound ^{125}I-(Tyr^4)bombesin by tumor cells. *Prostate* **1994**, *25*, 29–38. [CrossRef] [PubMed]

16

Synthesis and Initial In Vivo Evaluation of [11C]AZ683—A Novel PET Radiotracer for Colony Stimulating Factor 1 Receptor (CSF1R)

Sean S. Tanzey [1] , **Xia Shao** [2], **Jenelle Stauff** [2], **Janna Arteaga** [2], **Phillip Sherman** [2],
Peter J. H. Scott [1,2,*] and **Andrew V. Mossine** [2,*]

[1]   Department of Medicinal Chemistry, University of Michigan, Ann Arbor, MI 48109, USA;
     tanzeys@umich.edu

[2]   Department of Radiology, University of Michigan, Ann Arbor, MI 48109, USA; xshao@umich.edu (X.S.);
     jrstauff@umich.edu (J.S.); jannaa@umich.edu (J.A.); psherman@umich.edu (P.S.)

*   Correspondence: pjhscott@umich.edu (P.J.H.S.); avmossine@gmail.com (A.V.M.)

Abstract: Positron emission tomography (PET) imaging of Colony Stimulating Factor 1 Receptor (CSF1R) is a new strategy for quantifying both neuroinflammation and inflammation in the periphery since CSF1R is expressed on microglia and macrophages. AZ683 has high affinity for CSF1R (K_i = 8 nM; IC_{50} = 6 nM) and >250-fold selectivity over 95 other kinases. In this paper, we report the radiosynthesis of [11C]AZ683 and initial evaluation of its use in CSF1R PET. [11C]AZ683 was synthesized by 11C-methylation of the desmethyl precursor with [11C]MeOTf in 3.0% non-corrected activity yield (based upon [11C]MeOTf), >99% radiochemical purity and high molar activity. Preliminary PET imaging with [11C]AZ683 revealed low brain uptake in rodents and nonhuman primates, suggesting that imaging neuroinflammation could be challenging but that the radiopharmaceutical could still be useful for peripheral imaging of inflammation.

Keywords: neuroinflammation; microglia; carbon-11; radiochemistry; positron emission tomography

1. Introduction

Colony Stimulating Factor 1 Receptor (CSF1R, M-CSF, or cFMS) is a class III receptor tyrosine kinase [1] that regulates immune response by controlling the survival and activity of macrophages and macrophage-like cells [2]. Aberrant activity of CSF1R, or its endogenous ligands (CSF1 and IL-34), plays a role in many disorders that have an immune/inflammatory component [3]. Specifically, chronic inflammation caused by increased activity of macrophages due to increased CSF1R response is present in many autoimmune disorders such as rheumatoid arthritis, inflammatory bowel disease, and autoimmune nephritis, among others [4,5]. The contribution of CSF1R to symptomatic Alzheimer's Disease (AD) is also well known, due in part to its proliferative effects on microglia, which are associated with neuroinflammation, a hallmark clinical symptom of AD [6,7]. A mechanism for CSF1R involvement in inter-neuronal transmission of pathogenic tau protein by microglia was also recently elucidated [8]. Involvement of CSF1R in certain types of cancers, such as gliomas, also correlates with poor disease prognosis, as proliferation of CSF1R-controlled tumor-associated macrophages (TAMs) correlates with tumor angiogenesis and metastasis [4,9–11].

Consequently, CSF1R inhibitors (both small molecules and biologics) have been proposed as a means of controlling inflammation in this multitude of diseases and disorders via macrophage depletion/regulation [12]. Many CSF1R inhibitors, including some that are kinase-specific, can be found in both academic and patent literature [4,5,13], and several have proceeded to clinical trials for the treatment of RA [14] and various types of cancer [11]. However, not all macrophage populations are CSF1R-sensitive, necessitating that CSF1R involvement must be positively identified prior to the start of treatment. As CSF1R is a cell surface receptor, its upregulation is only present at the site of inflammation. Although blood biomarkers can be used to directly measure CSF1R involvement in certain diseases, such as lymphoma [11], methods of determining CSF1R involvement and quantifying CSF1R levels at loci not directly connected to the central circulatory system is difficult, particularly in the CNS, and employs either indirect means (i.e., measurement of CSF1 levels as a proxy for CSF1R [14]) or invasive procedures (i.e., immunohistochemistry using a biopsy sample or surgically excised tissue [15,16]). In fact, despite the implication of irregular CSF1R levels in numerous diseases [4], quantitative information on expression levels in disease is generally lacking from the literature. In part this is because CSF1R levels are constantly changing as, for example, macrophages are produced and/or cleared, but also because there is currently an unmet need for a non-invasive method that can positively identify and quantify CSF1R involvement in disease. This goal can be readily achieved with positron emission tomography (PET) imaging, wherein a CSF1R-selective radiolabeled ligand (radiopharmaceutical) would be used to detect changes in activity, expression levels, and localization of CSF1R in a minimally-invasive manner. Furthermore, a brain-penetrant CSF1R-selective PET imaging agent could be used to selectively image microglia, as they are the only cells in the brain that express CSF1R under normal conditions [17]. Microglia associate with amyloid beta plaques in the brain [18], and are implicated in pathological tau transmission [8] and neuroinflammation [6,7], both of which are important in the progression of neurodegenerative disorders.

The current method of choice for imaging macrophages/microglia is by targeting the translocator protein 18 kDa (TSPO). However, TSPO is not an ideal imaging target since it is expressed in various tissue types (in addition to immune cells). Moreover, a single nucleotide polymorphism (SNP) in the TSPO gene has been identified that leads to considerable variability in its expression levels between patients and, consequently, variability in the corresponding PET data [19]. Therefore, a CSF1R imaging agent selective for microglia is of considerable interest for using PET both to quantify CSF1R and as a surrogate biomarker for neuroinflammation (and peripheral inflammation).

Radiopharmaceuticals used in PET imaging are often structural analogs of existing pharmaceutical agents that have been labeled with a positron-emitting radionuclide such as ^{11}C, ^{18}F or ^{124}I. As such, the radiopharmaceutical can be expected to possess the same pharmacokinetic properties as its nonradioactive counterpart and behave accordingly in vivo. Fortunately, lead identification for CSF1R PET radiopharmaceutical development is relatively straightforward because recent interest in developing CSF1R inhibitors has led to hundreds of active compounds, several of which have also been translated into clinical trials (see Figure 1 for several leads) [4,5,13]. PET imaging agents for CSF1R have been reported [20,21], but none have seen widespread use to date. One is a mixed inhibitor of both CSF1R and tropomyosin receptor kinases B and C (Trk B/C) [20], while the second ([^{11}C]JHU11744) has shown promise in preliminary evaluation in rodent models of AD and neuroinflammation [21].

PET imaging of CSF1R therefore remains underdeveloped and herein we attempt to address this issue through development of [^{11}C]AZ683, a new radiopharmaceutical for CSF1R. AZ683 (Figure 1) was selected because it has >250-fold selectivity for CSF1R over 95 other kinases, low plasma protein binding, a good pharmacokinetic (PK) profile, and both fluorine and N-methyl moieties which are potential sites for radiolabeling with ^{18}F or ^{11}C, respectively [22–24]. Moreover, AZ683 has low nanomolar affinity for CSF1R ($K_i = 8$ nM; $IC_{50} = 6$ nM), making it ideal for PET studies which typically utilize nanomoles-picomoles of radiotracer, and the cLogP of the neutral (uncharged) compound is 3.1 which suggests that it should cross the BBB. Since N-methylation of the desmethyl precursor with [^{11}C]MeI (or [^{11}C]MeOTf) was envisioned to be simpler than ^{18}F-labeling of this scaffold, the synthesis and carbon-11 radiolabeling of [^{11}C]AZ683 was undertaken for initial evaluation and is described herein. We also report preliminary evaluation of the radiotracer as a CSF1R imaging agent in rodent and non-human primate PET imaging studies.

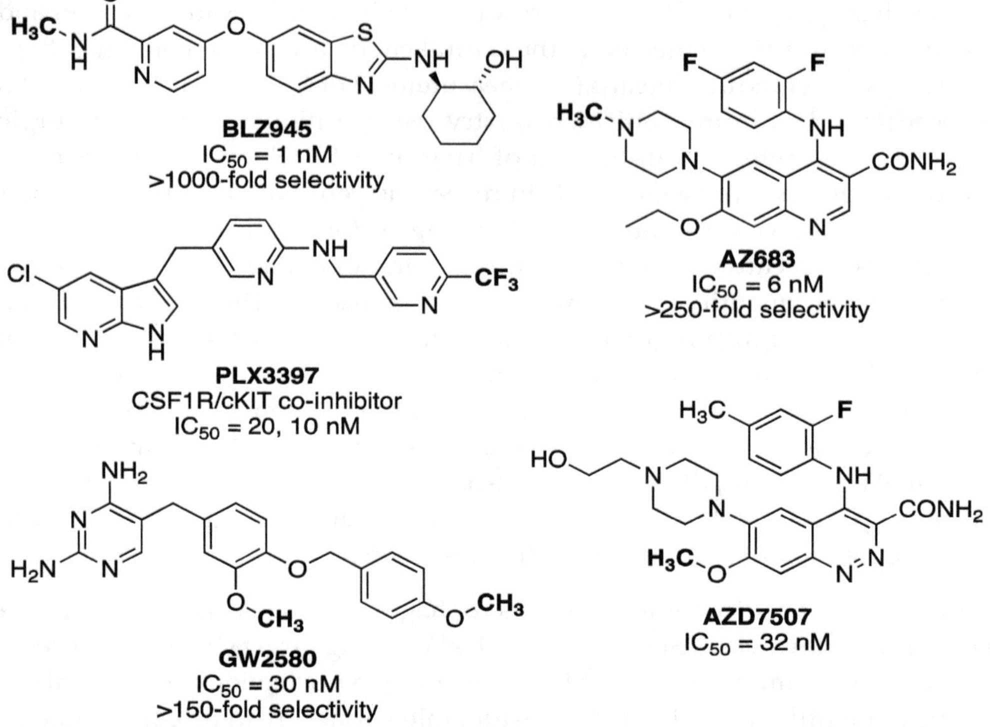

Figure 1. Potential lead compounds for CSF1R radiopharmaceutical development (proposed radiolabeling sites are shown in red).

2. Results and Discussion

2.1. Synthesis of Reference Standard and Precursor

AZ683 reference standard **6a** and *N*-desmethyl precursor **7** were synthesized via modified literature procedures in five and six steps, respectively (Scheme 1) [23]. Both syntheses diverged from a common intermediate **4**. This common intermediate was synthesized via condensation of 4-bromo-3-ethoxyaniline (**1**) with diethylethoxymethylenemalonate to yield **2**. This was followed by cyclization/chlorination with $POCl_3$ and tetrabutylammonium chloride to form chloroquinoline **3**. A subsequent S_NAr reaction with 2,4-difluoroaniline yielded intermediate **4**. Buchwald–Hartwig cross-coupling was then used to couple either *N*-Boc piperazine or *N*-methylpiperazine with **4**, yielding intermediates **5a** and **5b** for the reference standard and precursor, respectively. Amidation of the ethyl ester of **5** was performed using formamide/NaOEt to generate reference standard **6a** and *N*-Boc protected precursor **6b**. Final deprotection of the Boc group of **6b** with trimethylsilyl chloride in methanol furnished precursor **7**. Precursor **7** and reference standard **6a** were readily separable on analytical and semipreparative Phenomenex Luna C18 columns using a 30% ethanolic eluent buffered with sodium phosphate at a pH of 6.6 (see *Materials and Methods* for details).

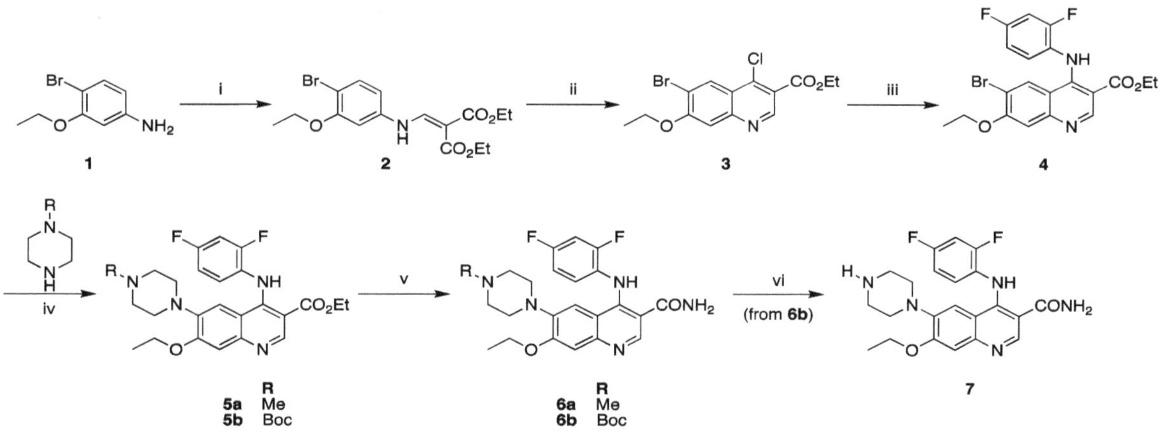

Scheme 1. Synthesis of precursor and reference standard for [^{11}C]AZ683. Reagents and conditions: (i) diethylethoxymethylenemalonate, K_2CO_3, MeCN, 70 °C (71%); (ii) $POCl_3$, TBACl, toluene, 130 °C (17%); (iii) 2,4-difluoroaniline, 20% AcOH, EtOH, 80 °C (66%); (iv) 1–5 mol % Pd_2(dba)$_3$, BINAP, Cs_2CO_3, toluene, 100 °C (**5a**: 54%; **5b**: 45%); (v) formamide, NaOEt, EtOH/THF, reflux (**6a**: 32%; **6b**: 30%); (vi) TMSCl, MeOH, room temp (100% from **6b**).

2.2. Radiosynthesis of [^{11}C]AZ683

Radiolabeling of [^{11}C]AZ683 was accomplished by treating precursor **7** with [^{11}C]MeOTf (Scheme 2). The labeling reaction was automated using a TRACERLab FX$_{C\text{-pro}}$ synthesis module and our standard carbon-11 procedures [25]. Following radiolabeling, [^{11}C]AZ683 was purified within the synthesis module via semipreparative HPLC and formulated for injection (0.9% saline solution containing 10% ethanol) using a Waters C18 1cc vac cartridge to trap/release the product. This resulted in an overall non-decay corrected activity yield of 1125 ± 229 MBq (3.0% based upon 37 GBq of [^{11}C]MeOTf), radiochemical purity >99%, and molar activity of 153 ± 38 GBq/µmol (n = 4), confirming doses were suitable for preclinical evaluation.

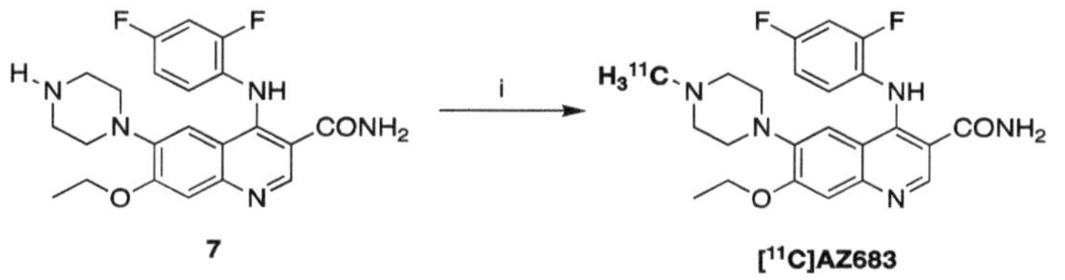

Scheme 2. Radiosynthesis of [^{11}C]AZ683. Reagents and conditions: (i) [^{11}C]MeOTF, DMF, rt, 3 min (3.0% activity yield).

2.3. Preclinical PET Imaging

Initial evaluation of the imaging properties of [^{11}C]AZ683 was undertaken in female Sprague–Dawley rat. [^{11}C]AZ683 was administered via intravenous tail vein injection and rodent brain imaging was conducted for 60 min. To our surprise, [^{11}C]AZ683 showed very little brain uptake but did show high uptake and retention in the pituitary and thyroid glands (Figure 2, left). Although both glands are known for expression of CSF1R protein (thyroid) and CSF1R RNA (thyroid and pituitary) [26], we assume the very high uptake is more likely indicative of non-specific binding associated with the lipophilic nature of the compound (Table 1). Since inter-species differences are sometimes apparent between rodents and non-human primates due to the higher metabolic rate in rodents and differing BBB efflux systems, imaging in rhesus macaque brain was also performed. The primate imaging results largely mirrored the rat data, with fairly poor brain influx during the early frames, followed by almost complete washout and little brain retention in a normal brain (Figure 2, right). There was some retention in the central region of the brain that was likely ventricular uptake and, as before, the pituitary gland could be observed in frame and showed a much greater degree of uptake than brain. Overall though, brain uptake in monkey was higher than in rat and there was perhaps some focal uptake in the monkey cerebellum (standardized uptake value (SUV) ~0.3–0.4 at late time points). Given that the cerebellum is an area of known CSF1R expression in humans [26], and CSF1R function is thought to be conserved between vertebrates [27], this signal could correspond to CSF1R, presumably associated with microglia found in the monkey cerebellum [28]. However, this will need to be confirmed in future in vitro experiments with primate brain sections. Target receptor density of CSF1R could ostensibly be low in a non-diseased control animal and would explain poor brain retention, but again normal CSF1R levels are challenging to quantify in vivo as they are transient and expected to fluctuate with the turnover of macrophages and microglia. However, low receptor density would not limit first pass brain influx and efflux which was also quite low. Overall these PET imaging data suggest imaging CSF1R associated with neuroinflammation using [^{11}C]AZ683 may be challenging, but that uptake in monkey could be sufficient to observe accumulation in a brain inflammation model. There is literature precedent for TSPO radiotracers with low brain uptake being used to successfully image inflammation in rat models [29,30]. Moreover, the present studies do not rule out labeling the scaffold with a longer-lived PET radionuclide (e.g., ^{18}F or ^{124}I) and using a prolonged infusion protocol so that sufficient radiotracer accumulates at sites of inflammation. [^{11}C]AZ683 could also possibly be used for imaging of peripheral CSF1R to evaluate its role in inflammation outside of the brain.

Given that [^{11}C]AZ683 possesses properties mostly consistent with BBB permeability (Table 1) [23,31,32], the lack of brain uptake was unexpected and the reasons for it are unclear. It is possible that [^{11}C]AZ683 is a substrate for an efflux transporter on the BBB and since, for example, P-glycoprotein transporter (P-gp) expression is higher in rodents than monkeys (and humans) [33], this could explain the 2–3-fold higher uptake of the radiotracer observed in monkey brain. Given the differences in type and expression levels of efflux transporters between species, monkeys are better for predicting the role of P-gp in limiting brain penetration of drugs in humans [33]. However, as we take a conservative view towards primate safety, methods to determine whether efflux activity is responsible for the low brain uptake of [^{11}C]AZ683 (e.g., cyclosporin A blockade of the P-gp transporter [34]) have not been pursued at this time. Alternatively, in this case, cLogP estimates (Table 1) may not be a good indicator of BBB permeability. [^{11}C]AZ683 has multiple groups containing nitrogen and oxygen atoms which are ionizable, corresponding to multiple pKa values (Figure 3 [32]). We do not expect the primary amide to limit BBB permeability since we conduct brain imaging with other primary amide-containing radiopharmaceuticals such as [^{11}C]LY2795050 [35]. Understanding the relationship between cLogP of charged species as a function of pH is complicated [31], but it is likely that AZ683 is charged at physiological pH and this could be the reason for poor brain uptake. The oxygen and nitrogen atoms in question also participate in hydrogen bonding, and cLogP—the total number of oxygen and nitrogen atoms in a drug molecule (N + O) offers information about logBBB. If cLogP—(N + O) >0, logBBB is likely to be positive and the drug has a good probability of entering the CNS [31]. In the case of AZ863, cLogP—(N + O) = −4, suggesting the number of oxygen and nitrogen atoms may be too high for good CNS penetration. All of these issues should be considered in the design of next generation CSF1R radiopharmaceuticals going forward.

Table 1. Properties of [^{11}C]AZ683 compared to a typical CNS drug.

Property	Preferred Value for Successful CNS Drugs [31]	[^{11}C]AZ683 [23,32]
Activity	Low nM	K_i = 8 nM; IC$_{50}$ = 6 nM
cLogP	<5 (Lipinski's Ro5 [29]) <2.7 (optimized [29])	3.1
tPSA	60–70 Å^2	83 Å^2
Molecular weight	≤450 g/mol	441 g/mol
H-bond donors	≤3	2
H-bond acceptors	≤7	6
Rotatable bonds	<8	8
Metabolic stability	$T_{1/2}$ > 3.1 h	2.1 h
Solubility	>60 µg/mL	128 µg/mL
pKa	7.5–10.5	6.5–7.5
cLogP—(N + O)	>0	−4

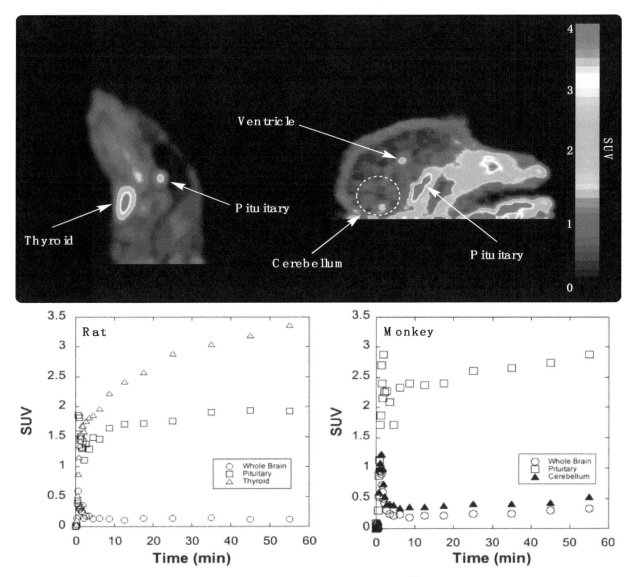

Figure 2. Summed rodent (left) and primate (right) PET images of [^{11}C]AZ683 (0–60 min after injection of the radiotracer) and associated time–radioactivity curves (SUV = standardized uptake value).

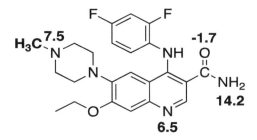

Figure 3. Multiple pKa values for AZ683 [32].

3. Materials and Methods

3.1. Synthesis

3.1.1. General Considerations

All the chemicals were purchased from commercially available suppliers and used without purification. Automated flash chromatography was performed with Biotage Isolera Prime system.

High-performance liquid chromatography (HPLC) was performed using a Shimadzu LC-2010A HT system. ^{1}H NMR spectra were acquired using a Varian 400 apparatus (400 MHz) in $CDCl_3$ or CD_3OD. δ are reported in ppm relative to tetramethylsilane ($\delta = 0$), J are given in Hz. Mass spectra were measured on an Agilent Technologies (Santa Clara CA, USA) Q-TOF HPLC-MS or Micromass (Manchester, UK) VG 70-250-S Magnetic sector mass spectrometer employing the electrospray ionization (ESI) method.

3.1.2. Compounds Synthesized

Diethyl 2-(((4-bromo-3-ethoxyphenyl)amino)methylene)malonate (**2**). To a solution mixture of 4-bromo-3-ethoxyaniline hydrochloride (**1**) (0.66 g, 3 mmol) and K_2CO_3 (1.68 g, 12.2 mmol) in MeCN (30 mL) was added diethyl-ethoxymethylene malonate (620 μL, 3 mmol). The reaction was heated to reflux and allowed to stir for 36 h, at which time it was cooled and vacuum filtrated through celite to remove potassium carbonate. The filtrate was purified by flash chromatography using a hexane-EtOAc gradient to yield **2** (0.84 g, 71%). ^{1}H-NMR (400 MHz, $CDCl_3$) δ 11.00 (d, $J = 13.5$ Hz, 1H), 8.45 (d, $J = 13.5$ Hz, 1H), 7.49 (d, $J = 8.5$ Hz, 1H), 6.63 (d, $J = 8.5$ Hz, 1H), 6.59 (d, $J = 2.4$ Hz, 1H), 4.33–4.22 (m, 4H), 4.09 (q, $J = 7.0$ Hz, 2H), 1.49 (t, $J = 7.0$ Hz, 3H), 1.38–1.31 (m, 6H). [M + H]$^+$: Expected 386.0598, Found 386.0604.

Ethyl 6-bromo-4-chloro-7-ethoxyquinoline-3-carboxylate (**3**). Compound **2** (0.84 g, 2.2 mmol) was dissolved in dry Toluene (2.5 mL). *Tert*-Butyl ammonium chloride (TBACl: 1.94 g, 7 mmol) was added, followed by $POCl_3$ (2 mL, 22 mmol) while stirring at room temperature for 5 min. The reaction mixture was then heated to reflux and stirred for 68 h. After this time the reaction was cooled, diluted with DCM (30 mL) and quenched with water (30 mL). The aq. layer was extracted with further DCM (30 mL) and the combined organic fractions were washed with brine (60 mL), dried (Na_2SO_4) and concentrated. The crude material was purified by flash chromatography using a hexane/EtOAc gradient to yield **3** (0.15 g, 17%). ^{1}H-NMR (400 MHz, $CDCl_3$) δ 9.16 (s, 1H), 8.61 (s, 1H), 7.42 (s, 1H), 4.48 (q, $J = 7.2$ Hz, 2H), 4.28 (dd, $J = 14.1, 7.0$ Hz, 2H), 1.58 (t, $J = 7.0$ Hz, 3H), 1.45 (t, $J = 7.2$ Hz, 3H). [M + H]$^+$: Expected 357.9840, Found 359.9820. Cl-37 accounts for difference in expected value.

Ethyl 6-bromo-4-((2,4-difluorophenyl)amino)-7-ethoxyquinoline-3-carboxylate (**4**). Compound **3** (0.15 g, 0.41 mmol) was dissolved in ethanol (10 mL). 20 mol % acetic acid (4.7 μL, 0.082 mmol) was added followed by 2,4-difluoroaniline (46 μL, 0.45 mmol, 1.1 eq.). The reaction was heated to reflux and stirred for 24 h. After this time the reaction was cooled and Et_3N (100 μL) was added to neutralize acetic acid. The crude reaction mixture was purified by flash chromatography to yield title compound **4** (0.11 g, 66%). ^{1}H-NMR (400 MHz, $CDCl_3$) δ 10.30 (s, 1H), 9.19 (s, 1H), 7.73 (s, 1H), 7.03 (s, 1H), 6.97–6.94 (m, 1H), 6.94–6.92 (m, 1H), 6.84 (t, $J = 8.3$ Hz, 1H), 4.43 (q, $J = 7.1$ Hz, 2H), 4.23 (q, $J = 7.0$ Hz, 2H), 1.53 (t, $J = 7.0$ Hz, 3H), 1.45 (t, $J = 7.1$ Hz, 3H). [M + H]$^+$: Expected 451.0463, Found 451.0463.

Ethyl 4-((2,4-difluorophenyl)amino)-7-ethoxy-6-(4-methylpiperazin-1-yl)quinoline-3-carboxylate (**5a**). Compound **3** (113 mg, 0.251 mmol) was dissolved in dry toluene (10 mL). To this solution, 1-methylpiperizine (33.4 μL, 0.301 mmol, 1.2 eq.) was added. This solution was aspirated with a syringe and added to a mixture of 2.5 mol % $Pd_2(dba)_3$ (5.75 mg, 0.007 mmol), 2.5 mol % BINAP (3.9 mg, 0.007 mmol) and 1.6 eq. of Cs_2CO_3 (0.13 g, 0.402 mmol) under Ar. The reaction was heated to 100°C and stirred for 60 h. After this time the reaction was cooled and quenched with satd. $KHCO_3$ (20 mL). The organic layer was washed with water (50 mL) and the water was extracted twice with EtOAc. The organic layers were combined, washed with brine (60 mL), concentrated and dried (Na_2SO_4). The residue was purified by flash chromatography using an EtOAc/MeOH gradient to yield compound **5a** (64 mg, 54%). ^{1}H-NMR (400 MHz, $CDCl_3$) δ 10.14 (s, 1H), 9.11 (s, 1H), 7.32 (s, 1H), 7.26 (s, 1H), 7.00–6.90 (m, 1H), 6.89 (s, 1H), 6.75 (t, $J = 8.4$ Hz, 1H), 4.42 (q, $J = 7.1$ Hz, 2H), 4.21 (q, $J = 6.9$ Hz, 2H), 2.83 (m, 4H), 2.55 (m, 4H), 2.30 (s, 3H), 1.51 (t, $J = 6.9$ Hz, 3H), 1.48–1.44 (m, 3H). [M + H]$^+$: Expected 471.2202, Found 471.2202.

Ethyl 6-(4-(tert-butoxycarbonyl)piperazin-1-yl)-4-((2,4-difluorophenyl)amino)-7-ethoxyquinoline -3-carboxylate (**5b**). The same procedure described for the synthesis of **5a** was also used to prepare **5b** (61 mg, 44.5%). ^{1}H-NMR (400 MHz, CDCl$_3$) δ 10.08 (s, 1H), 9.12 (s, 1H), 7.30 (s, 1H), 6.96–6.88 (m, 2H), 6.86 (s, 1H), 6.75 (t, J = 8.2 Hz, 1H), 4.43 (q, J = 7.1 Hz, 3H), 4.21 (q, J = 7.0 Hz, 2H), 3.53–3.45 (m, 4H), 2.75–2.67 (m, 4H), 1.52 (t, J = 7.0 Hz, 3H), 1.47 (s, 9H), 1.44 (d, J = 7.1 Hz, 3H). [M + H]$^+$: Expected 557.2571, Found 557.2571.

4-((2.,4-Difluorophenyl)amino)-7-ethoxy-6-(4-methylpiperazin-1-yl)quinoline-3-carboxamide (AZ683 Reference Standard **6a**). Compound **5a** (53 mg, 0.113 mmol) was dissolved in THF (0.1 mL) and formamide (22.4 µL, 0.563 mmol, 5 eq.) was added. To this solution, a 21% wt solution of NaOEt in EtOH (231 µL, 0.563 mmol, 5 eq.) was added. The reaction was heated to reflux and stirred for 16 h, after which time it was cooled and quenched with NH$_4$Cl (53 mg, 1 mmol). The reaction mixture was concentrated onto silica and purified by flash chromatography using an EtOAc/MeOH gradient to yield compound **6a** (16 mg, 32%). ^{1}H-NMR (400 MHz, CD$_3$OD) δ 8.78 (s, 1H), 7.27 (s, 1H), 7.16–7.06 (m, 3H), 6.95 (t, J = 8.6 Hz, 1H), 4.25 (q, J = 6.9 Hz, 3H), 3.10 (m, 4H), 2.73 (m, 4H), 1.96 (s, 3H), 1.51 (t, J = 6.9 Hz, 3H). [M + H]$^+$: Expected 442.2049, Found 442.2048.

tert-Butyl 4-(3-carbamoyl-4-((2,4-difluorophenyl)amino)-7-ethoxyquinolin-6-yl)piperazine-1-carboxylate (**6b**). The same procedure described for the synthesis of **6a** was used to prepare **6b** (18 mg, 30%). ^{1}H-NMR (400 MHz, CDCl$_3$) δ 10.44 (s, 1H), 8.76 (s, 1H), 7.27 (s, 1H), 6.94–6.88 (m, 2H), 6.87 (s, 1H), 6.74 (t, J = 8.3 Hz, 1H), 6.21 (br. s, 1H), 4.20 (q, J = 6.9 Hz, 2H), 3.48–3.47 (m, 4H), 2.73–2.71 (m, 4H), 1.51 (t, J = 6.9 Hz, 3H), 1.47 (s, 9H). [M + H]$^+$: Expected 528.2417, Found 528.2419.

4-((2,4-Difluorophenyl)amino)-7-ethoxy-6-(piperazin-1-yl)quinoline-3-carboxamide (**7**). Compound **6b** (18 mg, 0.034 mmol) was dissolved in dry MeOH (5 mL) and cooled to -78 °C for 5 min. Trimethylsilyl chloride (TMS-Cl, 43.3 µL, 0.341 mmol, 10 eq.) was added and the reaction was allowed to warm up to room temperature and was stirred until deprotection was complete as determined by TLC (~25 h). The reaction was quenched with water and concentrated to remove solvent and excess TMS-Cl. The concentrate was re-dissolved in MeOH and re-concentrated two more times to ensure complete removal of TMS-Cl. The product was further dried in a vacuum desiccator to yield compound **7** (15 mg, 100%). ^{1}H-NMR (400 MHz, CD$_3$OD) δ 8.80 (s, 1H), 7.56–7.50 (m, 1H), 7.38 (s, 1H), 7.34 (s, 1H), 7.26–7.18 (m, 1H), 7.14 (t, J = 8.4 Hz, 1H), 4.33 (q, J = 7.0 Hz, 2H), 3.39–3.33 (m, 4H), 3.22–3.20 (m, 4H), 1.55 (t, J = 7.0 Hz, 3H). [M + H]$^+$: Expected 428.1893, Found 428.1892.

3.2. Radiochemistry

3.2.1. General Considerations

All the chemicals (except for reference standard **6a** and precursor **7** noted above) were purchased from commercially available suppliers and used without purification: sodium chloride, 0.9% USP and Sterile Water for Injection, USP were purchased from Hospira; Dehydrated Alcohol for Injection, USP was obtained from Akorn Inc. (Lake Forest IL, USA) HPLC was performed using a Shimadzu (Kyoto, Japan) LC-2010A HT system equipped with a Bioscan B-FC-1000 radiation detector, and HPLC columns were acquired from Phenomenex (Torrance CA, USA). Other synthesis components were obtained as follows: sterile filters were acquired from MilliporeSigma (Burlington MA, USA); C18 Vac 1cc Sep-Paks were purchased from Waters Corporation (Milford MA, USA); Sep-Paks were flushed with 5 mL of ethanol followed by 10 mL of sterile water prior to use.

3.2.2. Radiosynthesis of [^{11}C]AZ683

[^{11}C]CO$_2$ was produced with a General Electric Healthcare (GE, Uppsala, Sweden) PETTrace cyclotron via the ^{14}N(p,α)^{11}C reaction. High purity N$_2$ (g) containing 0.5% O$_2$ was irradiated at 40 µA for 30 min to generate [^{11}C]CO$_2$ (~111 GBq), which was delivered to a GE TRACERLab FX$_{C-Pro}$ synthesis module and converted to [^{11}C]MeOTf (~37 GBq) as previously described [25]. [^{11}C]MeOTf was bubbled at 15 mL/min through a solution of precursor **7** (1 mg) in DMF (100 µL) at room temperature for 3 min. Following radiolabeling, the reaction mixture was diluted with HPLC mobile phase and purified by semipreparative HPLC (column: Phenomenex Luna C18, 10µ, 10 × 250 mm; mobile phase: 27% ethanol, 10 mM Na_2HPO_4, pH = 5.75; flow rate: 5 mL/min; see Figure 4 for a representative semipreparative HPLC trace). The peak corresponding to [^{11}C]AZ683 (t_R ~12–14 min) was collected, diluted in water (50 mL), and the resulting solution was passed through a Waters C18 1cc vac cartridge to trap the product. [^{11}C]AZ683 was eluted from the cartridge with ethanol (1 mL) and diluted with 0.9% saline solution (9 mL) to provide the formulated product in 10% EtOH. The dose was passed through a 0.22 µm sterile filter into a sterile dose vial. The overall non-decay corrected activity yield of [^{11}C]AZ683 was 1125 ± 229 MBq (3.0% based upon 37 GBq of [^{11}C]MeOTf) and quality control testing (see below) confirmed radiochemical purity >99%, and molar activity of 153 ± 38 GBq/µmol (n = 4), confirming doses were suitable for preclinical evaluation.

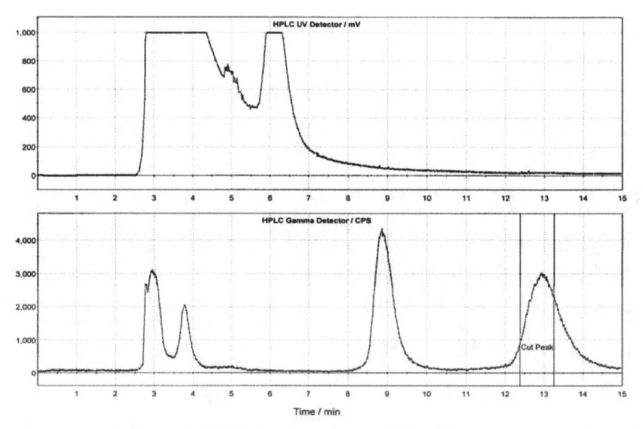

Figure 4. Typical semi-preparative HPLC trace for [^{11}C]AZ683.

3.2.3. Quality Control Testing of [^{11}C]AZ683

Visual inspection

Doses were visually examined and required to be clear, colorless, and free of particulate matter.

Dose pH

The pH of the doses was determined by applying a small amount of the dose to pH-indicator strips and determined by visual comparison to the scale provided. pH needs to be between 4.5 and 7.5, and the pH of each [^{11}C]AZ683 dose synthesized in this study was 5.0.

Analytical HPLC

Analytical HPLC was performed using a Shimadzu LC-2010A HT system equipped with a Bioscan B-FC-1000 radiation detector (column: Phenomenex Luna C18, 5µ, 4.6 × 150 mm; mobile phase: 27%

ethanol, 10 mM Na$_2$HPO$_4$, pH: 5.75; flow rate: 0.75 mL/min). Analysis confirmed radiochemical purity >99% (t$_R$ of [^{11}C]AZ683 ~6 min; see Figure 5 for a typical analytical HPLC trace) and coinjection with unlabeled reference standard **6a** confirmed radiochemical identity (see Figure 6 for a coinjection HPLC trace).

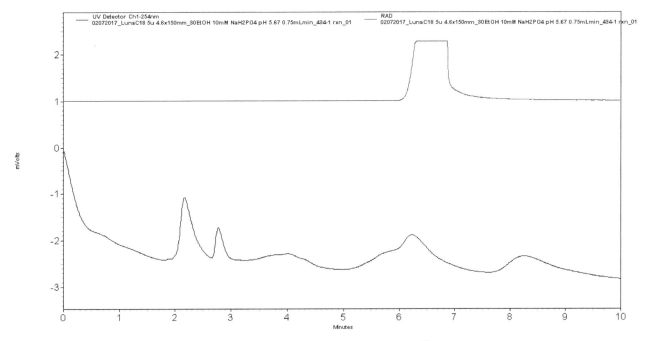

Figure 5. Analytical HPLC trace for formulated [^{11}C]AZ683 dose.

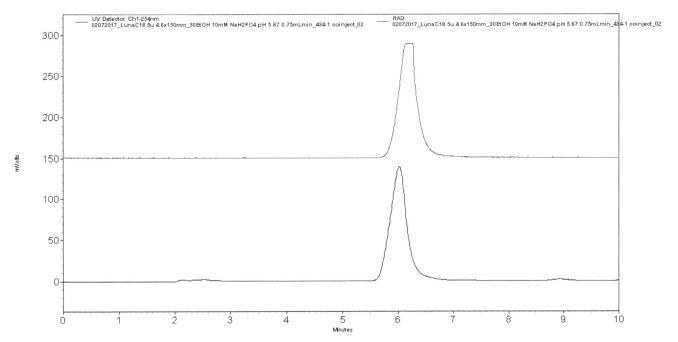

Figure 6. Analytical HPLC trace for formulated [^{11}C]AZ683 dose co-injected with AZ683 reference standard **6a**.

3.3. Preclinical PET Imaging

3.3.1. General Considerations

Rodent and primate imaging studies were performed at the Univiersity of Michigan (UM) using a Concorde (CTI-Concorde, Knoxville TN, USA) MicroPET P4 scanner. The University of Michigan is accredited by the Council on Accreditation of the Association for Assessment and Accreditation of Laboratory Animal Care (AAALAC International, Frederick MD, USA) and imaging studies were conducted in accordance with the standards set by the Institutional Animal Care and Use Committee (IACUC) at the University of Michigan (PRO00008103: Biodistribution and Pharmacokinetics of Radiolabeled Compounds; Approval date: 1/16/2018).

3.3.2. Animal Husbandry and Housing

Husbandry and housing for rodents and primates is provided by the University Laboratory for Animal Medicine (ULAM) at UM, and animal facilities are in compliance with the regulations defined by the US Department of Agriculture (USDA).

Monkeys: The University of Michigan PET Center has maintained 2 rhesus macaques for ~15 years and the monkeys are individually housed in adjacent steel cages (83.3 cm high × 152.4 cm wide × 78.8 cm deep) equipped with foraging boxes. They are currently housed in adjacent cages as repeated attempts to socially house them in the same cage have been unsuccessful due to aggressive incompatibility. Cages are metal and do contain gridded floors for radiation safety reasons (radioactive waste is contained to the gridded floor and is easier to clean). Temperature and humidity are carefully controlled, and the monkeys are kept on a 12 h light/12 h dark schedule. Monkeys are fed Lab Fiber Plus Monkey Diet (PMI Nutrition Intl. LLC, Shoreview MN, USA) that is supplemented with fresh fruit and vegetables daily. Water and enrichment toys (manipulanda and food-based treats) are available continuously in the home cage.

Rodents: Rats are housed in Allentown #3 micro ventilated cages (27 cm wide × 49 cm deep × 27 cm high, floor area 923 Sq cm) with animal housing densities set by ULAM and the Guide for the Care and Use of Laboratory Animals. Housing is located on ventilated racks with continuous water and air supply exchange. All animals are provided with LabDiet 5LOD as well as enrichment materials, and are on a light schedule of 12 h light/12 h dark.

3.3.3. Rodent Imaging Protocol

Rodent imaging studies were done using a female Sprague–Dawley rat (weight = 237 g, n = 1). The rat was anesthetized (isoflurane), intubated, and positioned in the PET scanner. Following a transmission scan, the animal was injected (via intravenous (*i.v.*) tail vein injection) with [^{11}C]AZ683 (14.8 MBq) as a bolus over 1 min, and the brain imaged for 60 min (5 × 1 min frames-2 × 2.5 min frames-2 × 5 min frames-4 × 10 min frames).

3.3.4. Primate Imaging Protocol

Primate imaging studies were done using a mature female rhesus monkey (weight = 9.4 kg, n = 1). The animal was anesthetized in the home cage with ketamine and transported to the PET imaging suite. The monkey was intubated for mechanical ventilation, and anesthesia was continued with isoflurane. Anesthesia was maintained throughout the duration of the PET scan. A venous catheter was inserted into one hind limb and the monkey was placed on the PET gantry with its head secured to prevent motion artifacts. Following a transmission scan, the animal was injected i.v. with [^{11}C]AZ683 (145.0 MBq) as a bolus over 1 min, and the brain imaged for 60 min (5 × 2 min frames-4 × 5 min frames-3 × 10 min frames).

3.3.5. PET Image Analysis

Emission data were corrected for attenuation and scatter, and reconstructed using the 3D maximum a priori (3D MAP) method. By using a summed image, regions of interest (ROI) were drawn on multiple planes, and the volumetric ROIs were then applied to the full dynamic data set to generate time-radioactivity curves.

4. Conclusions

In conclusion, we have developed a radiosynthesis of [^{11}C]AZ683 for PET imaging of CSF1R and neuroinflammation that provides doses suitable for preclinical use. However, preliminary preclinical PET imaging in rodents and nonhuman primates revealed low brain uptake of [^{11}C]AZ683. Overall, these PET imaging data suggest imaging CSF1R associated with neuroinflammation using [^{11}C]AZ683 could be challenging and emphasize that high affinity, good selectivity, and appropriate drug-like properties do not guarantee that a compound will make a good radiopharmaceutical for in vivo brain PET. Nevertheless, uptake in monkey could be sufficient to observe accumulation in a brain inflammation model. These studies also do not rule out labeling the scaffold with a longer-lived PET radionuclide (e.g., ^{18}F or ^{124}I) and using a prolonged infusion protocol to ensure that sufficient radiotracer accumulates at sites of inflammation for imaging and quantitation of CSF1R. [^{11}C]AZ683 could potentially also be used for imaging of peripheral CSF1R to evaluate its role in inflammation outside the brain. Future evaluation in animal models of inflammation appears warranted.

Author Contributions: Conceptualization: P.J.H.S. and A.V.M.; Investigation: S.S.T., X.S., J.S., J.A., P.S. and A.V.M.; Methodology: S.S.T., X.S. and A.V.M; Writing: S.S.T., P.J.H.S. and A.V.M.; Supervision: P.J.H.S.; Funding acquisition: P.J.H.S.

References

1. Verstraete, K.; Savvides, S.N. Extracellular assembly and activation principles of oncogenic class III receptor tyrosine kinases. *Nat. Rev. Cancer* **2012**, *12*, 753–766. [CrossRef] [PubMed]
2. Michell-Robinson Mackenzie, A.; Touil, H.; Healy Luke, M.; Durafourt Bryce, A.; Bar-Or, A.; Antel Jack, P.; Owen David, R.; Moore Craig, S. Roles of microglia in brain development, tissue maintenance and repair. *Brain* **2015**, *138 (Pt 5)*, 1138–1159. [CrossRef]
3. Nakamichi, Y.; Udagawa, N.; Takahashi, N. IL-34 and CSF-1: Similarities and differences. *J. Bone Miner. Metab.* **2013**, *31*, 486–495. [CrossRef] [PubMed]
4. El-Gamal, M.I.; Al-Ameen, S.K.; Al-Koumi, D.M.; Hamad, M.G.; Jalal, N.A.; Oh, C.-H. Recent advances of colony-stimulating factor-1 receptor (CSF-1R) kinase and its inhibitors. *J. Med. Chem.* **2018**, *61*, 5450–5466. [CrossRef] [PubMed]
5. Burns, C.J.; Wilks, A.F. c-FMS inhibitors: A patent review. *Expert Opin. Ther. Pat.* **2011**, *21*, 147–165. [CrossRef] [PubMed]
6. Spangenberg Elizabeth, E.; Lee Rafael, J.; Najafi Allison, R.; Rice Rachel, A.; Elmore Monica, R.P.; Blurton-Jones, M.; Green Kim, N.; West Brian, L. Eliminating microglia in Alzheimer's mice prevents neuronal loss without modulating amyloid-β pathology. *Brain* **2016**, *139 (Pt 4)*, 1265–1281. [CrossRef]
7. Olmos-Alonso, A.; Schetters Sjoerd, T.T.; Sri, S.; Askew, K.; Mancuso, R.; Perry, V.H.; Gomez-Nicola, D.; Vargas-Caballero, M.; Holscher, C. Pharmacological targeting of CSF1R inhibits microglial proliferation and prevents the progression of Alzheimer's-like pathology. *Brain* **2016**, *139 (Pt 3)*, 891–907. [CrossRef]
8. Asai, H.; Ikezu, S.; Tsunoda, S.; Medalla, M.; Luebke, J.; Haydar, T.; Wolozin, B.; Butovsky, O.; Kugler, S.; Ikezu, T. Depletion of microglia and inhibition of exosome synthesis halt tau propagation. *Nat. Neurosci.* **2015**, *18*, 1584–1593. [CrossRef]
9. Pyonteck, S.M.; Akkari, L.; Schuhmacher, A.J.; Bowman, R.L.; Sevenich, L.; Quail, D.F.; Olson, O.C.; Quick, M.L.; Huse, J.T.; Teijeiro, V.; et al. CSF-1R inhibition alters macrophage polarization and blocks glioma progression. *Nat. Med.* **2013**, *19*, 1264–1272. [CrossRef]
10. Coniglio, S.J.; Eugenin, E.; Dobrenis, K.; Stanley, E.R.; West, B.L.; Symons, M.H.; Segall, J.E. Microglial stimulation of glioblastoma invasion involves epidermal growth factor receptor (EGFR) and colony stimulating factor 1 receptor (CSF-1R) signaling. *Mol. Med.* **2012**, *18*, 519–527. [CrossRef]
11. von Tresckow, B.; Morschhauser, F.; Ribrag, V.; Topp, M.S.; Chien, C.; Seetharam, S.; Aquino, R.; Kotoulek, S.; de Boer, C.J.; Engert, A. An open-label, multicenter, phase I/II study of JNJ-40346527, a CSF-1R inhibitor, in patients with relapsed or refractory hodgkin lymphoma. *Clin. Cancer Res.* **2015** *21*, 1843–1850. [CrossRef]

12. Elmore Monica, R.P.; Lee Rafael, J.; Green Kim, N.; West Brian, L. Characterizing newly repopulated microglia in the adult mouse: Impacts on animal behavior, cell morphology, and neuroinflammation. *PLoS ONE* **2015**, *10*, e0122912. [CrossRef] [PubMed]

13. Patel, S.; Player, M.R. Colony-stimulating factor-1 receptor inhibitors for the treatment of cancer and inflammatory disease. *Curr. Top. Med. Chem.* **2009**, *9*, 599–610. [CrossRef] [PubMed]

14. Genovese Mark, C.; Hsia, E.; Belkowski Stanley, M.; Chien, C.; Masterson, T.; Thurmond Robin, L.; Manthey Carl, L.; Yan Xiaoyu, D.; Ge, T.; Franks, C.; et al. Results from a phase IIA parallel group study of JNJ-40346527, an oral CSF-1R inhibitor, in patients with active rheumatoid arthritis despite disease-modifying antirheumatic drug therapy. *J. Rheumatol.* **2015**, *42*, 1752–1760. [CrossRef] [PubMed]

15. Ries, C.H.; Cannarile, M.A.; Hoves, S.; Benz, J.; Wartha, K.; Runza, V.; Rey-Giraud, F.; Pradel, L.P.; Feuerhake, F.; Klaman, I.; et al. Targeting tumor-associated macrophages with anti-CSF-1R antibody reveals a strategy for cancer therapy. *Cancer Cell* **2014**, *25*, 846–859. [CrossRef] [PubMed]

16. Ota, T.; Urakawa, H.; Kozawa, E.; Ikuta, K.; Hamada, S.; Tsukushi, S.; Shimoyama, Y.; Ishiguro, N.; Nishida, Y. Expression of colony-stimulating factor 1 is associated with occurrence of osteochondral change in pigmented villonodular synovitis. *Tumor Biol.* **2015**, *36*, 5361–5367. [CrossRef] [PubMed]

17. Elmore, M.R.P.; Najafi, A.R.; Koike, M.A.; Dagher, N.N.; Spangenberg, E.E.; Rice, R.A.; Kitazawa, M.; Matusow, B.; Nguyen, H.; West, B.L.; et al. Colony-stimulating factor 1 receptor signaling is necessary for microglia viability, unmasking a microglia progenitor cell in the adult brain. *Neuron* **2014**, *82*, 380–397. [CrossRef] [PubMed]

18. Dagher, N.N.; Najafi, A.R.; Kayala, K.M.N.; Elmore, M.R.P.; White, T.E.; Medeiros, R.; Green, K.N.; West, B.L. Colony-stimulating factor 1 receptor inhibition prevents microglial plaque association and improves cognition in 3xTg-AD mice. *J. Neuroinflamm.* **2015**, *12*, 139. [CrossRef]

19. Turkheimer, F.; Rizzo, G.; Bloomfield, P.; Howes, O.; Zanotti-Fregonara, P.; Bertoldo, A.; Veronese, M. The methodology of TSPO imaging with positron emission tomography. *Biochem. Soc. Trans.* **2015**, *43*, 586–592. [CrossRef]

20. Bernard-Gauthier, V.; Schirrmacher, R. 5-(4-((4-[^{18}F]fluorobenzyl)oxy)-3-methoxybenzyl)pyrimidine-2, 4-diamine: A selective dual inhibitor for potential PET imaging of Trk/CSF-1R. *Bioorg. Med. Chem. Lett.* **2014**, *24*, 4784–4790. [CrossRef]

21. Naik, R.; Misheneva, V.; Minn, I.L.; Melnikova, T.; Mathews, W.; Dannals, R.; Pomper, M.; Savonenko, A.; Pletnikov, M.; Horti, A. PET tracer for imaging the macrophage colony stimulating factor receptor (CSF1R) in rodent brain. *J. Nucl. Med.* **2018**, *59* (Suppl. 1), 547.

22. Scott, D.A.; Balliet, C.L.; Cook, D.J.; Davies, A.M.; Gero, T.W.; Omer, C.A.; Poondru, S.; Theoclitou, M.-E.; Tyurin, B.; Zinda, M.J. Identification of 3-amido-4-anilinoquinolines as potent and selective inhibitors of CSF-1R kinase. *Bioorg. Med. Chem. Lett.* **2009**, *19*, 697–700. [CrossRef] [PubMed]

23. Scott, D.A.; Bell, K.J.; Campbell, C.T.; Cook, D.J.; Dakin, L.A.; Del Valle, D.J.; Drew, L.; Gero, T.W.; Hattersley, M.M.; Omer, C.A.; et al. 3-Amido-4-anilinoquinolines as CSF-1R kinase inhibitors 2: Optimization of the PK profile. *Bioorg. Med. Chem. Lett.* **2009**, *19*, 701–705. [CrossRef] [PubMed]

24. Scott, D.A.; Dakin, L.A.; Del Valle, D.J.; Diebold, R.B.; Drew, L.; Gero, T.W.; Ogoe, C.A.; Omer, C.A.; Repik, G.; Thakur, K.; et al. 3-Amido-4-anilinocinnolines as a novel class of CSF-1R inhibitor. *Bioorg. Med. Chem. Lett.* **2011**, *21*, 1382–1384. [CrossRef] [PubMed]

25. Shao, X.; Hoareau, R.; Runkle, A.C.; Tluczek, L.J.M.; Hockley, B.G.; Henderson, B.D.; Scott, P.J.H. Highlighting the versatility of the Tracerlab synthesis modules. Part 2: Fully automated production of [^{11}C]-labeled radiopharmaceuticals using a Tracerlab FXC-Pro. *J. Label. Compd. Radiopharm.* **2011**, *54*, 819–838. [CrossRef]

26. CSF1R. Available online: https://www.proteinatlas.org/ENSG00000182578-CSF1R/tissue (accessed on 26 November 2018).

27. Droin, N.; Solary, E. Editorial: CSF1R, CSF-1 and IL-34, a ménage à trois" conserved across vertebrates. *J. Leukoc. Biol.* **2010**, *87*, 745–747. [CrossRef] [PubMed]

28. Cammermeyer, J. The life history of the microglial cell: A light microscopic study. In *Neurosciences Research*, 1st ed.; Ehrenpreis, S., Solnitzky, O.C., Eds.; Academic Press: New York, NY, USA; London, UK, 1970; Volume 3, pp. 43–129.

29. Tiwari, A.K.; Ji, B.; Yui, J.; Fujinaga, M.; Yamasaki, T.; Xie, L.; Luo, R.; Shimoda, Y.; Kumata, K.; Zhang, Y.; et al. [^{18}F]FEBMP: Positron emission tomography imaging of TSPO in a model of neuroinflammation in rats, and in vivo autoradiograms of the human brain. *Theranostics* **2015**, *5*, 961–969. [CrossRef] [PubMed]

30. Sridharan, S.; Lepelletier, F.-X.; Trigg, W.; Banister, S.; Reekie, T.; Kassiou, M.; Gerhard, A.; Hinz, R.; Boutin, H. Comparative evaluation of three TSPO PET radiotracers in a LPS-induced model of mild neuroinflammation in rats. *Mol. Imaging Biol.* **2017**, *19*, 77–89. [CrossRef] [PubMed]

31. Pajouhesh, H.; Lenz, G. Medicinal chemical properties of succesful central nervous system drugs. *NeuroRX* **2005**, *2*, 541–553. [CrossRef] [PubMed]

32. cLogP and tSPA values were estimated using ChemDraw Professional 16.0 (PerkinElmer, Waltham, MA, USA) and pKa values were estimated using MarvinSketch (ChemAxon, Budapest, Hungary).

33. Chu, X.; Bleasby, K.; Evers, R. Species differences in drug transporters and implications for translating preclinical findings to humans. *Expert Opin. Drug Metab. Toxicol.* **2013**, *9*, 237–252. [CrossRef] [PubMed]

34. Fawaz, M.V.; Brooks, A.F.; Rodnick, M.E.; Carpenter, G.M.; Shao, X.; Desmond, T.J.; Sherman, P.; Quesada, C.A.; Hockley, B.G.; Kilbourn, M.R.; et al. High affinity radiopharmaceuticals based upon lansoprazole for PET imaging of aggregated tau in Alzheimer's disease and progressive supranuclear palsy: Synthesis, preclinical evaluation, and lead selection. *ACS Chem. Neurosci.* **2014**, *5*, 718–730. [CrossRef] [PubMed]

35. Yang, L.; Brooks, A.F.; Makaravage, K.J.; Zhang, H.; Sanford, M.S.; Scott, P.J.H.; Shao, X. Radiosynthesis of [^{11}C]LY2795050 for preclinical and clinical PET imaging using Cu(II)-mediated cyanation. *ACS Med. Chem. Lett.* **2018**, in press. [CrossRef]

17

2-Nitroimidazole-Furanoside Derivatives for Hypoxia Imaging—Investigation of Nucleoside Transporter Interaction, ^{18}F-Labeling and Preclinical PET Imaging

Florian C. Maier [1], Anna Schweifer [2,†], Vijaya L. Damaraju [3], Carol E. Cass [3], Gregory D. Bowden [1]◉, Walter Ehrlichmann [1], Manfred Kneilling [1,4], Bernd J. Pichler [1], Friedrich Hammerschmidt [2] and Gerald Reischl [1,*]

[1] Werner Siemens Imaging Center, Department of Preclinical Imaging and Radiopharmacy, Eberhard Karls University of Tübingen, Röntgenweg 13, 72076 Tübingen, Germany; florian.maier@med.uni-tuebingen.de (F.C.M.); gregory.bowden@med.uni-tuebingen.de (G.D.B.); walter.ehrlichmann@med.uni-tuebingen.de (W.E.); manfred.kneilling@med.uni-tuebingen.de (M.K.); bernd.pichler@med.uni-tuebingen.de (B.J.P.)

[2] Faculty of Chemistry, Institute of Organic Chemistry, University of Vienna, Währingerstraße 38, A-1090 Vienna, Austria; anna.schweifer@univie.ac.at (A.S.); friedrich.hammerschmidt@univie.ac.at (F.H.)

[3] Department of Oncology, University of Alberta, Edmonton, AB T6G 2R7, Canada; vd1@ualberta.ca (V.L.D.); ccass@ualberta.ca (C.E.C.)

[4] Department of Dermatology, Eberhard Karls University of Tübingen, 72076 Tübingen, Germany

* Correspondence: gerald.reischl@uni-tuebingen.de

† Deceased.

Abstract: The benefits of PET imaging of tumor hypoxia in patient management has been demonstrated in many examples and with various tracers over the last years. Although, the optimal hypoxia imaging agent has yet to be found, 2-nitroimidazole (azomycin) sugar derivatives—mimicking nucleosides—have proven their potential with [^{18}F]FAZA ([^{18}F]fluoro-azomycin-α-arabinoside) as a prominent representative in clinical use. Still, for all of these tracers, cellular uptake by passive diffusion is postulated with the disadvantage of slow kinetics and low tumor-to-background ratios. We recently evaluated [^{18}F]fluoro-azomycin-β-deoxyriboside (β-[^{18}F]FAZDR), with a structure more similar to nucleosides than [^{18}F]FAZA and possible interaction with nucleoside transporters. For a deeper insight, we comparatively studied the interaction of FAZA, β-FAZA, α-FAZDR and β-FAZDR with nucleoside transporters (SLC29A1/2 and SLC28A1/2/3) in vitro, showing variable interactions of the compounds. The highest interactions being for β-FAZDR (IC$_{50}$ 124 $\pm$ 33 µM for SLC28A3), but also for FAZA with the non-nucleosidic α-configuration, the interactions were remarkable (290 $\pm$ 44 µM {SLC28A1}; 640 $\pm$ 10 µM {SLC28A2}). An improved synthesis was developed for β-FAZA. For a PET study in tumor-bearing mice, α-[^{18}F]FAZDR was synthesized (radiochemical yield: 15.9 $\pm$ 9.0% (n = 3), max. 10.3 GBq, molar activity > 50 GBq/µmol) and compared to β-[^{18}F]FAZDR and [^{18}F]FMISO, the hypoxia imaging gold standard. We observed highest tumor-to-muscle ratios (TMR) for β-[^{18}F]FAZDR already at 1 h p.i. (2.52 $\pm$ 0.94, n = 4) in comparison to [^{18}F]FMISO (1.37 $\pm$ 0.11, n = 5) and α-[^{18}F]FAZDR (1.93 $\pm$ 0.39, n = 4), with possible mediation by the involvement of nucleoside transporters. After 3 h p.i., TMR were not significantly different for all 3 tracers (2.5–3.0). Highest clearance from tumor tissue was observed for β-[^{18}F]FAZDR (56.6 $\pm$ 6.8%, 2 h p.i.), followed by α-[^{18}F]FAZDR (34.2 $\pm$ 7.5%) and [^{18}F]FMISO (11.8 $\pm$ 6.5%). In conclusion, both isomers of [^{18}F]FAZDR showed their potential as PET hypoxia tracers. Differences in uptake behavior may be attributed to a potential variable involvement of transport mechanisms.

Keywords: tumor hypoxia; PET; small animal imaging; azomycin nucleosides; [^{18}F]FMISO

1. Introduction

Nowadays, the value of tumor hypoxia imaging for patient stratification, targeted and individualized therapy, and the monitoring thereof is undeniable [1–6]. The presence of tumor hypoxia is associated with increased tumor-aggressiveness, invasiveness, and therapy resistance [1,7,8]. While considerable effort has been made in the past decades, the full potential of hypoxia imaging, especially using specific tracers for positron emission tomography (PET) still has to be unraveled, as detection sensitivity, PET tracer target specificity, and the underlying molecular mechanisms by which these can be achieved are not entirely clear. Thus, there is still the need for optimization of hypoxia tracers; the mechanistic questions of the underlying principles of PET hypoxia tracer uptake and image contrast need to be answered as well. Of the numerous hypoxia tracer classes that have evolved, we investigated the class of 2-nitroimidazoles in the past, with a specific focus on ^{18}F-labeled 1-(5′-deoxy-5′-fluoro-α-D-arabinofuranosyl)-2-nitroimidazole ([^{18}F]FAZA) [9–13]. To date, the uptake mechanism of e.g. [^{18}F]FAZA has not been identified in detail, yet it is assumed to be via passive diffusion, as an alpha-configurated nucleoside derivative should not be transported actively. It has been conceptualized in the past [13–16] that uptake and retention of 2-nitroimidazole-sugars in hypoxic tumor tissue can be altered by permutation of both, sugar moiety and stereochemistry at the anomeric carbon atom (2-nitroimidazole linked)—with the rationale to take advantage of transport mechanisms involving nucleoside transporters. Involvement of nucleoside transporters in the tissue uptake-process of 2-nitroimidazole-sugars was only investigated recently with β-allofuranose as C_6-sugar [15]. Transport of nucleosides and nucleoside analog drugs is mediated by two unrelated protein families in humans, the SLC28 family of concentrative nucleoside transporters (hCNTs) and the SLC29 family of equilibrative nucleoside transporters (hENTs) [17]. The SLC28 family has three concentrative (hCNT1/2/3) members and the SLC29 family four equilibrative members (hENT1/2/3/4), respectively. The roles of human nucleoside transporters (hNTs) in transport of nucleosides and nucleoside drugs are summarized in recent reviews [18,19].

Here, we aimed at a systematic investigation of the interaction of selected 2-nitroimidazole-furanoses, resembling nucleoside analogs, with each of the five recombinant hNTs produced in a yeast model system (hENT1/2 and hCNT1/2/3). Transporters that may play a role in uptake of these nitroimidazoles into hypoxic tumor cells or normoxic control tissue like e.g. the muscle should be identified. The four compounds chosen for evaluation of their interaction with nucleoside transporters are found in Table 1, together with references to published data and the work list for the actual study. Besides the transporter interaction investigation, for β-FAZA, a novel synthesis route should be developed and for 1′-α-[2′,5′-dideoxy-5′-[^{18}F]fluoro-D-ribofuranosyl]-2-nitroimidazole (α-[^{18}F]FAZDR) ^{18}F-radiolabeling should be established. In subsequent small animal PET imaging in a well-established tumor hypoxia model (colon carcinoma mouse model), α-[^{18}F]FAZDR should be compared with [^{18}F]FMISO, the gold standard in PET imaging of hypoxia [20,21] and β-[^{18}F]FAZDR, of which positive PET imaging results have been recently obtained [13]. The *mouse* colon carcinoma model could be chosen, as mouse transporters exhibit close similarity to human nucleoside transporters [22]. With this comparative study, we sought to gain further insight into the importance and influence of the sugar moiety and configuration of 2-nitroimidazole at the anomeric carbon atom on tracer uptake and image contrast.

Table 1. 2-Nitroimidazole arabinose (FAZA) or deoxyribose (FAZDR) α-, β-derivatives with references to published data or to be investigated in this study (*), regarding transporter interaction, ^{18}F-radiolabeling and small animal PET imaging.

Compound	Transporter Interaction	^{18}F-Radiolabeling	PET *In Vivo* Data (^{18}F-Labeled; Small Animal Studies)
FAZA	*	[12]	[9–13]
β-FAZA	*	[14]	[14]
α-FAZDR	*	*	*
β-FAZDR	*	[13]	[13] and *

2. Results

2.1. Organic Chemistry

FAZA [23,24], α-FAZDR and β-FAZDR [13] were prepared by known procedures; for β-FAZA, a novel synthesis route was developed, although β-FAZA is a known compound [14]. Figure 1 gives the structures of the non-radioactive fluorinated 2-nitroimidazole sugars that were synthesized and evaluated for their interaction with human nucleoside transporters (see Section 2.3).

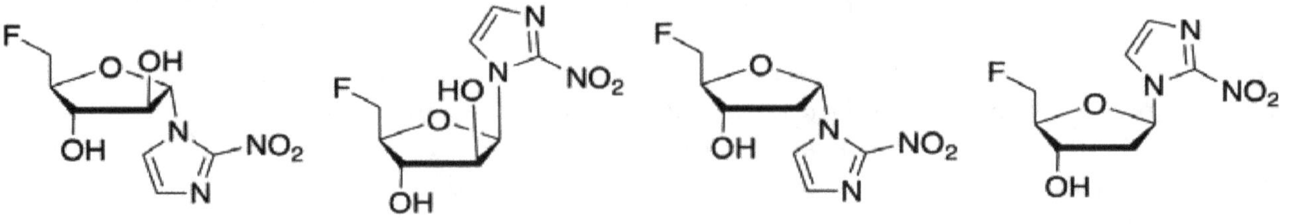

Figure 1. Chemical structures of the fluorinated 2-nitroimidazole C_5-sugars FAZA, β-FAZA and α-, β-FAZDR, synthesized and used in the investigation of their interaction with human nucleoside transporters.

An improved synthesis of the β-arabinose-derived nucleoside analog β-FAZA from the known starting material β-**1** (prepared as described by Kumar et al. [25]) was developed (Scheme 1). Selective silylation of the primary hydroxyl group at C-5′ with TBDMSCl/imidazole in pyridine, followed by acetylation, furnished crystalline and fully protected nucleoside β-**2** (80%). Bis(2-methoxyethyl)aminosulfur trifluoride [26] (Deoxo-Fluor®) converted it to 5′-fluoro nucleoside β-**3** in 80% yield. Deprotection with MeONa in MeOH gave the desired arabinose-derived nucleoside β-FAZA in 75%. β-FAZA was recently prepared by a different approach [14]. Here, we were able to improve the overall process compared to [14] by a reduction of synthetic steps (for initial reaction steps from the commercially available 1-β-D-(ribofuranosyl)-2-nitroimidazole, see [14,25]), overall reaction times, and an increase in yield to 48% for the three steps shown in Scheme 1, compared to 21% for the last three steps in [14]. The improvement was obviously due to the utilization of the commercial fluorination agent, Deoxo-Fluor®, in the penultimate step.

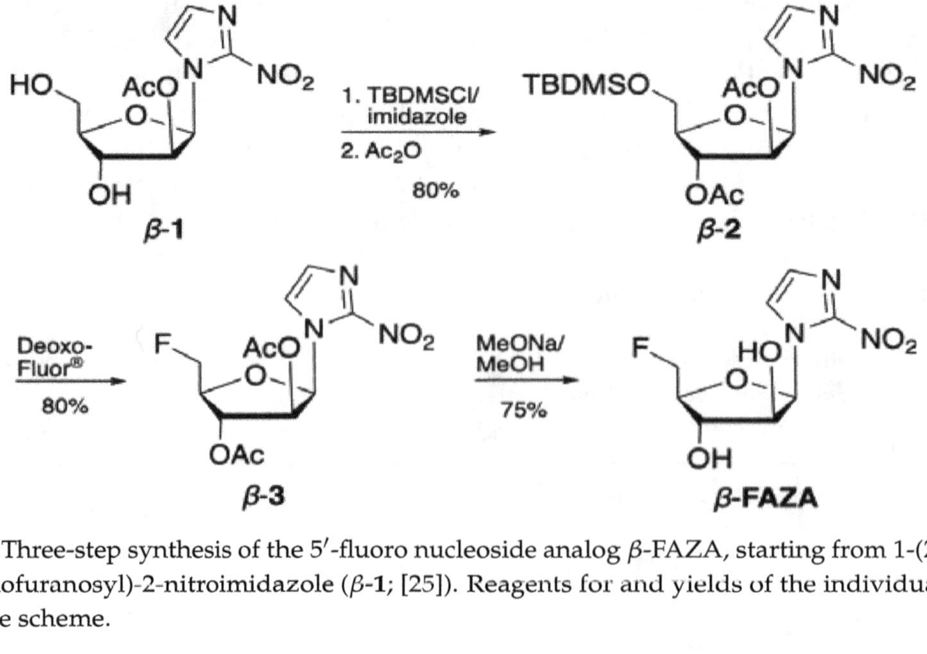

Scheme 1. Three-step synthesis of the 5′-fluoro nucleoside analog β-FAZA, starting from 1-(2′-O-acetyl-β-D-arabinofuranosyl)-2-nitroimidazole (β-**1**; [25]). Reagents for and yields of the individual steps are given in the scheme.

2.2. Radiochemistry

For a direct comparison with gold standard hypoxia PET imaging agent [^{18}F]FMISO and the recently evaluated beta-isomer β-[^{18}F]FAZDR [13] in a small-animal imaging study, alpha-ribofuranoside α-[^{18}F]FAZDR was synthesized.

Radiolabeling, hydrolysis, and purification were carried out similar to the synthesis of β-[^{18}F]FAZDR (Scheme 2). Radiochemistry was performed on the same automated synthesis module (TRACERlab FX$_{F-N}$, GE, non-cassette based) as for the other two PET tracers. Radiochemical yields were 15.9 $\pm$ 9.0% (n = 3) with higher variations compared to β-[^{18}F]FAZDR (10.9 $\pm$ 2.4%, n = 4, uncorrected for decay [13]). Maximum yield obtained was 10.3 GBq at the end of the synthesis. As these amounts were sufficient for the planned mouse experiments and quality of the product was also satisfactory, the process and reaction parameters were not optimized further.

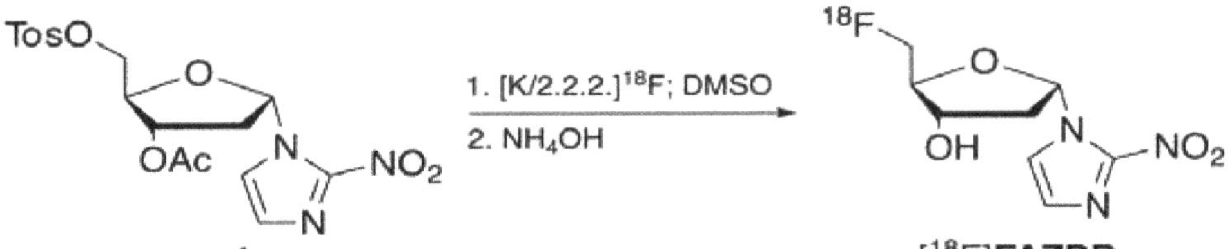

Scheme 2. Radiosynthesis of α-[^{18}F]FAZDR by nucleophilic substitution from the tosyl precursor α-1 and subsequent hydrolysis with NH$_4$OH.

Radiochemical (RCP) and chemical purity (CP) were determined using HPLC and TLC. The latter method showed RCP of α-[^{18}F]FAZDR of > 97%; in HPLC radiochromatograms, only the product peak was visible, corresponding to > 98% of RCP. With UV detection at 220 nm, only matrix peaks were visible (< 5 min retention time), with no other chemical impurities above the detection limit. The product solutions were always clear, colorless, and free of visible particles with a pH of 6.7 and a molar activity > 50 GBq/μmol.

2.3. Transporter Studies in Saccharomyces cerevisiae

The interaction of 2-nitroimidazole sugars with nucleoside transporters was determined by ability of the 2-nitroimidazole sugars to inhibit [^{3}H]uridine uptake in yeast cells producing recombinant human nucleoside transporters and results expressed as IC$_{50}$ values. Among the four compounds tested, only the β-sugar compounds inhibited hENT1 and hENT2 (SLC29A1/2), but at high concentrations. For FAZA and α-FAZDR, no interaction was detected. β-FAZDR inhibited hCNT1 (SLC28A1) and hCNT3 (SLC28A3) potently with IC$_{50}$ values of 269 $\pm$ 4 μM and 124 $\pm$ 33 μM, respectively. FAZA inhibited hCNT1 with an IC$_{50}$ value of 290 $\pm$ 44 μM and FAZA was the only compound to show considerable inhibitory activity against hCNT2 (SLC28A2) with an IC$_{50}$ value of 640 $\pm$ 10 μM. Individual IC$_{50}$ values for all compounds and investigated transporters are summarized in Table 2.

In summary, FAZA inhibited [^{3}H]uridine transport by hCNT1 and hCNT2, in contrast to the commonly accepted theory of FAZA entering cells by passive diffusion. Although some of the compounds inhibited [^{3}H]uridine uptake by nucleoside transporters, transporter interaction does not necessarily imply transport through the cell membrane. To confirm this uptake, experiments with the corresponding radioactive compounds needed to be undertaken, which was not possible here, due to their lack of availability. Keeping this in mind, it is nevertheless possible that our results challenge the current understanding of FAZA image contrast, as tumor-type dependent transporter expression might especially alter the early-phase uptake in tumor tissue and contribute to PET signal heterogeneity. This should be clarified in additional studies in the future. In contrast to FAZA, β-FAZA with the nucleosidic β-configuration showed weak interaction with the nucleoside transporters. Among the tested compounds, β-FAZDR showed best inhibition of uridine uptake by hCNT1 and hCNT3, while

α-FAZDR showed no interaction with any transporter. Thus, both the deoxyribose sugar moiety and the β-configuration of the 2-nitroimidazole at the anomeric carbon atom are important molecular properties, if nucleoside transporter mediated uptake is envisaged in order to obtain higher TMR at early imaging time-points.

Table 2. Inhibition of [^{3}H]uridine transport by the 2-nitroimidazole sugar compounds in yeast cells producing each of the five recombinant hNTs in concentration-effect experiments, as described in Methods. IC_{50} values (calculated from dose-response curves) are presented as the mean $\pm$ SE for $n = 2$–3 experiments. (NI = no interaction).

Compound	hENT1 (SLC29A1)	hENT2 (SLC29A2)	hCNT1 (SLC28A1)	hCNT2 (SLC28A2)	hCNT3 (SLC28A3)
			IC_{50} (μM)		
FAZA	NI	NI	290 ± 44	640 ± 10	1385 ± 100
β-FAZA	2070 ± 50	>3000	>3000	>3000	2309 ± 352
β-FAZDR	NI	>3000	269 ± 4	NI	124 ± 33
α-FAZDR	NI	NI	NI	NI	NI

2.4. PET Hypoxia Imaging of CT26 Colon Carcinoma Bearing Mice

To build upon both, the obtained results from transporter studies in *Saccharomyces cerevisiae* and our recently published data on β-[^{18}F]FAZDR PET imaging, we subsequently performed small animal hypoxia imaging with α-[^{18}F]FAZDR and β-[^{18}F]FAZDR in comparison with the clinical gold standard [^{18}F]FMISO in CT26 colon carcinoma bearing BALB/c mice, a well-characterized tumor model for imaging hypoxia ([9,11,13], Figure 2A). Here, we were especially interested in the direct comparison of α-[^{18}F]FAZDR and β-[^{18}F]FAZDR, as the 2-nitroimidazole position at the anomeric carbon atom of 2-deoxyribofuranoside proved to be of importance for nucleoside transporter interaction.

First, we quantified [^{18}F]FMISO uptake in hypoxic tumor tissue and in normoxic muscle tissue. While [^{18}F]FMISO uptake was not significantly different at 1 h p.i. between tumor and muscle tissue (tumor: 2.49 ± 0.88 %ID/cc, muscle: 1.81 ± 0.58 %ID/cc), also reflected by the low TMR at 1 h p.i. (1.37 ± 0.11, $n = 5$), we obtained significantly higher uptake in tumors at 2 h and 3 h p.i. (Figure 2B,C). In direct comparison, we then investigated α-[^{18}F]FAZDR (Figure 2A), where we expected hypoxia targeting in tumor tissue, but no major involvement of nucleoside transporters regarding tissue uptake. α-[^{18}F]FAZDR-TMR at 1 h p.i. were higher (however, not significantly different) compared to TMR of [^{18}F]FMISO at 1 h p.i. (α-[^{18}F]FAZDR: 1.93 ± 0.39, $n = 4$; [^{18}F]FMISO: 1.37 ± 0.11, $n = 5$; Figure 2B). Furthermore, α-[^{18}F]FAZDR showed a significantly higher uptake in tumor tissue at 1 h, 2 h and at 3 h p.i. (1 h p.i. tumor: *1.90 ± 0.48 %ID/cc, muscle: *1.01 ± 0.32 %ID/cc; 3 h p.i. tumor: *0.88 ± 0.42 %ID/cc, muscle: *0.31 ± 0.15 %ID/cc; $n = 4$, * $p < 0.05$, Figure 2D). While the washout from both, tumor and muscle tissue of [^{18}F]FMISO was limited, we observed an increased washout for α-[^{18}F]FAZDR from both, tumor and muscle tissue (Figure 2D).

Next, we investigated β-[^{18}F]FAZDR uptake and TMR. In good accordance with data recently published by us [13], we could again show a substantial washout of β-[^{18}F]FAZDR from both, tumor and muscle tissue (Figure 2E). Furthermore, β-[^{18}F]FAZDR was characterized by a significantly higher TMR in comparison to [^{18}F]FMISO at 1 h p.i. (Figure 2B). From 0.40 ± 0.07 %ID/cc at 1 h p.i., the tumor uptake decreased to 0.18 ± 0.06 %ID/cc at 2 h p.i. and to 0.12 ± 0.05 %ID/cc at 3 h p.i., while normoxic muscle uptake decreased from the initially measured 0.17 ± 0.03 %ID/cc at 1 h p.i. to 0.07 ± 0.01 %ID/cc at 2 h p.i. and to 0.04 ± 0.01 %ID/cc at 3 h p.i. ($n = 4$, Figure 2E). This reproduced the results obtained in [13], also with regards to the TMR, which were 2.52 ± 0.94 at 1 h p.i., 2.65 ± 0.87 at 2 h p.i. and 2.91 ± 1.01 at 3 h p.i. ($n = 4$).

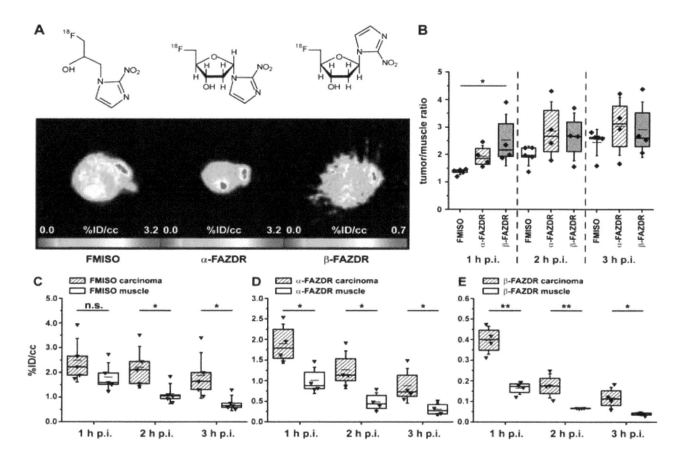

Figure 2. Exemplary structures and PET images of [^{18}F]FMISO, α-[^{18}F]FAZDR and β-[^{18}F]FAZDR in carcinoma tissue 1 h p.i. (**A**), calculated tumor-to-muscle ratios (TMR) are shown in **B**. β-[^{18}F]FAZDR (n = 4) displayed significantly higher TMR in comparison to [^{18}F]FMISO (n = 5) 1 h p.i. (**B**), while α-[^{18}F]FAZDR-TMR (n = 4) were not significantly different at any time-point. [^{18}F]FMISO displayed significantly higher uptake in carcinomas vs. muscles only at 2 h and 3 h p.i. (**C**), while α-[^{18}F]FAZDR and β-[^{18}F]FAZDR at all measured time-points (1 h, 2 h and 3 h p.i.). * p < 0.05, ** p < 0.01 (**D,E**).

To get a deeper understanding of this body of data, we also calculated tumor and muscle clearance for [^{18}F]FMISO, α-[^{18}F]FAZDR and β-[^{18}F]FAZDR at 2 h and 3 h p.i. relative to 1 h p.i. Tumor clearance for [^{18}F]FMISO was calculated to 11.8 $\pm$ 6.5% at 2 h p.i. (muscle clearance at 2 h p.i. 37.2 $\pm$ 4.3%) and to 26.9 $\pm$ 10.1% at 3 h p.i. (muscle clearance at 3 h p.i. 58.6 $\pm$ 3.3%, n = 5, Figure 3A); tumor clearance was significantly lower than muscle clearance for [^{18}F]FMISO (p < 0.01). In direct comparison to [^{18}F]FMISO, we observed higher tumor and muscle clearance rates for α-[^{18}F]FAZDR (Figure 3B). Tumor clearance for α-[^{18}F]FAZDR amounted to 34.2 $\pm$ 7.5% at 2 h p.i. (muscle clearance at 2 h p.i. 53.3 $\pm$ 8.3%) and to 55.3 $\pm$ 8.3% at 3 h p.i. (muscle clearance at 3 h p.i. 70.3 $\pm$ 5.5%, n = 4, Figure 3B) with significantly higher clearance rates from normoxic muscle tissue (p < 0.05). Finally, we quantified clearance rates for β-[^{18}F]FAZDR, which turned out to be not significantly different between tumor and muscle tissue, reproducing our previously published results [13]. Overall, β-[^{18}F]FAZDR tumor clearance was 56.6 $\pm$ 6.8% at 2 h p.i. (muscle clearance at 2 h p.i. 58.4 $\pm$ 8.2%) and 71.5 $\pm$ 7.0% at 3 h p.i. (muscle clearance at 3 h p.i. 75.3 $\pm$ 6.4%, n = 4, Figure 3C).

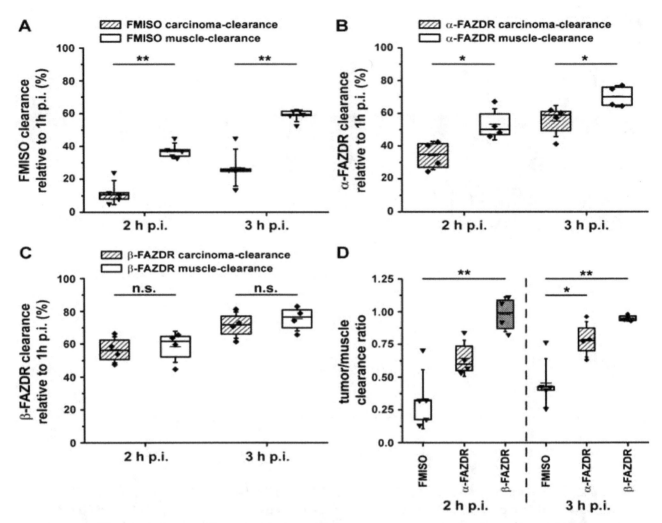

Figure 3. [^{18}F]FMISO clearance was significantly different from carcinoma and muscle tissue ($n = 5$, **A**), however lower in comparison to clearance rates from both tissues for α-[^{18}F]FAZDR ($n = 4$, **B**) and β-[^{18}F]FAZDR ($n = 4$, **C**). Tumor/muscle-clearance ratios were significantly lower for [^{18}F]FMISO in comparison to β-[^{18}F]FAZDR at 2 h p.i. and to both, α-[^{18}F]FAZDR and β-[^{18}F]FAZDR at 3 h p.i. * $p < 0.05$, ** $p < 0.01$ (**D**).

Next, we calculated clearance ratios for tumor relative to muscle tissue at 2 h and 3 h p.i. for a direct comparison between [^{18}F]FMISO, α-[^{18}F]FAZDR and β-[^{18}F]FAZDR. Here, clearance ratios well below unity indicate higher clearance from muscle tissue, unity indicates equal clearance rates for both tumor and muscle tissue, and clearance ratios bigger than unity indicate higher clearance rates from tumor tissue. The latter case was not expected, as this would likely be the case for a rather hypoxia-unspecific tracer. Fitting the results of tracer-specific uptake behavior, TMR and clearance rates, [^{18}F]FMISO showed the lowest clearance ratios (*, **0.45 ± 0.17, $n = 5$, 3 h p.i.), followed by α-[^{18}F]FAZDR (*0.79 ± 0.12, $n = 4$, 3 h p.i.) and β-[^{18}F]FAZDR with unitary clearance ratios (**0.95 ± 0.02, $n = 4$, 3 h p.i., * $p < 0.05$, ** $p < 0.01$, Figure 3D).

Conclusively, we observed the highest TMR for β-[^{18}F]FAZDR at 1 h p.i. in comparison to [^{18}F]FMISO and α-[^{18}F]FAZDR, most probably mediated by the involvement of nucleoside transporters (Figure 2B). However, β-[^{18}F]FAZDR was also characterized by the lowest net uptake in both tumor and muscle tissue in direct comparison with [^{18}F]FMISO and α-[^{18}F]FAZDR (Figure 2C–E), while [^{18}F]FMISO- and α-[^{18}F]FAZDR-uptake were comparable. Further confirming these findings, clearance rates from tumor tissue (and tumor-to-muscle clearance ratios) were lowest for [^{18}F]FMISO, followed by α-[^{18}F]FAZDR and β-[^{18}F]FAZDR.

3. Discussion

While a lot of effort has been put in the development of hypoxia specific PET tracers (based on 2-nitroimidazole as hypoxia-selective moiety), and a wealth of studies indicate both hypoxia specificity and added value for patient stratification and treatment monitoring [1–6]; the exact image contrast generating mechanisms are still poorly understood. While the commonly accepted underlying theory assumes trapping of 2-nitroimidazole-based PET tracers in hypoxic tissue and washout from normoxic control tissue [12,23,27], a plethora of studies (both clinical and preclinical) have demonstrated that this is most probably not the only mechanism explaining the obtained image contrast for various 2-nitroimidazole-based PET tracers in diverse tumor-entities [9,13,28–31]. Especially, the fact that PET tracer kinetics of 2-nitroimidazole-based compounds can indicate both reversible or irreversible uptake in patients with the selfsame tumor type, e.g. head and neck cancer, challenges the concept of hypoxia-selective trapping [31]. This ambiguous behavior was also observed by others in both mouse and man [28,32,33]. Substantial tumor and muscle washout could recently be observed by us for both $[^{18}F]$FAZA [9] and β-$[^{18}F]$FAZDR [13]. While rapid washout from normoxic control tissue (in this case muscle tissue) was anticipated, we were again struck by the high washout rates from hypoxic tumor tissue, especially for β-$[^{18}F]$FAZDR, and also, to a lesser extent, α-$[^{18}F]$FAZDR. However, for both α-$[^{18}F]$FAZDR and $[^{18}F]$FMISO, the clearance ratios indicate lower tumor clearance, fitting the common theory of the underlying principle of a hypoxia-detecting PET tracer. But, although the unitary clearance ratios imply it, this does not conclude that β-$[^{18}F]$FAZDR is not a valid hypoxia marker. In fact, we could recently prove the tumor hypoxia specificity of β-$[^{18}F]$FAZDR [13]. Thus, one could conclude from this body of data that hypoxia tracer image contrast consists of three different components, which are theoretically influenced by the contribution of nucleoside transporters (detailed analysis of hypoxia tracer kinetic modeling complexity can be found in [30]): (i) Free tracer in tissue or in the fractional blood volume of target and reference tissue, (ii) non-specifically bound in target and reference tissue, and (iii) specifically bound or trapped in target tissue. Looking at all examined time-points (1 h, 2 h and 3 h p.i.), the in vivo behavior of the 2-nitroimidazole tracers we used in this study, ($[^{18}F]$FMISO, α-$[^{18}F]$FAZDR and β-$[^{18}F]$FAZDR), could be explained by reversible kinetics. However, theoretically, if the sum of free and non-specifically bound tracer in target tissue is higher than the actual specific binding in target tissue, the observed clearance could be dominated by the washout of the non-specific or free tracer, while the specific fraction of the PET signal does not necessarily need to be reversible to generate the observed contrast; this could also be caused by a smaller fraction of irreversible binding. In addition, nucleoside transporters actively contribute to early and, thus also to late PET image contrast. While we cannot draw conclusions on the dominance of free, non-specific or specific fractions, we can conclude that nucleoside transporters definitely influence image contrast, especially early image contrast, here at 1 h p.i. Furthermore, the hypoxia specificity of α-$[^{18}F]$FAZDR could be indirectly proven in this manuscript, as α-$[^{18}F]$FAZDR-uptake perfectly resembled β-$[^{18}F]$FAZDR-uptake in the same tumor, imaged on consecutive days (Figure 2A).

We additionally validated this finding by an exemplary scan of one CT26 colon carcinoma bearing mouse with $[^{18}F]$FAZA, α-$[^{18}F]$FAZDR and β-$[^{18}F]$FAZDR on three consecutive days (Figure 4), displaying very similar uptake patterns. This can be concluded as the hypoxia selectivity of β-$[^{18}F]$FAZDR, as recently shown by us [13], while $[^{18}F]$FAZA hypoxia selectivity was shown by us and others in a plethora of publications [1,5,7,9,10,12,13,28,29,31]. In perfect concordance with the transporter data from this study, TMR at 1 h p.i. were highest for β-$[^{18}F]$FAZDR, probably due to the involvement of nucleoside transporters.

Conclusively, the exact mechanism generating 2-nitroimidazole PET hypoxia tracer image contrast is still elusive, while we add knowledge on stereochemistry-dependent involvement of nucleoside transporters regarding both early and late PET signals of 2-nitroimidazole-sugars. For the first time, we could show an interaction of FAZA with nucleoside transporters, thus cellular FAZA-uptake may not solely be attributable to passive diffusion—although our results still need to be taken with caution, as interaction might not necessarily be related to active transport. These findings open up novel avenues for hypoxia imaging and might help clarifying the underlying principles of hypoxia imaging.

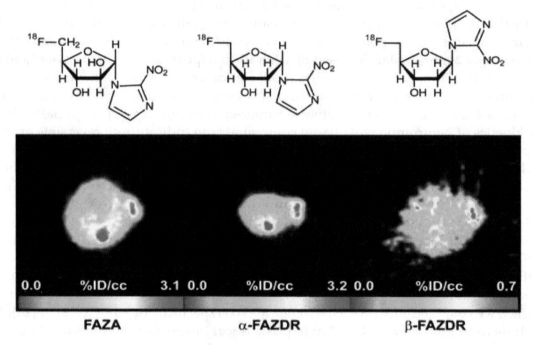

Figure 4. Exemplary scan of one CT26 colon carcinoma-bearing mouse with [18F]FAZA, α-[18F]FAZDR and β-[18F]FAZDR on three consecutive days, along with structures of used hypoxia tracers.

4. Materials and Methods

4.1. General

Acetonitrile for azeotropic drying before 18F-radiolabeling was from Merck (DNA synthesis grade, Darmstadt, Germany). Dimethylsulfoxide (DMSO, dried over molecular sieves) as solvent for labeling was used from Fluka (Germany). Kryptofix 2.2.2. was purchased from Merck.

FAZA [23,24], the precursor [13] for radiosynthesis of α-[18F]FAZDR (1-(3′-O-acetyl-2′-deoxy-5′-O-p-toluenesulfonyl-α-D-ribofuranosyl)-2-nitroimidazole (α-1)), α-FAZDR and β-FAZDR [13] were prepared by known procedures. All other chemicals and solvents (either Fluka or Merck) were of the highest purity available and used as received. Deuterated solvents were ordered from Eurisotop GmbH (Saarbrücken, Germany).

1H and 13C NMR spectra (J-modulated except for 2-nitroimidazole derivatives) were obtained from compounds dissolved in CDCl3, acetone-d6, and MeOH-d4 at 300 K using a Bruker AV 400 (1H: 400.13 MHz and 13C: 100.61 MHz) spectrometer. Chemical shifts were referenced to residual CHCl3 ($\delta_H = 7.24$), CDCl3 ($\delta_C = 77.00$), residual CHD2C(O)CD3 ($\delta_H = 2.05$), CD3C(O)CD3 ($\delta_C = 30.50$), residual CHD2OD ($\delta_H = 3.31$) and CD3OD ($\delta_C = 49.00$). IR spectra were measured of films on a silicon disk [34] or in ATR mode on a Bruker VERTEX 70 IR spectrometer. Optical rotations were measured at 20 °C on a PerkinElmer 351 polarimeter in a 1 dm cell. TLC was carried out on 0.25 mm thick precoated Merck plates; silica gel 60 F_{254}. Flash (column) chromatography was performed with Merck silica gel 60 (230–400 mesh). Spots were visualized by UV and/or dipping the plate into a solution of $(NH_4)_6Mo_7O_{24} \cdot 4H_2O$ (23.0 g) and of $Ce(SO_4)_2 \cdot 4H_2O$ (1.0 g) in 10% aqueous H_2SO_4 (500 mL), followed by heating with a heat gun. Melting points were determined on a Reichert Thermovar instrument and were uncorrected.

4.2. Synthesis of 1-(5'-Deoxy-5'-fluoro-β-D-arabinofuranosyl)-2-nitroimidazole (β-FAZA)

1-(5'-tert.-Butyldimethylsilyl-2',3'-di-O-acetyl-β-D-arabinofuranosyl)-2-nitroimidazole (β-2): A solution of TBDMSCl (0.068 g, 0.45 mmol, 1.1 equiv.) in dry pyridine (1.43 mL) was added to a mixture of 1-(2'-O-acetyl-β-D-arabinofuranosyl)-2-nitroimidazole (β−1; [25]) (0.118 g, 0.41 mmol) and imidazole (0.056 g, 0.82 mmol, 2 equiv.) at –20 °C under argon atmosphere. The mixture was stirred and allowed to warm to room temperature in the cooling bath within 18 h before Ac_2O (0.27 mL) was added. After 1 h and addition of water (10 mL) and stirring for 15 min, the reaction mixture was extracted with EtOAc (3 × 7 mL). The combined organic layers were dried ($MgSO_4$) and concentrated under reduced pressure. The residue was dried at 0.5 mbar and flash chromatographed (hexanes/EtOAc = 2:1, R_f = 0.56) to yield silylated and acetylated nucleoside β-2 (0.145 g, 80%) as colorless crystals; mp. 93–94 °C (iPr_2O, cooling from +50 °C to +4 °C); $[\alpha]_D^{20}$ = +77.8 (c = 1.07, acetone). IR (Si): ν = 2931, 2858, 1754, 1542, 1482, 1370, 1239, 1098 cm^{-1}; ^1H NMR (400.13 MHz, $CDCl_3$): δ = 7.79 (d, J = 1.1 Hz, 1H), 7.13 (d, J = 1.1 Hz, 1H), 6.79 (d, J = 5.3 Hz, 1H), 5.73 (dd, J = 5.3, 4.3 Hz, 1H), 5.36 (dd, J = 5.8, 4.3 Hz, 1H), 4.11 (td, J = 5.8, 3.4 Hz, 1H), 3.92 (AB part of ABX system, J_{AB} = 11.4 Hz, J_{AX} = J_{BX} = 3.4 Hz, 2H), 2.08 (s, 3H), 1.79 (s, 3H), 0.92 (s, 9 H), 0.11 (s, 3H), 0.106 (s, 3H) ppm; ^{13}C NMR (100.61 MHz, $CDCl_3$): δ = 169.6, 168.6, 144.4, 128.1, 123.2, 86.7, 82.3, 75.0, 73.9, 61.3, 25.8 (3C), 20.6, 20.0, 18.3, −5.5, −5.6 ppm. Analysis calcd for $C_{18}H_{29}N_3O_8Si$ (443.53): C, 48.75%; H, 6.59%; N, 9.47%: Found: C, 48.73%, H, 6.49%; N, 9.42%.

1-(2',3'-Di-O-acetyl-5'-O-deoxy-5'-fluoro-β-D-arabinofuranosyl)-2-nitroimidazole (β-3): A solution of 1-(5'-tert.-butyldimethylsilyl-2',3'-di-O-acetyl-β-D-arabinofuranosyl)-2-nitroimidazole (β-2) (0.117 g, 0.264 mmol) and Deoxo-Fluor® (0.22 mL, 0.528 mmol, 2 equiv., 50% in toluene) in dry 1,2-dichloroethane (0.23 mL) was stirred and heated at 75–80 °C under argon for 2 h. The mixture was cooled at 0 °C, diluted with a saturated aqueous solution of $NaHCO_3$ (10 mL) and extracted with EtOAc (3 × 10 mL). The combined organic layers were dried (Na_2SO_4) and concentrated under reduced pressure. The residue was flash chromatographed (hexanes/EtOAc = 2:1, R_f = 0.23) to give 5'-fluoro nucleoside β-3 (0.070 g, 80%) as colorless needles; mp. 113–114 °C ($CHCl_3$/iPr_2O, +50 °C to −27 °C) (lit.: 112–114 °C [14]); $[\alpha]_D^{20}$ = +62.4 (c = 0.75, acetone). IR (Si): ν = 3163, 2992, 1758, 1542, 1483, 1369, 1232, 1055 cm^{-1}. The NMR spectroscopic data are in agreement with those in the literature [14]. Analysis calculated for $C_{12}H_{14}FN_3O_7$ (331.26): C, 43.51%; H, 4.26%; N, 12.69. Found: C, 43.59%, H, 4.13%; N, 12.60%.

1-(5'-Deoxy-5'-fluoro-β-D-arabinofuranosyl)-2-nitroimidazole (β-FAZA): A solution of MeONa in MeOH (1.7 mL, 0.2 M) was added to a solution of protected fluoro arabino nucleoside β-3 (0.061 g, 0.184 mmol) in dry MeOH (2.7 mL) under argon at −20 °C. After stirring for 45 min at that temperature, the solution was neutralized with AcOH and concentrated under reduced pressure. The residue was flash chromatographed (hexanes/EtOAc = 1:2, R_f = 0.34) to furnish fluoro nucleoside β-FAZA (0.034 g, 75%) as yellowish crystals; mp. 148 °C decomp. (MeOH/iPr_2O, cooling to −18 °C); $[\alpha]_D^{20}$ = +142.2 (c = 0.69, MeOH). IR (ATR): ν = 3175, 1536, 1482, 1352, 1250, 1158, 1098, 1075, 1043, 1021 cm^{-1}. The NMR spectroscopic data are in agreement with those in the literature [14]. Analysis calcd for $C_8H_{10}FN_3O_5$ (247.18): C, 38.87%; H, 4.08%; N, 17.00%. Found: C, 38.89%, H, 3.95%; N, 16.94%.

4.3. Radiosynthetic Procedures

[18F]FMISO was synthesized according to [35] and [18F]FAZA, β-[18F]FAZDR following [13].

For synthesis of α-[18F]FAZDR, a TRACERlab FX_{F-N} automated system (GE Healthcare, Münster, Germany) was used. [18F]Fluoride was produced at a PETtrace cyclotron (GE Healthcare, Uppsala, Sweden) in a niobium target body from [18O]water (Rotem, Israel) via the $^{18}O(p,n)^{18}F$ nuclear reaction and beam currents of 35 μA. The [18F]fluoride was trapped on a Sep-Pak Light Accell Plus QMA anion exchange cartridge (Waters, USA, preconditioning: 10 mL 1 N aqueous $NaHCO_3$, 10 mL H_2O, 5 mL acetonitrile, 10 mL air). Subsequently, radioactivity was eluted with a mixture of 900 μL of acetonitrile and 100 μL of water containing 3.5 mg (25 μmol) of potassium carbonate and 15 mg (40 μmol) of Kryptofix 2.2.2. The solvent was evaporated (vacuum ca. 12 mbar) at 70 °C for 7 min and then at

120 °C for another 7 min. Labeling was carried out after addition of 5 mg of precursor (α-1) in 1 mL of DMSO at 70 °C for 5 min. After cooling to ca. 40 °C, 1 mL of 0.2 N NH$_4$OH was added for hydrolysis (10 min). The reaction mixture was neutralized using 0.5 mL of 0.2 N NaH$_2$PO$_4$ and injected onto the semi-preparative HPLC column for purification. A Luna C18(2) 250 × 10 mm, 5 µm (Phenomenex, Aschaffenburg, Germany) and a mixture of 8% ethanol in 10 mM Na$_2$HPO$_4$ (v/v) as eluent were used. The product was eluted with a retention time of 24 min (k' = 9.8; flow rate 5 mL/min), detected by UV (220 nm) and a radio detector. Product volume was ca. 5–7 mL. Finally, the product was sterile filtered through a 0.22 µm filter (Millex-GS, Millipore, USA). Overall synthesis time was 65 min. Activity was determined and a sample taken for quality control.

Identity, radiochemical and chemical purity of α-[^{18}F]FAZDR were determined using an analytical HPLC system with a Phenomenex Luna C18(2) column (250 × 4.6 mm, 5 µm); eluent was 5% acetonitrile in water (v/v) and flow rate 2 mL/min. HPLC eluate was monitored by radio- and UV detector (220 nm) in series. In this system, the product eluted with a retention time of 27 min (k' = 26). Radio-TLC was performed on silica gel plates (POLYGRAM SIL G/UV$_{254}$, 40 × 80 mm, Macherey&Nagel, Düren, Germany) with ethylacetate as eluent. For analysis, a phosphor imager (Cyclone Plus, PerkinElmer, Rodgau, Germany) was used, showing an R$_f$-value between 0.57–0.64 for the product.

4.4. Transporter Studies in Saccharomyces cerevisiae

Saccharomyces cerevisiae yeast was separately transformed with plasmids (pYPhENT1, pYPhENT2, pYPhCNT1, pYPhCNT2, or pYPhCNT3) encoding hNTs (hENT1, hENT2, hCNT1, hCNT2, or hCNT3, respectively) as described elsewhere [36,37]. Uptake of 1 µmol/L [^{3}H]uridine (Moravek Biochemicals) into yeast was measured as previously described [37,38] using a semi-automated cell harvester (Micro96 HARVESTER; Skatron Instruments, Tranby, Norway). Yeast was incubated at room temperature with 1 µmol/L [^{3}H]uridine in yeast growth media (pH 7.4) in the presence or absence (uninhibited controls) of graded concentrations (0-3 mM) of test compounds. The following compounds were used for transporter experiments: FAZA, β-FAZA, α-FAZDR, β-FAZDR. Uridine self-inhibition was used to determine maximum inhibition of mediated transport. Concentration–effect curves were subjected to nonlinear regression analysis using Prism software (version 4.03; GraphPad Software Inc.) to obtain the concentration of test compound that inhibited uridine uptake by 50%, relative to that of untreated cells (IC$_{50}$ values). Each IC$_{50}$ value determination was conducted with nine concentrations and four replicates per concentration and experiments were repeated two to three times.

4.5. Cell Culture

CT26 mouse colon carcinoma cells were cultured as previously described [9], and mycoplasma infections were checked once a month. The cells were a kind gift of Prof. Dr. med. Ralph Mocicat (Institute of Molecular Immunology, German Research Center for Environmental Health, Munich, Germany).

4.6. Animals

The above-described CT26 mouse colon carcinoma cells were subcutaneously inoculated in the right shoulder of female BALB/c mice (1 × 10^6 cells in phosphate-buffered saline, PBS). Subsequently, the carcinomas were allowed to grow for a period of 13 days, reaching approximately 0.3 cm^3. PET imaging experiments were conducted within day 14-16 post tumor inoculation. All animal experiments were conducted according to guidelines for the use and care of laboratory research animals under the German Animal Protection Law, and approved by local authorities (Regierungspräsidium Tübingen).

4.7. PET Imaging

[^{18}F]FMISO (11.8 ± 1.2 MBq, $n = 5$), α-[^{18}F]FAZDR (12.6 ± 1.3 MBq, $n = 4$) and β-[^{18}F]FAZDR (11.7 ± 0.9 MBq, $n = 4$) were intravenously injected (via the tail vein) in female CT26 colon carcinoma bearing BALB/c mice 14–16 days post tumor inoculation. One animal was scanned on three consecutive days with [^{18}F]FAZA, α-[^{18}F]FAZDR and β-[^{18}F]FAZDR; all other animals were scanned with only one PET tracer (either [^{18}F]FMISO, α-[^{18}F]FAZDR or β-[^{18}F]FAZDR). All experiments were done using medical air as carrier gas for isoflurane anesthesia (1.5% isoflurane during PET scans, flow rate 0.4 L/min), including tracer injections, with a specialized vaporizer (Vetland, Louisville, KY, USA). Subsequent to the tracer injections, the animals were allowed to freely move in their home cages for an uptake period of 55 min, thus, breathing room air. After the uptake period, static 10 min PET scans were acquired at 1 h post injection (p.i.), 2 h p.i. and 3 h p.i. PET scans were performed with a Siemens Inveon dedicated PET (DPET, Siemens Healthcare, Knoxville, TN, USA). PET scans were then reconstructed with a two-dimensional ordered subset expectation maximization algorithm (OSEM2D with 16 subsets and 4 iterations). Image zoom was set to 1 and matrix size to 128 × 128 yielding a final PET image spatial resolution of 0.79 × 0.79 × 0.80 mm^3. PET data were manually corrected for radioactive decay of ^{18}F.

PET image analysis was performed using the PMOD 3.2_base 64 image viewing tool (PMOD Technologies, Zürich, Switzerland). Standardized volumes-of-interest (VOI, spheres with a diameter of 2 mm) were placed over the maximal activity in the carcinoma tissue (hypoxic target tissue), while the VOI placement in the shoulder muscle tissue (contralateral to carcinomas, normoxic control tissue) was done according to studies previously performed by our group [11,13]. Finally, PET data were expressed as percent injected dose per cubic-centimeter (%ID/cc) or tumor-to-muscle ratio (TMR).

4.8. Statistical Analysis

All statistical data analysis was preceded by tests for homoscedasticity and normality of PET data. These tests were performed using the Brown-Forsythe and the Shapiro-Wilk test with the Origin 8.0 Pro Software Package (OriginLab, Northhampton, USA). Normally distributed data were analyzed for statistically significant differences with the two-sample Student's t-test, done with the JMP 11.1.1 software package (SAS Institute GmbH, Böblingen, Germany). Multi-group comparisons were performed with p-values adjusted according to the number of groups (Tukey Kramer correction). Data are shown as the arithmetic mean ± one standard deviation (SD), unless otherwise mentioned; box plots contain all individual data points, the 25th, 50th and 75th percentile, as well as the arithmetic mean and one standard deviation (indicated by whiskers). For all tests, except for multi-group comparisons, p-values below 0.05 were considered as statistically relevant.

Author Contributions: A.S. and F.H. planned and carried out syntheses of organic compounds. V.L.D. and C.E.C. conceptualized and performed transporter studies. W.E. performed radiosyntheses. F.C.M., M.K., B.J.P. and G.R. conceptualized in vivo studies. F.C.M. carried out in vivo studies, analyzed in vivo data and performed statistical analysis. F.C.M., G.D.B., F.H., V.L.D., C.E.C. and G.R. drafted the manuscript. G.R. conceptualized radiolabeling procedures and edited the manuscript. B.J.P. helped design and coordinate all studies, edited the manuscript and reviewed the data. All authors read and approved the final manuscript.

Acknowledgments: The authors thank Susanne Felsinger for recording the NMR spectra, Johannes Theiner for the combustion analysis, and Funda Cay and Daniel Bukala for excellent technical assistance during all in vivo experiments.

References

1. Stieb, S.; Eleftheriou, A.; Warnock, G.; Guckenberger, M.; Riesterer, O. Longitudinal PET imaging of tumor hypoxia during the course of radiotherapy. *Eur. J. Nucl. Med. Mol. Imaging* **2018**, *45*, 2201–2217. [CrossRef] [PubMed]

2. Xu, Z.; Li, X.F.; Zou, H.; Sun, X.; Shen, B. (18)F-Fluoromisonidazole in tumor hypoxia imaging. *Oncotarget* **2017**, *8*, 94969–94979. [CrossRef] [PubMed]

3. Colliez, F.; Gallez, B.; Jordan, B.F. Assessing Tumor Oxygenation for Predicting Outcome in Radiation Oncology: A Review of Studies Correlating Tumor Hypoxic Status and Outcome in the Preclinical and Clinical Settings. *Front. Oncol.* **2017**, *7*, 10. [CrossRef] [PubMed]

4. Kim, M.M.; Parolia, A.; Dunphy, M.P.; Venneti, S. Non-invasive metabolic imaging of brain tumours in the era of precision medicine. *Nat. Rev. Clin. Oncol.* **2016**, *13*, 725–739. [CrossRef] [PubMed]

5. Vordermark, D.; Horsman, M.R. Hypoxia as a Biomarker and for Personalized Radiation Oncology. *Recent Results Cancer Res.* **2016**, *198*, 123–142. [PubMed]

6. O'Connor, J.P.; Rose, C.J.; Waterton, J.C.; Carano, R.A.; Parker, G.J.; Jackson, A. Imaging intratumor heterogeneity: Role in therapy response, resistance, and clinical outcome. *Clin. Cancer Res.* **2015**, *21*, 249–257. [CrossRef] [PubMed]

7. Widmer, D.S.; Hoek, K.S.; Cheng, P.F.; Eichhoff, O.M.; Biedermann, T.; Raaijmakers, M.I.G.; Hemmi, S.; Dummer, R.; Levesque, M.P. Hypoxia Contributes to Melanoma Heterogeneity by Triggering HIF1α-Dependent Phenotype Switching. *J. Investig. Dermatol.* **2013**, *133*, 2436–2443. [CrossRef] [PubMed]

8. Wu, M.Z.; Chen, S.F.; Nieh, S.; Benner, C.; Ger, L.P.; Jan, C.I.; Ma, L.; Chen, C.H.; Hishida, T.; Chang, H.T.; et al. Hypoxia Drives Breast Tumor Malignancy through a TET-TNFalpha-p38-MAPK Signaling Axis. *Cancer Res.* **2015**, *75*, 3912–3924. [CrossRef] [PubMed]

9. Maier, F.C.; Kneilling, M.; Reischl, G.; Cay, F.; Bukala, D.; Schmid, A.; Judenhofer, M.S.; Röcken, M.; Machulla, H.J.; Pichler, B.J. Significant impact of different oxygen breathing conditions on noninvasive in vivo tumor-hypoxia imaging using [^{18}F]-fluoro-azomycinarabino-furanoside ([^{18}F]FAZA). *Radiat. Oncol.* **2011**, *6*, 165. [CrossRef] [PubMed]

10. Souvatzoglou, M.; Grosu, A.L.; Röper, B.; Krause, B.J.; Beck, R.; Reischl, G.; Picchio, M.; Machulla, H.J.; Wester, H.J.; Piert, M. Tumour hypoxia imaging with [^{18}F]FAZA PET in head and neck cancer patients: A pilot study. *Eur. J. Nucl. Med. Mol. Imaging* **2007**, *34*, 1566–1575. [CrossRef] [PubMed]

11. Mahling, M.; Fuchs, K.; Thaiss, W.M.; Maier, F.C.; Feger, M.; Bukala, D.; Harant, M.; Eichner, M.; Reutershan, J.; Lang, F.; et al. A Comparative pO2 Probe and [^{18}F]Fluoro-Azomycinarabino-Furanoside ([^{18}F]FAZA) PET Study Reveals Anesthesia-Induced Impairment of Oxygenation and Perfusion in Tumor and Muscle. *PLoS ONE* **2015**, *10*, e0124665. [CrossRef] [PubMed]

12. Piert, M.; Machulla, H.J.; Picchio, M.; Reischl, G.; Ziegler, S.; Kumar, P.; Wester, H.J.; Beck, R.; McEwan, A.J.; Wiebe, L.I.; et al. Hypoxia-specific tumor imaging with 18F-fluoroazomycin arabinoside. *J. Nucl. Med.* **2005**, *46*, 106–113. [PubMed]

13. Schweifer, A.; Maier, F.C.; Ehrlichmann, W.; Lamparter, D.; Kneilling, M.; Pichler, B.J.; Hammerschmidt, F.; Reischl, G. [^{18}F]Fluoro-azomycin-2-deoxy-beta-d-ribofuranoside—A new imaging agent for tumor hypoxia in comparison with [^{18}F]FAZA. *Nucl. Med. Biol.* **2016**, *43*, 759–769. [CrossRef] [PubMed]

14. Kumar, P.; Roselt, P.; Reischl, G.; Cullinane, C.; Beiki, D.; Ehrlichmann, W.; Binns, D.; Naimi, E.; Yang, J.; Hicks, R.; et al. beta-[^{18}F]Fluoro Azomycin Arabinoside (beta-[^{18}F]FAZA): Synthesis, Radiofluorination and Preliminary PET Imaging of Murine A431 Tumors. *Curr. Radiopharm.* **2017**, *10*, 93–101. [CrossRef] [PubMed]

15. Wanek, T.; Kreis, K.; Krizkova, P.; Schweifer, A.; Denk, C.; Stanek, J.; Mairinger, S.; Filip, T.; Sauberer, M.; Edelhofer, P.; et al. Synthesis and preclinical characterization of 1-(6'-deoxy-6'-[^{18}F]fluoro-beta-d-allofuranosyl)-2-nitroimidazole (beta-6'-[^{18}F]FAZAL) as a positron emission tomography radiotracer to assess tumor hypoxia. *Bioorg. Med. Chem.* **2016**, *24*, 5326–5339. [CrossRef] [PubMed]

16. Schweifer, A.; Malová Křižková, P.; Mereiter, K.; Hammerschmidt, F. Preparation of Nonradioactive Standards and a Precursor for a Hypoxia 18F PET Tracer Derived from 1-(β-D-Galactopyranosyl)-2-nitroimidazole. *Synthesis* **2017**, *49*, 2933–2938.

17. Young, J.D.; Yao, S.Y.; Baldwin, J.M.; Cass, C.E.; Baldwin, S.A. The human concentrative and equilibrative nucleoside transporter families, SLC28 and SLC29. *Mol. Asp. Med.* **2013**, *34*, 529–547. [CrossRef] [PubMed]

18. Damaraju, V.L.; Sawyer, M.B.; Mackey, J.R.; Young, J.D.; Cass, C.E. Human nucleoside transporters: Biomarkers for response to nucleoside drugs. *Nucleosides Nucleotides Nucleic Acids* **2009**, *28*, 450–463. [CrossRef] [PubMed]

19. Zhang, J.; Visser, F.; King, K.M.; Baldwin, S.A.; Young, J.D.; Cass, C.E. The role of nucleoside transporters in cancer chemotherapy with nucleoside drugs. *Cancer Metastasis Rev.* **2007**, *26*, 85–110. [CrossRef]

20. Hendrickson, K.; Phillips, M.; Smith, W.; Peterson, L.; Krohn, K.; Rajendran, J. Hypoxia imaging with [F-18]FMISO-PET in head and neck cancer: Potential for guiding intensity modulated radiation therapy in overcoming hypoxia-induced treatment resistance. *Radiother. Oncol.* **2011**, *101*, 369–375. [CrossRef]

21. Boeke, S.; Thorwarth, D.; Monnich, D.; Pfannenberg, C.; Reischl, G.; La Fougère, C.; Nikolaou, K.; Mauz, P.S.; Paulsen, F.; Zips, D.; et al. Geometric analysis of loco-regional recurrences in relation to pre-treatment hypoxia in patients with head and neck cancer. *Acta Oncol.* **2017**, *56*, 1571–1576. [CrossRef] [PubMed]

22. Damaraju, V.L.; Damaraju, S.; Young, J.D.; Baldwin, S.A.; Mackey, J.; Sawyer, M.B.; Cass, C.E. Nucleoside anticancer drugs: The role of nucleoside transporters in resistance to cancer chemotherapy. *Oncogene* **2003**, *22*, 7524–7536. [CrossRef] [PubMed]

23. Kumar, P.; Stypinski, D.; Xia, H.; McEwan, A.J.B.; Machulla, H.-J.; Wiebe, L.I. Fluoroazomycin arabinoside (FAZA): Synthesis, ^{2}H and ^{3}H-labelling and preliminary biological evaluation of a novel 2-nitroimidazole marker of tissue hypoxia. *J. Label. Compd. Radiopharm.* **1999**, *42*, 3–16. [CrossRef]

24. Zanato, C.; Testa, A.; Zanda, M. Improved synthesis of the hypoxia probe 5-deutero-5-fluoro-5-deoxy-azomycin arabinoside (FAZA) as a model process for tritium radiolabeling. *J. Fluor. Chem.* **2013**, *155*, 110–117. [CrossRef]

25. Kumar, P.; Ohkura, K.; Beiki, D.; Wiebe, L.I.; Seki, K. Synthesis of 1-beta-D-(5-deoxy-5-iodoarabinofuranosyl)-2-nitroimidazole (beta-IAZA): A novel marker of tissue hypoxia. *Chem. Pharm. Bull.* **2003**, *51*, 399–403. [CrossRef] [PubMed]

26. Al-Maharik, N.; O-Hagan, D. Organofluorine chemistry: Deoxyfluorination reagents for C-F bond synthesis. *Aldrichim. Acta* **2011**, *44*, 65–79.

27. Fujibayashi, Y.; Taniuchi, H.; Yonekura, Y.; Ohtani, H.; Konishi, J.; Yokoyama, A. Copper-62-ATSM: A new hypoxia imaging agent with high membrane permeability and low redox potential. *J. Nucl. Med.* **1997**, *38*, 1155–1160. [PubMed]

28. Busk, M.; Munk, O.L.; Jakobsen, S.; Wang, T.; Skals, M.; Steiniche, T.; Horsman, M.R.; Overgaard, J. Assessing hypoxia in animal tumor models based on pharmocokinetic analysis of dynamic FAZA PET. *Acta Oncol.* **2010**, *49*, 922–933. [CrossRef]

29. Busk, M.; Horsman, M.R.; Jakobsen, S.; Bussink, J.; van der Kogel, A.; Overgaard, J. Cellular uptake of PET tracers of glucose metabolism and hypoxia and their linkage. *Eur. J. Nucl. Med. Mol. Imaging* **2008**, *35*, 2294–2303. [CrossRef]

30. Li, F.; Joergensen, J.T.; Hansen, A.E.; Kjaer, A. Kinetic modeling in PET imaging of hypoxia. *Am. J. Nucl. Med. Mol. Imaging* **2014**, *4*, 490–506.

31. Shi, K.; Souvatzoglou, M.; Astner, S.T.; Vaupel, P.; Nüsslin, F.; Wilkens, J.J.; Ziegler, S.I. Quantitative assessment of hypoxia kinetic models by a cross-study of dynamic 18F-FAZA and ^{15}O-H$_2$O in patients with head and neck tumors. *J. Nucl. Med.* **2010**, *51*, 1386–1394. [CrossRef] [PubMed]

32. Verwer, E.E.; Bahce, I.; van Velden, F.H.P.; Yaqub, M.; Schuit, R.C.; Windhorst, A.D.; Raijmakers, P.; Hoekstra, O.S.; Lammertsma, A.A.; Smit, E.F.; et al. Parametric Methods for Quantification of 18F-FAZA Kinetics in Non–Small Cell Lung Cancer Patients. *J. Nucl. Med.* **2014**, *55*, 1772–1777. [CrossRef] [PubMed]

33. Verwer, E.E.; van Velden, F.H.P.; Bahce, I.; Yaqub, M.; Schuit, R.C.; Windhorst, A.D.; Raijmakers, P.; Lammertsma, A.A.; Smit, E.F.; Boellaard, R. Pharmacokinetic analysis of [^{18}F]FAZA in non-small cell lung cancer patients. *Eur. J. Nucl. Med. Mol. Imaging* **2013**, *40*, 1523–1531. [CrossRef] [PubMed]

34. Mikenda, W. Solid films and layers deposited on silicon—A versatile infrared sampling technique. *Vib. Spectrosc.* **1992**, *3*, 327–330. [CrossRef]

35. Patt, M.; Kuntzsch, M.; Machulla, H.J. Preparation of [^{18}F]fluoromisonidazole by nucleophilic substitution on THP-protected precursor: Yield dependence on reaction parameters. *J. Radioanal. Nucl. Chem.* **1999**, *240*, 925–927. [CrossRef]

36. Vickers, M.F.; Kumar, R.; Visser, F.; Zhang, J.; Charania, J.; Raborn, R.T.; Baldwin, S.A.; Young, J.D.; Cass, C.E. Comparison of the interaction of uridine, cytidine, and other pyrimidine nucleoside analogues with recombinant human equilibrative nucleoside transporter 2 (hENT2) produced in Saccharomyces cerevisiae. *Biochem. Cell Biol.* **2002**, *80*, 639–644. [CrossRef] [PubMed]

37. Zhang, J.; Visser, F.; Vickers, M.F.; Lang, T.; Robins, M.J.; Nielsen, L.P.; Nowak, I.; Baldwin, S.A.; Young, J.D.; Cass, C.E. Uridine binding motifs of human concentrative nucleoside transporters 1 and 3 produced in Saccharomyces cerevisiae. *Mol. Pharmacol.* **2003**, *64*, 1512–1520. [CrossRef] [PubMed]

38. Vickers, M.F.; Zhang, J.; Visser, F.; Tackaberry, T.; Robins, M.J.; Nielsen, L.P.; Nowak, I.; Baldwin, S.A.; Young, J.D.; Cass, C.E. Uridine recognition motifs of human equilibrative nucleoside transporters 1 and 2 produced in Saccharomyces cerevisiae. *Nucleosides Nucleotides Nucleic Acids* **2004**, *23*, 361–373. [CrossRef] [PubMed]

Permissions

List of Contributors

Nils Erik Halvorsen and Ole Heine Kvernenes
Center for Nuclear medicine/PET, Department of Radiology, Haukeland University Hospital, Jonas Lies vei 65, N-5021 Bergen, Norway

Alessandra Boschi
Department of Morphology, Surgery and Experimental Medicine, University of Ferrara, Ferrara 44121, Italy

Petra Martini
Department of Morphology, Surgery and Experimental Medicine, University of Ferrara, Ferrara 44121, Italy Italy and Legnaro National Laboratories, Italian National Institute for Nuclear Physics (LNL-INFN), Legnaro (PD) 35020, Italy

Nina Pfannkuchen, Marian Meckel and Frank Rösch
Institute of Nuclear Chemistry, Johannes Gutenberg University Mainz, Fritz-Strassmann-Weg 2, 55128 Mainz, Germany

Ralf Bergmann
Helmholtz-Zentrum Dresden-Rossendorf, Institute of Radiopharmaceutical Cancer Research, Bautzner Landstrasse 400, 01328 Dresden, Germany

Michael Bachmann
Helmholtz-Zentrum Dresden-Rossendorf, Institute of Radiopharmaceutical Cancer Research, Bautzner Landstrasse 400, 01328 Dresden, Germany University Cancer Center (UCC) Carl Gustav Carus, Tumorimmunology, Technical University Dresden, Fetscherstr. 74, 01307 Dresden, Germany

Chandrasekhar Bal
Department of Nuclear Medicine & PET, All India Institute of Medical Sciences, Ansari Nagar, New Delhi 110029, India

Mike Sathekge
Department of Nuclear Medicine, University of Pretoria & Steve Biko Academic Hospital, Private Bag X169, Pretoria 0001, South Africa

Wolfgang Mohnike
Diagnostisch Therapeutisches Zentrum, DTZ am Frankfurter Tor, Kadiner Straße 23, 10243 Berlin, Germany

Richard P. Baum
Department of Nuclear Medicine, Center for PET/CT, Zentralklinik Bad Berka, Robert-Koch-Allee 9, 99438 Bad Berka, Germany

Adrienne Müller Herde, Silvan D. Boss, Yingfang He and Simon M. Ametamey
Center for Radiopharmaceutical Sciences of ETH, PSI, and USZ, Department of Chemistry and Applied Biosciences of ETH, 8093 Zurich, Switzerland

Roger Schibli and Linjing Mu
Center for Radiopharmaceutical Sciences of ETH, PSI, and USZ, Department of Chemistry and Applied Biosciences of ETH, 8093 Zurich, Switzerland Department of Nuclear Medicine, University Hospital Zurich, 8091 Zurich, Switzerland

Ana Claudia R. Durante
Department of Physiological Sciences, School of Medical Sciences, Santa Casa de Sao Paulo, Rua Cesario Mota Junior 61, Sao Paulo 01221-020, Brazil Hospital Israelita Albert Einstein, Avenida Albert Einstein 627/701, Sao Paulo 05652-900, Brazil

Danielle V. Sobral and Luciana Malavolta
Department of Physiological Sciences, School of Medical Sciences, Santa Casa de Sao Paulo, Rua Cesario Mota Junior 61, Sao Paulo 01221-020, Brazil

Ana Claudia C. Miranda, Érika V. de Almeida, Leonardo L. Fuscaldi and Marycel R. F. F. de Barboza
Hospital Israelita Albert Einstein, Avenida Albert Einstein 627/701, Sao Paulo 05652-900, Brazil

Melchiore Giganti and Licia Uccelli
Department of Morphology, Surgery and Experimental Medicine, University of Ferrara, Ferrara 44121, Italy

Micòl Pasquali
Department of Physic and Earth Science, University of Ferrara, Ferrara 44122, Italy

Claudio Trapella, Alessandro Massi, Adriano Duatti, Remo Guerrini, Vinicio Zanirato, Anna Fantinati and Erika Marzola
Department of Chemical and Pharmaceutical Sciences, University of Ferrara, Ferrara 44121, Italy

Tais Basaco
Department of Chemistry and Biochemistry, University of Bern, 3012 Bern, Switzerland Laboratory of Radiochemistry, Paul Scherrer Institute (PSI), 5232 Villigen PSI, Switzerland

Stefanie Pektor and Matthias Miederer
Clinic for Nuclear Medicine, University Medical Center Mainz, 55131 Mainz, Germany

Josue M. Bermudez, Niurka Meneses, Stefan Schürch and Andreas Türler
Department of Chemistry and Biochemistry, University of Bern, 3012 Bern, Switzerland

Manfred Heller
Department for Biomedical Research (DBMR), University of Bern, 3010 Bern, Switzerland

José A. Galván
Institute of Pathology, University of Bern, 3010 Bern, Switzerland

Kayluz F. Boligán and Stephan von Gunten
Institute of Pharmacology (PKI), University of Bern, 3010 Bern, Switzerland

Chrysoula Vraka, Verena Pichler, Neydher Berroterán-Infante, Tim Wollenweber, Anna Pillinger, Maximilian Hohensinner, Lukas Fetty, Xiang Li, Cecile Philippe and Marcus Hacker
Division of Nuclear Medicine, Department of Biomedical Imaging and Image-guided Therapy, Medical University of Vienna, 1090 Vienna, Austria

Dietrich Beitzke
Department of Biomedical Imaging and Image-guided Therapy, Division of Cardiovascular and Interventional Radiology, Medical University of Vienna, 1090 Vienna, Austria

Katharina Pallitsch
Institute of Organic Chemistry, University of Vienna, 1090 Vienna, Austria

Markus Mitterhauser
Division of Nuclear Medicine, Department of Biomedical Imaging and Image-guided Therapy, Medical University of Vienna, 1090 Vienna, Austria
Ludwig-Boltzmann-Institute Applied Diagnostics, 1090 Vienna, Austria

Wolfgang Wadsak
Division of Nuclear Medicine, Department of Biomedical Imaging and Image-guided Therapy, Medical University of Vienna, 1090 Vienna, Austria
Center for Biomarker Research in Medicine, CBmed GmbH, 8010 Graz, Austria

Alicia Vall-Sagarra and Carmen Wängler
Biomedical Chemistry, Department of Clinical Radiology and Nuclear Medicine, Medical Faculty Mannheim of Heidelberg University, Theodor-Kutzer-Ufer 1-3, 68167 Mannheim, Germany

Shanna Litau
Biomedical Chemistry, Department of Clinical Radiology and Nuclear Medicine, Medical Faculty Mannheim of Heidelberg University, Theodor-Kutzer-Ufer 1-3, 68167 Mannheim, Germany
Molecular Imaging and Radiochemistry, Department of Clinical Radiology and Nuclear Medicine, Medical Faculty Mannheim of Heidelberg University, Theodor-Kutzer-Ufer 1-3, 68167 Mannheim, Germany

Björn Wängler
Molecular Imaging and Radiochemistry, Department of Clinical Radiology and Nuclear Medicine, Medical Faculty Mannheim of Heidelberg University, Theodor-Kutzer-Ufer 1-3, 68167 Mannheim, Germany

Gert Fricker
Institute of Pharmacy and Molecular Biotechnology, University of Heidelberg, Im Neuenheimer Feld 329, 69120 Heidelberg, Germany

Ralf Schirrmacher, Justin J. Bailey and Esther Schirrmacher
Department of Oncology, Division of Oncological Imaging, University of Alberta, Edmonton, Alberta T6G 2R3, Canada

Andrew V. Mossine
Division of Nuclear Medicine, Department of Radiology, The University of Michigan Medical School, Ann Arbor, MI, 48109, USA

Peter J. H. Scott
Division of Nuclear Medicine, Department of Radiology, The University of Michigan Medical School, Ann Arbor, MI, 48109, USA
The Interdepartmental Program in Medicinal Chemistry, University of Michigan, Ann Arbor, MI 48109, USA

Lena Kaiser, Peter Bartenstein and Simon Lindner
Department of Nuclear Medicine, Ludwig-Maximilians-University of Munich, Marchioninistrasse 15, Munich 81377, Germany

David R. Kaplan
Program in Neurosciences and Mental Health, Hospital for Sick Children and Department of Molecular Genetics, University of Toronto, Toronto, ON, Canada

Alexey Kostikov and Jean-Paul Soucy
McConnell Brain Imaging Centre, Montreal Neurological Institute, McGill University, 3801 University Street, Montreal, QC H3A 2B4, Canada

Gert Fricker and Anne Mahringer
Institute of Pharmacy and Molecular Biotechnology, University of Heidelberg, Heidelberg 69120, Germany

Pedro Rosa-Neto
Translational Neuroimaging Laboratory, McGill Centre for Studies in Aging, Douglas Mental Health University Institute, Montreal, QC H4H 1R3, Canada

Alexander Thiel
McConnell Brain Imaging Centre, Montreal Neurological Institute, McGill University, 3801 University Street, Montreal, QC H3A 2B4, Canada
Jewish General Hospital, Lady Davis Institute, Montreal, QC HT3 1E2, Canada

Vadim Bernard-Gauthier
Azrieli Centre for Neuro-Radiochemistry, Research Imaging Centre, Centre for Addiction and Mental Health, Toronto, ON M5T 1L8, Canada
Department of Psychiatry, University of Toronto, Toronto, ON M5T 1R8, Canada

Dominik Summer, Sonja Mayr and Clemens Decristoforo
Department of Nuclear Medicine, Medical University Innsbruck, Anichstrasse 35, A-6020 Innsbruck, Austria

Milos Petrik
Institute of Molecular and Translational Medicine, Faculty of Medicine and Dentistry, Palacky University, CZE-77900 Olomouc, Czech Republic

Katia Schoeler
Biocenter—Division of Developmental Immunology, Medical University of Innsbruck, Innrain 80/82, A-6020 Innsbruck, Austria

Lisa Vieider and Barbara Matuszczak
Institute of Pharmacy, Pharmaceutical Chemistry, University of Innsbruck, Center for Chemistry and Biomedicine (CCB), Innrain 80/82, A-6020 Innsbruck, Austria

Roswitha Tönnesmann
Department of Nuclear Medicine, University Medical Center Freiburg, Faculty of Medicine, University of Freiburg, 79106 Freiburg, Germany

Philipp T. Meyer, Matthias Eder and Ann-Christin Baranski
Department of Nuclear Medicine, University Medical Center Freiburg, Faculty of Medicine, University of Freiburg, 79106 Freiburg, Germany
Division of Radiopharmaceutical Development, German Cancer Consortium (DKTK), partner site Freiburg, and German Cancer Research Center (DKFZ), 69120 Heidelberg, Germany

Maximilian Klingler, Christine Rangger, Piriya Kaeopookum and Elisabeth von Guggenberg
Department of Nuclear Medicine, Medical University of Innsbruck, Anichstrasse 35, A-6020 Innsbruck, Austria

Hassan Elsaidi
Department of Oncology, Cross Cancer Institute, Faculty of Medicine and Dentistry, University of Alberta, 11560 University Avenue, Edmonton, AB T6G 1Z2, Canada
Department of Pharmaceutical Chemistry, Faculty of Pharmacy, University of Alexandria, El Sultan Hussein St. Azarita, Alexandria 21521, Egypt

Fatemeh Ahmadi
Centre for Probe Development and Commercialization, 1280 Main Street West, Hamilton, ON L8S 4K1, Canada

Leonard I. Wiebe
Department of Oncology, Cross Cancer Institute, Faculty of Medicine and Dentistry, University of Alberta, 11560 University Avenue, Edmonton, AB T6G 1Z2, Canada
Joint Appointment to Faculty of Pharmacy and Pharmaceutical Sciences, University of Alberta, Edmonton, AB T6G 2E1, Canada

Piyush Kumar
Department of Oncology, Cross Cancer Institute, Faculty of Medicine and Dentistry, University of Alberta, 11560 University Avenue, Edmonton, AB T6G 1Z2, Canada

Aikaterini Kaloudi, Emmanouil Lymperis, Panagiotis Kanellopoulos, Berthold A. Nock and Theodosia Maina
Molecular Radiopharmacy, INRASTES, NCSR "Demokritos", 15310 Athens, Greece

Beatrice Waser and Jean Claude Reubi
Cell Biology and Experimental Cancer Research, Institute of Pathology, University of Berne, CH-3010 Berne, Switzerland

Marion de Jong
Department of Radiology & Nuclear Medicine Erasmus MC, 3015 CN Rotterdam, The Netherlands

Eric P. Krenning
Cytrotron Rotterdam BV, Erasmus MC, 3015 CN Rotterdam, The Netherlands

Sean S. Tanzey
Department of Medicinal Chemistry, University of Michigan, Ann Arbor, MI 48109, USA

Xia Shao, Jenelle Stauff, Janna Arteaga and Phillip Sherman
Department of Radiology, University of Michigan, Ann Arbor, MI 48109, USA

Florian C. Maier, Gregory D. Bowden, Walter Ehrlichmann, Bernd J. Pichler and Gerald Reischl
Werner Siemens Imaging Center, Department of Preclinical Imaging and Radiopharmacy, Eberhard Karls University of Tübingen, Röntgenweg 13, 72076 Tübingen, Germany

Anna Schweifer and Friedrich Hammerschmidt
Faculty of Chemistry, Institute of Organic Chemistry, University of Vienna, Währingerstraße 38, A-1090 Vienna, Austria

Vijaya L. Damaraju and Carol E. Cass
Department of Oncology, University of Alberta, Edmonton, AB T6G 2R7, Canada

Manfred Kneilling
Werner Siemens Imaging Center, Department of Preclinical Imaging and Radiopharmacy, Eberhard Karls University of Tübingen, Röntgenweg 13, 72076 Tübingen, Germany
Department of Dermatology, Eberhard Karls University of Tübingen, 72076 Tübingen, Germany

Index

Printed in the USA
CPSIA information can be obtained
at www.ICGtesting.com
JSHW051407091023
49903JS00006B/319

9 781646 466351